Men Who Sell Sex

Social Aspects of AIDS
Series Editor: Peter Aggleton
(Institute of Education, University of London)

AIDS is not simply a concern for scientists, doctors and medical researchers, it has important social dimensions as well. These include individual, cultural and media responses to the epidemic, stigmatization and discrimination, counselling, care and health promotion. This series of books brings together work from many disciplines including psychology, sociology, cultural and media studies, anthropology, education and history. The titles will be of interest to the general reader, those involved in education and social research, and scientific researchers who want to examine the social aspects of AIDS.

Recent titles include:

Power and Community: Organizational and Cultural Responses to AIDS
Dennis Altman

Moral Threats and Dangerous Desires: AIDS in the News Media
Deborah Lupton

Last Served? Gendering the HIV Pandemic
Cindy Patton

Crossing Borders: Migration, Ethnicity and AIDS
Edited by Mary Haour-Knipe

Bisexualities and AIDS: International Perspectives
Edited by Peter Aggleton

Sexual Interactions and HIV Risk: New Conceptual Perspectives in European Research
Edited by Luc Van Campenhoudt, Mitchell Cohen, Gustavo Guizzardi and Dominique Hausser

AIDS: Activism and Alliances
Edited by Peter Aggleton, Peter Davies and Graham Hart

AIDS as a Gender Issue
Edited by Lorraine Sherr, Catherine Hankins and Lydia Bennett

Drug Injecting and HIV Infection: Global Dimensions and Local Responses
Edited by Gerry Stimson, Don C. Des Jarlais and Andrew Ball

Sexual Behaviour and HIV/AIDS in Europe: Comparisons of National Surveys
Edited by Michel Hubert, Nathalie Bajos and Theo Sandfort

Men Who Sell Sex: International Perspectives on Male Prostitution and AIDS
Edited by Peter Aggleton

Men Who Sell Sex
International Perspectives on
Male Prostitution and AIDS

Edited by

Peter Aggleton

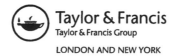

Taylor & Francis
Taylor & Francis Group

LONDON AND NEW YORK

First published in 1999 by UCL Press

Reprinted 2003 by Taylor & Francis
11 New Fetter Lane
London, EC4P 4EE

British Library Cataloguing-in-Publication Data
A CIP catalogue record for this book is available from the
British Library.

**Library of Congress Cataloging-in-Publication Data are
available**

ISBNs: 1-85728-862-9 HB
        1-85728-863-7 PB

Printed and bound by Antony Rowe Ltd, Eastbourne, East Sussex.

Contents

Contents

Acknowledgements

Without the support and encouragement of numerous friends, it would never have been possible to prepare this book. I am especially grateful to chapter authors for their willingness to document some of the many ways in which men exchange sex for money and other kinds of material benefit. I would also like to thank Helen Thomas and Paula Hassett for liaising with contributors and preparing the manuscript for publication, and Paula Hassett and Sylver Kerhel for assistance with translation. Finally, we owe an immense debt to the men whose lives are described here, for their willingness to talk openly about their experiences, and for providing insight into some of the complexity surrounding male sex work today.

Social Aspects of AIDS
Series Editor: Peter Aggleton
Institute of Education, University of London

Editorial Advisory Board

Notes on Contributors

Peter Aggleton is Professor in Education, Director of the Thomas Coram Research Unit and Associate Director of the Health and Education Research Unit at the Institute of Education, University of London. He has worked internationally in HIV/AIDS health promotion since the mid-1980s. His publications include *Health* (Routledge, 1990); *AIDS: Safety, Sexuality and Risk* (Ed. with Peter Davies and Graham Hart, Taylor & Francis, 1995), *Bisexualities and AIDS: International Perspectives* (Taylor & Francis, 1996), *AIDS: Activism and Alliances* (with Peter Davies and Graham Hart, Taylor & Francis, 1997) and *Success in HIV Prevention* (AVERT, 1997).

Dan Allman is a Canadian sociologist who works within the HIV Social, Behavioural and Epidemiological Studies Unit of the University of Toronto, Canada.

Dennis Altman is Professor of Politics at La Trobe University, Melbourne, and author of nine books, including *Homosexual: Oppression and Liberation* (Avon Books, 1971) and *Power and Community: Organizational and Cultural Responses to AIDS* (Taylor & Francis, 1994).

Amine Boushaba is a worker with the Association Marocaine de Lutte contre le SIDA in Casablanca.

Kendra E. Burchfiel is a research associate in the Department of Paediatric Infectious Diseases at Tulane University. She is the project director of a CDC funded multi-site collaborative study of injecting drug users. Her current research also includes the functioning of HIV positive mothers and their uninfected children.

Carlos F. Cáceres teaches and conducts research at the Department of Public Health, the Institute of Population Studies and the Institute of Tropical Medicine at Universidad Cayetano Heredia in Lima. He has extensive quantitative/ qualitative research experience in sexual and reproductive health, particularly with regard to the social epidemiology of HIV/AIDS and socio-cultural aspects of gender and sexuality.

Peter Davies is Professor in the Sociology of Health at the University of Portsmouth and Director of Sigma Research. He has been involved, since 1986, in research into the impact of HIV/AIDS on sexual behaviour as well as on policy for HIV prevention. He is the co-author of *Sex, Gay Men and AIDS* (Falmer Press, 1993), and editor with Peter Aggleton and Graham Hart of the Social Aspects of AIDS series of books.

Rayah Feldman is Principal Lecturer in Primary and Community Health Research at South Bank University. She was involved in the evaluation of the Landmark Centre and in research on local services for people with HIV/AIDS in east London. She is currently working on a comparative international study of reproductive rights for the International Community of Women Living with HIV/AIDS.

Rafael García is Professor and Head of the Graduate Programme at the Human Sexuality Institute of the Universidad Autónoma de Santo Domingo, and Director of the National Commission on AIDS (CONASIDA) in the Dominican Republic. His background is in psychiatry and sexology. With Antonio de Moya, he contributed a chapter to *Bisexualities and AIDS: International Perspectives* (Taylor & Francis, 1996).

Hakima Himmich is Director of the Association Marocaine de Lutte contre le SIDA in Casablanca.

Latéfa Imane is a worker with Association Marocaine de Lutte contre le SIDA in Casablanca.

Oscar G. Jiménez studied sociology at the Pontificia Universidad Católica del Perú (PUCP) in Lima. He has participated in various studies on health, sexuality and sexual risk taking, particularly among young men. He is currently involved in a study of sexual and preventive practices among young men and women in Peru, and another about social factors related to maternal mortality.

Shivananda Khan is the founder and chief executive of the Naz Foundation working on sexuality and sexual health issues in South Asian countries, and enabling the development of sexual health services for men who have sex with men.

Patrick Larvie is a doctoral candidate at the University of Chicago. He has worked as a research associate at the Institute for Social Medicine at the State University of Rio de Janeiro. His doctoral research is on the Brazilian National AIDS Program, focusing most closely on prevention initiatives.

Lindinalva Laurindo da Silva was a researcher at the Secretariat of Health in São Paulo, Brazil during the 1980s, where she carried out research on the different lifestyles of gay men and AIDS. Later, she worked in France with CERMES on research concerning male sex work and HIV, the experience of living with AIDS, and the relationship of patients to AIDS treatment.

Ana Luisa Liguori is country co-ordinator for the Population Programme in Mexico of the John T. and Catherine D. MacArthur Foundation. She has conducted research on Mexican sexual culture and on gender and AIDS. She is a member of the Editorial Boards of *Health and Human Rights* and *SIDA/ETS*, the Mexican National AIDS Council's quarterly publication.

Edward V. Morse is an Associate Professor of Sociology at Tulane University. Current research includes a CDC funded collaborative, multi-site study of young injecting drug users, a CDC funded study of HIV infected women and their uninfected children, and recruitment, retention and compliance in HIV-related clinical trial programmes. He is a consultant to the President of the United States on behavioural medicine issues, HIV transmission through the use of needles and compliance with medical treatment.

E. Antonio de Moya is research associate at the Human Sexuality Institute of the Universidad Autónoma de Santo Domingo, and Research Consultant at the Centro de Orientación e Investigación Integral (COIN), in the Dominican Republic. He headed the Research Department of the Dominican Republic National AIDS Program from 1985 to 1993. His current work focuses primarily on the social construction of masculinity as well as on family and community responses to HIV/AIDS. With Rafael García, he contributed a chapter to *Bisexualities and AIDS: International Perspectives* (Taylor & Francis, 1996).

Ted Myers is Director of the HIV Social, Behavioural and Epidemiological Studies Unit of the Faculty of Medicine, University of Toronto. He has worked and studied extensively in the field of addictions, mental and community health and is involved with a variety of community-based AIDS/HIV prevention initiatives. He has published numerous articles and presented papers at international and national conferences.

Nandasena Ratnapala teaches sociology and anthropology at the University of Sri Jayawardenepura, Nugegoda, Sri Lanka. He is author of a number of books in Sinhala and English, and he is a well known novelist, poet, essayist and researcher in sociology, anthropology and criminology. His publications include *Modification of Behaviour Among Commercial Sex Workers in Sri Lanka* (Colombo: Dipanee Press, 1995), *The Beggar in Sri Lanka* (Colombo: World Vision, 1996), *Buddhist Sociology* (New Delhi: Sri Satguru Publications, 1995), *Manual of Research* (Chandigar: Commonwealth Secretariat, Asia Centre, 1995) and *Crime and Punishment in the Buddhist Tradition* (New Delhi: Mittal, 1993).

Jacobo Schifter was born in San José, Costa Rica. He has written books on the Costa Rican Civil War and on United States–Central American relations during the Second World War. His main interest shifted to AIDS in the 1980s and he has written extensively on the epidemic and its impact in Central America. His most well known books are *The Formation of a Counterculture: AIDS and Homosexuality in Costa Rica* (1989), *Men who Love Men* (1992), and *Psychiatry and Homophobia* (1997). He is currently Regional Director of ILPES (Instituto Latinamericano de Prevención en Salud).

Patricia M. Simon is Associate Professor of Psychiatry at Louisiana State University School of Medicine. She has published extensively in the area of HIV/AIDS and its impact on various populations, including male sex workers, their clients, homeless people and African American women and children. Currently, she is a co-principal investigator of a CDC funded multi-site collaborative study of HIV and young injecting drug users, and a co-principal investigator of a CDC funded study of HIV infected women and their uninfected children.

Graeme Storer is completing a doctorate in Applied Linguistics in the School of English, Language and Media Studies at Macquarie University, Australia. His research interests include the application of critical discourse analysis to social science research and, in particular, to studies of homosexually active men. He works as a freelance consultant to non-governmental organizations in Asia, providing management and human resource development training and workshop facilitation.

Michael L. Tan is an anthropologist. He is Executive Director of the Health Action Information Network and Associate Professor at the University of the Philippines. He is a member of the Philippine National AIDS Council, a presidential advisory body.

Oussama Tawil is an Inter-Country Adviser with the Joint United Nations Programme on HIV/AIDS (UNAIDS) in Abidjan, Côte d'Ivoire.

Wim Zuilhof works for the SAD–Schorer Foundation, a national organization for care, health promotion and services for lesbian women and gay men. He has worked in the field of HIV prevention since 1987, and has designed and coordinated outreach projects for men who have sex with men. Since 1991 he has managed a national programme on HIV and STD prevention for young male sex workers. This includes chairing a national network for field-workers and the co-ordination of pilot projects for young men working as escorts, and for their clients.

Foreword

Dennis Altman

To speak of male sex work is to break several taboos simultaneously and to bring together discussion of (at least) two topics, namely homosexual desire and prostitution, whose very existence most governments and many ideology makers would prefer to deny. I say at least two because, as many of the following chapters make clear, much male prostitution also involves various forms of transgender identity/performance/desire, so that the boundary of 'male' sex work is itself problematic, just as the line between being paid for sex and receiving presents from a lover suggests an uncomfortable blurring of the distinction between the paid and the unpaid.

It is not that male prostitution has been universally ignored. It has a rich literature (indeed much of it from antiquity); in the past 30 years one thinks of the widely read writings of, say, Jean Genet, John Rechy and Robin Maugham. As 'hustlers' or 'gigolos', male prostitutes show up in a surprising number of films, though there is a major divide (largely class-based) between William Holden in *Sunset Boulevard* and Jon Voight in *Midnight Cowboy* or the boys who work/walk Santa Monica Boulevard in Bruce LaBruce's *Hustler White*. Recently a number of accounts of life as a male sex worker have appeared, for example Charles Isherwood's (1997) life of Joey Stefano and Scott O'Hara's (1996) *Autopornography*. By contrast there has been little serious academic recognition of the male sex worker, and what there is has often been overlain with a portentous mix of moralism and voyeurism.

While the onset of HIV meant that grudging attention came to be paid to both 'men who have sex with men' (a clumsy phrase adopted to overcome the confusion of identity with behaviour) and 'commercial sex workers', a certain resistance seemed to persist in recognizing that these two 'at risk' populations were not mutually exclusive. Indeed some gay organizations were themselves uncomfortable in acknowledging that sex workers and their clients were an essential part of their community, preferring an image of a world which ran smoothly on the grease of equally reciprocal desire.

But if there was comparatively little frank acknowledgement of the existence of commercial male sex, two dominant scripts tended to dominate the informal knowledge that has influenced AIDS policy makers internationally. The first is one that sees sex work as the product of economic necessity, either within or between nations (in its international version it places great emphasis on the development of sex tourism). This script places great stress on the fact that many sex workers are not 'really' homosexual, thus fuelling one of the great panics of the epidemic, namely the fear that male prostitutes would be 'vectors' of infection from the 'gay' to the 'general' community. The second is a far more romantic account, one which by contrast sees the sex worker as 'really' homosexual, who uses the sale of his body as a form of legitimation for what is otherwise unacknowledgeable. It is commonly argued by gay men of a particular age and class that there are a number of cultures where 'all' men can be had for the right amount.

Part of the romantic account is a belief that homosexual sex work is inherently less exploitative than heterosexual sex work, that the interactions between two men makes for a certain mutual equality which is missing in most transactions between a male client and a female seller. I am not sure if this assertion has ever been tested, and I am doubtful of its universal validity. Nonetheless the proposition that gender affects the relationships of commercial sex is a persuasive one, and well worth testing.

The various chapters in this book demonstrate remarkably clearly the complexities involved in talking about male sex work as if we were dealing with homogeneous populations or simple causal factors. It is a fact that money will be involved in a great many sexual encounters in almost any cash economy, and that the great majority of such transactions will not involve people who identify themselves as professional sex workers. This is why we should be skeptical of those studies which claim to tell us that 36 per cent of sex workers are positive/negative/use condoms or whatever: they assume a fixed population which is a fiction. It seems useful to think of sex work not as a fixed state or identity, but rather as a continuum ranging from organized prostitution through brothels, escort agencies, and so on, through to unmedited transactions resulting from chance encounters of the sort described in a number of the chapters. Recent Australian evidence suggests that a fifth to a quarter of all men who identify as gay may have accepted money for sex at some time in their life (Perkins and Bennett, 1985).

What is exciting about this book is that it crosses so many boundaries, bringing together as it does accounts from every continent and from a wide range of disciplines. The various authors seek to situate sex work within a range of frameworks: sociological and psychological, but also historical (Sri Lanka), economic (Britain and the United States), political (Brazil), legal (Canada), even linguistic (Thailand). Unfortunately the editor was unable to persuade someone to write a chapter on the gay pornographic industry that is now booming in parts of Eastern Europe, and its absence reminds us just how strong are the taboos which surround the discussion of commercial sex. There is another story to be told, too, about the relationship between HIV among gay men and the developing technologies of pornography, such as 'chat lines' or the Minitel in France, which would also raise questions about the commercialization of sex, even as it might question the easy distinction between 'paid' and 'unpaid' services.

Equally one finds here a diversity of political and moral positions: contrast, for example, the ways in which the British and American experiences are described, where the difference in language deployed is as revealing as the explicit judgements of the authors. By crossing these borders, the accounts in *Men Who Sell Sex* highlight both cultural specificities and the degree of similarity between countries with enormously different cultural and economic systems. In both rich and poor countries sex work is almost always the trade of the marginal (although there are more middle-class sex workers, often working as 'masseurs' and 'escorts' out of private apartments in the ritzy areas of large cities, than these accounts suggest). The murder of designer Gianni Versace by Andrew Cunanan led to a flurry of media stories about 'gay gigolos' (Fisher, 1997). There is less acknowledgement of men who provide paid services to women, although this is not uncommon in certain tourist destinations, and a number of chapters (for example on Sri Lanka and the Dominican Republic) do acknowledge these in passing.

One hears voices from many very different societies and cultures, but the stories are often remarkably similar. Thus in Shivanada Khan's recounting of sex work in the parks and streets of south Asia one comes across men who find pleasure as well as money in their encounters. In the study of Costa Rican workers, pleasure is seen 'as a major threat to a predominantly heterosexual identity'. In Lima one respondent, who could equally be found in Sydney, Montreal or Bangkok, says: 'When I am there it's to meet people, and when I meet them I don't think about whether they will pay me or not ... If they give me a tip it's very welcome.' As Zuilhof concludes for the Netherlands: 'Frequently clients are regarded as their friends, lovers, social workers or providers of sleeping accommodation. At times, sex with them can be pure lust, but it can also be a bad exchange, giving much more than one gets, or purely a cry for support or attention.'

There is a range of evidence in this book: in some cases there are numerous studies to draw on, in others these chapters are the first piece of writing on male sex work in a particular society. On all occasions the writers have tried to let the voices of the men themselves be heard (although only in a couple of cases do we hear the voices of their clients). But even this is not as unproblematic as current interest in 'qualitative' research might suggest. The chapter by Schifter and Aggleton on Costa Rica reminds us in very telling ways of the different strategies available to informants to compartmentalize their lives and describe feelings and behaviour which seem contradicted by other evidence. At the same time, one of the strengths of the book is the very specificity of some of the studies, and the richness of the ethnographic observations. The description of sexual transactions in the bath houses of Mexico City, of interactions within parks in Delhi, of life in the brothels of San José, are vivid reminders of the value of detailed ethnographic description in helping the reader understand and empathize with what can too easily be dismissed as alien and perhaps distasteful. The chapter on Morocco reminds us just how strong are the taboos against *acknowledging* homosexual behaviours, even where they are generally known to be widespread.

And Gay Identities

A number of the chapters seek to relate male sex work to arguments about sexual and gender identity. In most countries there seems to be an important distinction between 'macho' and 'transvestite' workers – in France between *travestis* and *garçons*; in Mexico between *travestis* and *masajistas*; in Peru between *activos* and *pasivos* – although as some of the contributors suggest (see the chapters on Thailand and the Dominican Republic) this is better understood as a continuum than as a clear dichotomy. In the same way some workers have a sense of themselves as gay while others, not necessarily immediately distinguishable, strongly deny any such identity. Each culture has somewhat different ways of conceptualizing sexuality and gender and their interconnection; Storer's discussion of identities in the Thai context draws attention to the fact that the dominant dichotomies implied by both North Atlantic and Latin American views of active/passive (John Rechy's 'real men' and 'queens') may not be appropriate elsewhere.

What is striking, although not always explicitly drawn out by the authors, is that for many men sex work becomes a way of coming to terms with being homosexual. As Kruks (1991) has argued: 'Contrary to a popular belief that most males involved in homosexual prostitution are heterosexuals, data collected by Children's Hospital Los Angeles shows that 72 per cent of males involved in survival sex identify themselves as gay or bisexual.' Almost all the contributors to this book point out the ways in which prostitution can be a way for a young man to come to terms with homosexual desires which social pressures would deny.

The chapter by Patrick Larvie on Brazil is the most explicit in linking the particularities of sex work to homophobia. His suggestion of an 'erotics of the closet' offers a way of understanding the particular ways in which sex work allows for homosexual encounters for both client and worker while maintaining existing boundaries around race, class, age and permissible behaviour. It is rewarding to read many of the other chapters in this book against Larvie's comment that 'For many males the act of prostitution may actually be more akin to a ritualized form of sexual transgression than the kind of sex-for-money transaction which occurs commonly among female and transvestite sex workers.' Moya and Garcia echo this in their description of some aspects of sex work in Santo Domingo. On the other hand, Liguori and Aggleton, in their discussion of sex work in Mexico City, suggest other links with homophobia, emphasizing the violence experienced by some male sex workers and the widespread neglect within HIV prevention programmes.

And HIV/AIDS?

The epidemiological history of AIDS is related to the patterns of global movement which typify the end of the twentieth century. While tourism is a relatively small part of the total picture, sex tourism has helped shape particular epidemics and spread particular ways of being homosexual, as the chapter on the Dominican Republic makes clear. A recent example, mentioned in the chapter on the Netherlands, is the movement of young Eastern Europeans across the former Iron Curtain, with often little means of support other than their bodies. In Berlin, Vienna and Paris young Poles, Czechs and Romanians often use saunas as places to find clients. In Kuala Lumpur, I have been told, one can pay for sex with young Bosnian refugees who have been admitted to Malaysia as a result of Islamic solidarity.

Without the HIV/AIDS epidemic most of the studies described in this book would not have occurred. Gradually policy makers have come to acknowledge the extent of male sex work, though I doubt if the government would even consider the assertion by Khan that there are as many men as women in sex work in Bangladesh. One early attempt by governments to estimate the numbers of male commercial sex workers concluded there were 'none' in China or Zambia; of the governments who responded only France, Colombia and the Czech Republic acknowledged men might make up 10 per cent or more of 'commercial workers' (Mann, Tarantola and Netter, 1996, p. 376). It is not surprising that male workers often remain stigmatized and ignored in programmes directed either at 'MSMs' or at 'prostitutes'.

Most of the authors in this book have been directly involved in HIV prevention work, and many of the chapters (for example France, Costa Rica, Brazil, India, Morocco) grow out of the experience of particular prevention programmes. AIDS, too, has furthered the development of political organization among sex workers, both men and women, although relatively few of the chapters in this book focus explicitly on this (but see Allman and Myers on Canada). All the contributors stress the general neglect of male sex workers in HIV programmes, and the need to develop specific programmes which will address their particular circumstances. The political organization and empowerment of sex workers in at least some countries (Australia, New Zealand, the Netherlands, South Africa) has been a significant development of the past decade, and has had some impact in developing countries such as Brazil, the Philippines and Thailand.

Conclusions

We need to analyze sex work on a number of levels, respecting both the extent to which the worker is often a more autonomous agent than his/her 'victim' status suggests, while not losing sight of the moral indignation with which Khan reminds us that 'For the vast majority of people sex work . . . is a survival strategy. For most it is a practice enforced by poverty, degradation, homelessness, hunger and powerlessness, a form of slavery to economic, social and cultural deprivation, stigmatization and marginalization . . .'.

At the same time, as Khan also reminds us (and as the chapters on the United States and France eloquently echo), sex work can also be a way of finding companionship and support. Peter Davies and Rayah Feldman write: 'These young men are evidently often seeking friendship and support as well as sex from their punters.' If there is a political economy to sex work there is an equally important libidinal and emotional economy at play/work. Nor is sex work *per se* either unsafe or dangerous; the Canadian chapter quotes sex work activist, Danny Cockerline, as saying: 'Most people who become infected with HIV are getting it for free.' The real threat of the male sex worker is that he destabilizes assumptions about gender, sexuality, desire and affection, and the temptation is always there to stereotype sex work as a simple transaction without larger social meanings.

This book sets the stage for continuing analysis of male sex work, which would both expand on the political and the libidinal economies explored by some of the authors. There is a need for some exploration of the erotic charge of paying and being paid, suggested in the common term 'to spend' for male orgasm. Edmund White (1997, p. 245) has written that 'Johns resent having to pay. Even if the idea of paying (and controlling) someone excites them in advance, after they come they feel insulted.' There is room for a whole new set of studies focusing on those who buy rather than those who sell sex, as well as on the quite extensive use of homosexual pornography and its relationship to HIV prevention.

To read *Men Who Sell Sex* is to find one's stereotypes constantly challenged, often within individual chapters as the authors struggle to come to terms with the complexities of their subject. The strength of this book is its very provisionality: that is, it reports a whole set of works in progress, attempts to make sense of complex questions which involve both the individual psyche and large global structures. Useful social research in an unfolding epidemic needs to combine the individual and the structural, to provide both conceptual frameworks and personal understandings. This *Men Who Sell Sex* does, in ways which are both challenging and moving.

References

FISHER, M. (1997) 'Cunanan fit the pattern of "preppy gigolo"', *International Herald Tribune*, 26 July.

ISHERWOOD, C. (1997) *Wonder Bread and Ecstasy: The Life and Death of Joey Stefano*, Los Angeles: Allison.

KRUKS, G. (1991) 'Gay and lesbian homeless/street youth: special issues and concerns', *Journal of Adolescent Health*, **12**, 7, pp. 515–18.

MANN, J., TARANTOLA, D. and NETTER, T. (Eds) (1996) *AIDS In the World*, Harvard University Press.

O'HARA, S. (1996) *Autopornography: A Life in the Lust Lane*, Binghampton: Haworth.

PERKINS, R. and BENNETT, G. (1985) *Being a Prostitute*, Sydney: Allen & Unwin.

WHITE, E. (1997) *The Farewell Symphony*, London: Chatto & Windus.

Chapter 1

Selling Sex in Cardiff and London

Peter Davies and Rayah Feldman

The advent of AIDS in the early 1980s found a scientific community sorely lacking in recent and reliable information about a number of the populations primarily affected, none more so than male sex workers, a group marginal not only to mainstream society, but to other marginal groups. The small literature that existed before the 1980s nevertheless paints a picture which incorporates:

> two compelling stereotypes: that of the straight hustler and that of the teenage runaway prostitute. These two portraits, often merged in a single, sorry account, dominate contemporary sociological descriptions and fuel popular and journalistic stereotypes. (Davies and Simpson, 1990, p. 109)

These images derive primarily from the work of Reiss (1961), Butts (1947) and, in Britain, Harris (1973) and Lloyd (1979). Of these, Reiss has certainly been the most influential. He describes a group of heterosexually identified young men engaging in sex work and characterizes the norms which allow them to reconcile a heterosexual self-image with homosexual activity. These include an emphasis on the financial rewards of the work and a denial of physical pleasure from the sex; a disdain and even hatred for the punter; and a restriction of sexual activity to the insertive, masculine role in oral intercourse.

Three aspects of this analysis are relevant here. First, we note a reluctance to believe that the rent boy can be homosexual by preference. Indeed, such a figure is strikingly absent from the literature. In policy terms, this presupposition manifests itself in the implicit goal of most interventions, removing the young men involved from sex work, and in the absence of sex work from interventions targeted on, or indeed developed by, the gay community.

Second, it seems taken for granted that no young man would rationally choose sex work as a means of living. It is sufficient at this point simply to note that sex work can, in many circumstances, be a relatively lucrative and attractive alternative to repetitive and demoralizing factory work or the ill-paid harum-scarum of the fast-food empires.

Third, child sexual abuse features prominently in early discussions of male sex work. On the one hand, there are those who take the youth of the men involved in sex work as *a priori* evidence that prostitution is little more than formally structured abuse (Lloyd, 1979). On the other hand, sexual abuse also appears as a key feature of the suggested etiology of the 'prostitute personality'. The late Richie McMullen has argued strongly that there is a 'logical process' from receiving gifts and/or money as 'reward' for suffering abuse as a child, through a process of self-legitimation in which he persuades himself of his complicity in and enjoyment of the abuse, to a position which 'allows him to abuse others and/or set himself up for further abuse' (McMullen, 1988, p. 40). West's work (1992) has, however, failed to find empirical support for this contention, and elsewhere we have doubted the logic of the argument (Robinson and Davies, 1991).

At the heart of this traditional discourse of male prostitution is the figure of the powerless prostitute. An alternative view of sex work has emerged from within feminism. At the heart of this new discourse is an attempt to replace discussion of 'prostitution' with the idea of sex work. In so doing it emphasizes the economic aspect of sex work, what people do, rather than the pathological or proto-psychiatric aspect, what they are.

Shorn of its feminist specificities, this perspective makes a distinction between sex work and destitution. It recognizes and highlights the fact that the literature and most discussion of male sex work concentrates on the conjunction of these two features, looking only at the homeless, drifting or otherwise 'chaotic' young man on the streets of the large cities. It then contrasts this with the existence of a flourishing market in sex supplied by individuals who in no way correspond to this stereotype (see Davies and Simpson, 1990; Robinson and Davies, 1991; Hickson *et al.*, 1994; also Marotta, Waldorf and Murphy, 1988, for American examples). Noting that there are many who carry out sex work in congenial circumstances and with control over their lives and work, it argues that this is a possible goal for all those who find themselves involved in sex work. Better, they argue, to work from a flat with the ability to choose customers than from the street-corners with desperation.

With this basic perspective, a different set of policy preferences from those associated with the traditional view emerges. These seek the decriminalization of sex work and, more broadly, its rescue from stigmatization. More specifically, it identifies the need to make sex workers better at their jobs (see Kooistra and Hazenkamp, 1992). This involves a number of specific agendas. First, it rejects removal from sex work as the only or the best solution in all cases. Second, it recognizes the importance of punter-free spaces as a means for workers to organize their own work in as congenial a manner as possible. Third, it recognizes that the aim of programmes for and by sex workers is to exploit the market position that they have. This involves the further development of existing skills and the empowerment of individuals.

Sex Work and HIV

The emergence of AIDS and the identification of the modes of transmission of HIV have led to a great deal of research on rates of HIV infection among female and, to a lesser extent, male sex workers in various cities around the world (Tirelli *et al.*, 1988; Coutinho, van Andel and Rijsdijk, 1988; Chiasson *et al.*, 1988; Elifson *et al.*, 1988). We refrain from detailed comment on these findings, since it seems a dubious and unscientific undertaking to compare the rates of HIV positivity in populations that are culturally diverse, from samples that vary in representativeness and in countries at different stages of the epidemic, as if the label 'prostitute' were a universal category with specific physical potentials for infection rather than a socially and culturally bound and constrained set of social and sexual practices and relationships.

Rather than this futile comparison, a recognition that sex workers may be presumed to be at risk of acquiring HIV through their work is needed and, thus, a valid aim of public policy is to assess the level of that risk and to take steps to enable those involved to minimize their exposure to infection.

Sex Work and Safer Sex

Many, if not most, health promotion projects promote the idea that unsafe sex consists of a particular behaviour or set of behaviours which have to be eradicated from the repertoire. When men having sex with men are concerned, anal intercourse is the behaviour most frequently and, given its high risk of transmission, rightly targeted activity. However, as we have elsewhere sought to argue (Davies and Weatherburn, 1991, Davies and Project SIGMA, 1992), at the individual level, such monolithic assessments of risk are neither actual nor realistic, nor always helpful features of sexual behaviour. While some individuals always and in every circumstance choose to avoid high risk behaviour, many others choose not to do so.

Despite this, most behavioural scientists recommend programmes which will ensure that the individuals avoid the behaviours entirely. We prefer a different approach, believing that individuals make complex assessments of the risk involved in a particular encounter or within a particular relationship, not on the basis of a sterile weighting of the benefits of sex in that context against the likelihood of infection and the disadvantages attendant upon it, but rather on the basis of a number of heuristic, contingent weightings, some of which may be more appropriate than others. In general, we believe that many gay and bisexual men have evolved risk minimization strategies that involve rational, well-informed and sophisticated decisions about their behaviour (for a detailed discussion of these points see Davies *et al.*, 1993, Chapter 5).

The actual risk for a particular sex worker will, of course, vary with the pattern of his sexual behaviour. In general, the greater the number of times he has anal intercourse, particularly in the receptive mode, the greater the risk. The use of condoms for anal intercourse, while reducing the risk to both partners, does not eradicate the risk. Smaller risks attach to the ingestion of semen, while a pattern of work that consisted solely of masturbation would seem to carry little or no risk of infection, however many clients were involved. The degree of exposure of an individual will depend on the actual mix of practices in his repertoire.

Methods

The complexity of male sex work as a lived experience demands an appropriately complex set of methods for understanding what is involved. The study described in this chapter used observation techniques and unstructured interviews within a broadly ethnographic approach as well as more structured, formal interviews. Ethnographic methods have been successfully employed in researching social groups or subcultures which have either withdrawn and/or have been excluded from mainstream society (Humphreys, 1970; Whyte, 1943). Ethnographic research is premised on exploring research subjects and their activities in their 'natural' setting.

This chapter reports on findings from ethnographic fieldwork and interviews carried out in 1992–93 with two groups of male sex workers. The first group came from the West End of London where we found a large street scene, with complex, intrinsic social organization. The second came from Cardiff, where there is a small street scene with a degree of intrinsic social organization, but mainly symbiotic within a larger 'street corner' society. A total of 130 young men participated in the study.

Numbers and Backgrounds

Formal interviews were carried out with 81 young men in Cardiff and 49 in London. While we are confident that the Cardiff sample includes nearly all the workers regularly selling sex in the area, this is not the case in London, where the majority of our contacts came from the charity Streetwise, which provides a range of services for this group of young men.

The average age of the Cardiff group was slightly under 18, with a range from 15 to 23. The average age of the young men interviewed in London was slightly higher than those in South Wales at 20, with a range from 16 to 29. Although the reported ages may be different from real ages, there did not seem to be large numbers of young boys involved in either scene. The majority of the sample was white and British. Four black men (two in each site) were interviewed, and 11 of the London group were from Western Europe or the white Commonwealth, reflecting the capital's international attraction.

The Cardiff group lived in a number of towns in the city's industrial hinterland. Some of these young men worked in their home towns while others preferred to travel to the more anonymous city. This tends to confirm evidence from our fieldwork that there is migration along the main train routes. Thus, there is a natural movement within the area to Cardiff, the largest city, and from the area as a whole to other cities, including London. There is also some movement to Amsterdam, and while this is organized, we have had no evidence of coercion.

In London, nearly all those in the sample were homeless and the remainder had precarious living arrangements with friends or in squats. By contrast, nearly half of the young men in Cardiff (47 per cent) lived with their parents and another 17 (21 per cent) with a male partner in a flat or house. Sixteen (20 per cent) lived alone in a flat or bedsit and six (7 per cent) in shared accommodation. Only three were living in squats.

In the London group, the level of formal education was minimal, whereas in Cardiff 15 of the workers were still at school and a further 15 had no qualifications, forty-one had CSE qualifications and eight GCSEs, two of whom were studying for A levels. There were five with A levels, two of whom were students in higher education. While the Cardiff group seems to reflect fairly well the class composition of the city, the London group was clearly drawn from the most deprived section of the community.

All the workers interviewed in South Wales laid claim to either a gay or bisexual identity, whereas in London, the picture was less clear-cut. Seventeen of the 48 (35 per cent) regarded themselves as gay, one as homosexual and two as queer (total 20: 41 per cent). Only four (8 per cent) regarded themselves as straight or heterosexual and a further 14 (28 per cent) as bisexual. Most made some qualification about the inability of these broad terms to confine or limit their potential or actual experience.

Thirteen (26 per cent) of the London group had a regular boyfriend at the time of interview and six (12 per cent) had a girlfriend. Two of these had children. In addition, 25 (51 per cent) said that they had had casual non-paying male sexual partners, but only two had had casual female partners. Five (11 per cent) reported both male and female non-paying partners. Company, trust and stability were stressed by many as the positive aspects of these relationships and a small but significant number reported having a boyfriend or girlfriend with whom they had not (yet) had sex. Yet others, in the early stages of a relationship, reported that they were very sexual. In South Wales, 23 (28 per cent) had a boyfriend and only six (7 per cent) a girlfriend. Fifty-nine (73 per cent) reported a non-paying male partner in the month before interview while only eight (10 per cent) reported a female partner who did not pay for sex.

Careers

Interviews did not deal in detail with personal histories or moral careers. Participants were asked, however, to recall their first experience with a punter, that is to recall their entry into sex work. Replies were recorded from 63 young men. Only five (6 per cent) of the respondents reported abuse at ages ranging from seven to 14. Another nine refused to answer this question, and in some cases the terms in which this was done suggests a traumatic memory. Nevertheless, the predominant figure in the recollections of the first experience is the recognition of an economic opportunity, though the dimensions of this are many. For a small number, a conscious decision is taken to work. For example,

> We had recently moved into a flat together and were finding we could afford rent, gas, electricity, food but we had little left for going out or saving for a holiday. So we discussed how we could earn extra money and as a joke at first said let's go on the game. We discussed this further and said we'd give it a try but wanking only. The first night we tried we did three punters each – that was £30 in total. Now we try to do five or six and we are saving for a holiday in Tunisia.

Some found out about the possibilities of earning money from others who earned money in that way:

> When I was 16 I went to a pub with a pal and he kept going to the toilet and coming back with money. He told me he was wanking old queens for £5 a go. He said it was easy money so I had a go.

Many, however, recall their 'first time' as part of the experimentation of youth. Central to this set of responses is the realization that what gave pleasure could also earn cash or goods.

> I was 14 years old and was out fishing with an older boy . . . He said he'd give me 10 Embassy [cigarettes] if I wanked him off. I agreed. I suppose indirectly he was my first punter as prior to that I'd done it for nothing.

Also noticeable is the fact that the first punter is often of the same age, or slightly older than the boy himself. Respondents spoke frequently of 'a boy', 'an older boy', 'older boys in school' and son on. Others have been approached by older men, usually referred to as 'old queens':

> I used to visit an older guy (about 55) and he used to give me money to touch me up. I think he's dead now.

> I was 16 years old. An old queen came up to me and I thought 'If he wants it badly enough he can pay for it.' I told him it would cost him £5 for a wank. Silly old bugger gave me £5 and I wanked him off.

While these were clearly significant events for the young men involved, it is important not to attribute causal force to them without further discussion.

Doubtless, many other boys and young men have been given or offered money for sex at one time or another. These young men have developed their insight, and made use of that knowledge in a particular way. Their choice to become sex workers, and to exploit that opportunity, is a logically separate decision.

Lifestyles and Social Networks

Despite the different demographic profile, life for the two groups was very similar. For these young men, sex work formed part of a street lifestyle in which the passing of time becomes an end in itself. They had few dependable long-term relationships even though they were acquainted with a wide range of people. The absence of employment, often few and weak family ties (which is typical of many young men of this age) enabled them to move freely from place to place in response to new opportunities. Furthermore, because many of them were also engaged in other kinds of illegal activities such as burglary and car theft, they sometimes needed to move house or even to leave town to lie low.

Most of them worked only spasmodically and left sex work for long or short periods, for instance to work abroad or in another town, because they had acquired a new sugar daddy, because they had a job, because they went to live with a girlfriend, and so on. This pattern was more evident in Cardiff where the financial rewards of sex work were less attractive. As an example, of 18 young men observed working in Cardiff in September 1990, and 13 in March 1991, only three of those working in September were also observed the following March.

Social relationships between the young men themselves were generally casual, depending on their presence at common meeting places. They also revolved around certain activities such as drinking, smoking dope, playing fruit machines, car thefts (joy-riding), and other kinds of theft such as shoplifting, burglary or stealing from cars. Socializing and making money were very much linked activities. They would meet at a café or a cottage, hang about, go off with a punter to make some money, and then come back and go to the pub with some of the others.

Although the workers used their earnings from sex work for basic necessities such as food, they also used them for social spending such as drinking. Their style of life may mean that they often spent money on cigarettes or drink rather than on food. This kind of spending helped to establish social position within the group. It is striking that on every occasion on which the field-worker lent a worker some money, he recorded hours or a day or two later that the money was repaid, or he was invited to have a drink with the worker in question. In other words, having money established a worker's independence and competence.

When possible, income from male street sex work is directed to the maintenance of 'street cred' among a particular group of young men, so that when a sex worker has money he will want to display this to his friends, including other sex workers. In practice the young men have little to display unless they thieve. One sex worker, Gerry, turned up one evening on his new mountain bike and chatted to the field-worker about fast cars and expensive bike gear and clothes. He seemed to disappear from the scene about a month after that, but three months later the field-worker recorded that Gerry was in prison on remand for theft. Mostly, however, having money is a fantasy. The study observed far more instances of the young men begging on the street, and borrowing, than of extravagance. Money was sought for very immediate and specific ends.

The 'macho' and erratic character of this lifestyle, and the fact that as a lifestyle it is not at all exclusive to gay young men, militate against the development of overtly close relationships (sexual or non-sexual). Extracts from the field diary express this contrast between sometimes intensive social interaction on the one hand, accompanied by secrecy and ambivalence about their sexuality on the other. As workers chose to withdraw from this kind of street-corner life, so they also may have tended to give up sex work. For instance one young man was now living with his pregnant girlfriend and said that he did not do many punters these days as he stays at home with his girlfriend most nights.

Like many other young men of this age, sex workers often maintain quite separate ongoing relationships with parents and family, which they keep well out of their street life. Sex work therefore appears within a wider lifestyle and culture, where self-image and self-esteem are created by interaction within a wide range of fleeting relationships: with state agencies, with members of mainstream society and with others who share the lifestyle.

Relationships with Punters

Contrary to the popular stereotype, male sex workers do not cater solely for the anonymous, married, 'respectable' man who wants quick gratification on his way home from work. In this stereotype, prostitution involves little more than casual and anonymous coupling, and the relationship between the client and the sex worker is so transient as to be unproblematic, at least in affective terms. Indeed the fact that sex becomes a depersonalized cash transaction is the basis of at least part of the moral opprobrium attached to prostitution.

In practice, sex workers distinguish clearly and consequentially between casual and regular clients. Participant observation also revealed varied, complex, long-term and even caring relationships between some punters and the young men whom they paid for sex. Some were friendly with their regulars:

He's a nice guy, I go drinking with him, he knows my Mum.

I like him, he's a nice chap. I spend the evening with him, go out for dinner, not just sex.

Most, however, were realistic about the relationships, with varying degrees of affection mixed with a healthy appreciation of their essentially mercenary quality.

I reckon he's a great guy. He knows I phone him to get paid. I don't mind him saying 'No' coz next time he might say 'Yes'. I like him.

Known him for eight years. Met at Comptons (gay pub). I have his phone number. We are really good friends. He is a source of income.

Takes me out for dinner, buys drinks and gives me coke. He is vile, I do it for the money.

Opinions were fairly evenly divided over the merits and demerits of regular and casual punters. On the one hand there were those who stressed the predictability and safety of the regular client:

I prefer regulars, you know what's expected. With casuals, I try to negotiate sex beforehand but there is a fear of rape.

I prefer regular, you know what's going to happen.

while others saw the time spent in 'socializing' as wasted:

Prefer casual, regulars start to feel something for you and I don't want that.

Some preferred casual punters for the speed with which their money could be extracted:

Find them anywhere. I get stopped in the street. Prefer the casuals, I can do them and forget about them. As little sex as possible for the most money. I try and figure out how much they can afford before I open my mouth.

Prefer casuals: go with them, fuck off and get more money.

while recognizing the difficulties involved in always making new contacts and the greater potential for something to go wrong:

Will only pick up a punter on the street if I am strapped for cash. Will go out on the street anyway to be with my friends. Never know what

> you're going to expect. Element of danger around the atmosphere, for both the punter and you. But it has to be done. Never know what they are like.

> Given up on the Dilly [Piccadilly Circus]. Most of the guys there are just looking for 16-year-olds. Us old hens just can't hack it.

More than half of the London sample claimed at some time to have had a sugar daddy or to have lived with a punter for some period of time. The sugar-daddy relationship is often problematic. One of the respondents summed up his relationship with a sugar daddy by saying that he had received from him 'gifts and grief'. This feeling that the older/richer man was seeking to buy commitment, to manipulate a financial into an affective relationship, was a common one.

> Met him at my usual pitch. He really fancied me and I thought 'Oh well'. He said I was too honest to be a rent boy. Nothing but trouble and a lot of money. Don't know what he got out of it, sexual satisfaction and a huge overdraft.

> We met two or three years ago at the Dilly. He was passing through. We never went out but I lived with him for year and a half. I was on the street at the time, there was something about me that he liked. I was with him because of his personality. He was really stupid. If I saw clothes I liked he bought them for me. It felt like he was buying my love.

Another respondent sought to describe the strange nature of the relationship as:

> Like my big brother, but we had sex.

Many were at pains to stress the lack of sexual contact in the relationship:

> He's an ex-rent boy. No sex. He's a really nice guy, I like him, I would never nick off him.

> What emerges most clearly in the comments both on regular punters and sugar daddies is the ambivalence: not only towards individual clients, about whom the respondents have mixed feelings, but also towards punters as a class.
> Some punters who know each other also refer workers to one another. These kinds of connections, if they are not coercive (and there is no evidence to suggest that they are), must involve some trust and affection between the individuals involved.

These young men evidently often seek friendship and support as well as sex from their punters. Alternatively, in some cases they see sex with punters as the price they pay for being looked after in some way. This price might sometimes be too high. One sex worker, John, had a job on the Isle of Wight arranged for him by a punter, Derek, but John did not want to sleep with Derek, and was not prepared to go unless he could have his own accommodation.

Both punters and most sex workers are very vulnerable to the aggression and dishonesty of a small number of workers. Although the style of fieldwork was biased in favour of information about more regular sex workers and punters, known venues also attract occasional punters and sex workers. The destruction of established venues, whether because of police zeal, gay bashers, or violent and dishonest sex workers, actually makes the task of outreach work among sex workers more difficult.

However, a significant minority of the sex workers were not well known to the field-worker or, evidently, to regular sex workers. In Cardiff, many connections were observed between older men unknown to the field-worker, and young men were seen loitering at the venues. For instance, a field-worker described seeing a young man whom he did not know get on the bus with a punter 'after lurking for about an hour' at the bus station. On other occasions workers would disappear into a multi-storey car park following or followed by a man. Such connections were frequently all that was observed, and one must assume that some of the workers and men were occasional players on the scene. Often both were keen to preserve anonymity.

On the other hand, a few men spent several hours each day at the sex working venues. They seemed to enjoy not only watching out for potential sexual partners, but also merely surveying the workers on the scene. They would stop and chat with other punters, free-trade cottagers and sex workers outside the cottages [public urinals] or in neighbouring cafés. Sometimes they would meet a regular sex worker at a pre-arranged spot, and after having sex, and/or going out for a meal or drink, they would come together to the pub or a café where punters and sex workers met.

Knowledge and Attitudes

Major differences were found in knowledge about and attitudes towards HIV and safer sex in the South Wales and London samples. In South Wales, there was a general vagueness about sources of information on HIV and AIDS, with most workers (38: 47 per cent) saying that all the listed sources were useful and eight (10 per cent) saying that none were. Of the single sources, outreach programmes were specifically mentioned by nine (11 per cent) of the workers. Only three (4 per cent) mentioned other sex workers and none mentioned punters. This suggests that outreach work is currently useful, even though there was not, at the time, a targeted programme in the area.

Even when specifically questioned about punters as a source of information on HIV and AIDS, only one of the participants said that a punter (or several punters) had given him information about HIV and safer sex. Similarly, only one reported that he gave information to his punters. These responses can be interpreted in two ways: either that safer sex is taken for granted as part of the culture and need not be talked about, or that the punter/worker relationship is not the place where such conversations take place. It seems, however, from the data on sexual behaviour (below) that the former is more likely.

In London, by contrast, general awareness of issues surrounding HIV and AIDS was widespread. This may reflect the influence of the Streetwise Project, the source of most of the respondents, which ran an effective set of HIV prevention programs. Only one respondent said that he 'didn't know' about safer sex (and he may have been being awkward). None of the accounts we were given of safer sex were seriously out of kilter with current understandings or guidelines.

Since many studies have shown that the link between knowledge and behaviour is weak, the importance of accurate knowledge must not be over-emphasized. Knowledge is, at best, a necessary condition for safer sex. At worst, it may be completely irrelevant, for example in the case where there is a demand for unsafe sex or where the factors encouraging the unsafe behaviour greatly outweigh those which discourage it.

Asked to voice their concerns about HIV, the respondents produced a range of answers which differ on two dimensions: personal relevance and degree of concern. A few made anodyne comments about the epidemic, which marked both its distance from them and its impersonal character:

Quite sad, epidemic, now out of control.

I am concerned about it but not personally.

Another group evinced concern, but at an impersonal level:

Really worried, [there are] so many ignorant people out there.

That it's on the increase but through the centuries things like the black plague burn themselves out. I hope AIDS will, coz wearing a condom is like having a sock on your dick.

Others felt it to be a matter which touched them personally, but which elicited little concern or relevance, either because of fatalism:

As long as I don't get it I don't give a shit.

or because of the choices made about safer sex:

Hopefully that I am not going to get it which is why I don't screw with casual punters.

I think I am in a low risk category as I always use condoms and lube. Work out what kind of person he is. Never cum inside a punter. Make sure I am safe.

Most, however, recognized its personal impact and relevance and some linked this concern to their behaviour, though with varying degrees of perceived efficacy:

I do think about it so I try to take a condom if I know I am doing a punter but it's more at the back of my mind than at the front. I know there's a danger but often I need the money.

I'm always careful. My partner has HIV so I have to be careful.

The majority in this group, however, interpreted the question as an invitation to volunteer the information that they had had an HIV antibody test. This suggests a degree of fatalism which, although understandable and indeed rational in the circumstances, is nonetheless sad. It is difficult to remain unmoved when one respondent volunteered:

If I was to catch it, I wouldn't be that worried. I would only get it from a boyfriend and love is more important than life. I've got really lonely: a couple of my friends committed suicide.

It is important to recognize that this sentiment marks not this young man's need for education, attitude change or even empowerment, but a rational reaction to a set of circumstances within which he finds himself. Changes in his view of the world will come only when those circumstances change. This points to a more general conclusion from this set of evidence, that is the importance of recognizing that for these young men HIV is just one problem among the many that confront them daily. It may be neither the most important nor the most immediate and it is both arrogant and dismissive for health educators to assume that it should be.

HIV Antibody Status

Respondents were also asked to say what they felt to be the advantages and disadvantages of knowing their antibody status. Most gave both advantages and disadvantages of a diagnosis, and all showed a high degree of awareness of the complexity of the issues involved. Unsurprisingly, accounts of the disadvantages centred on the certainty of an early death:

Knowing that you are dying. Problems with other people's attitudes.

A lot of people think you will have a short life. Nobody will want me, bang goes my sex life. Basically it's a worry and the more you worry the more your T-cell count goes down.

A very small number were fatalistic about the prospect:

Don't know – live your life. Don't get too upset.

If I got AIDS I would just go out and get off my face every night.

Many said that a positive result would spur them on to take greater care of themselves and others:

You can sort your shit out and do something for other people.

You are not going to pass it on to anyone. It would stop a lot of paranoia.

This was confirmed by one young man who had recently received a positive diagnosis:

It was a shock. I hadn't had unsafe sex. I will keep myself more healthy [and be] more conscious of risks to partners.

Most poignantly, a number of the young men remarked that a positive diagnosis would give them access to state benefits that they were now denied:

You can get a flat if you're positive and more sickness benefits and travelling expenses.

You get more money, sickness, mobility, attendance etc. . . .

Benefits, get a flat straight away.

I'd get a bus pass.

One respondent told us:

A lot of my friends have gone out of their way to catch it to get benefits. At least you can get on with your life.

And while we came across no direct evidence to corroborate this statement, it must be admitted that the course of action is rational.

Sexual Behaviour and HIV Risk

Detailed information on sexual practices in the week preceding interview was collected in the form of a diary. In London, 40 of the respondents reported 134 sexual sessions. Twenty-five of these were with regular punters, 40 with casual punters, 16 with regular non-paying male partners and three with regular non-paying female partners. A further 44 were with casual male partners who did not pay, and one with a casual female partner. In the following discussion we consider only those sessions involving paying partners.

In South Wales, 78 (96 per cent) of the young men interviewed had had sex with a punter in the month before interview. Of those that had done so, the average number of punters in the month before interview was 31, about one per day on average. Separately, participants were asked to recount in detail where and when they had had sex in the previous week. The total number of sessions was 523 for 80 people. The average number is thus almost exactly seven, one per day.

In London, 18 of the 134 sessions (13 per cent) involved only masturbation. The minimum charge reported was £25, the maximum £200 (which even the respondent regarded as unusual – and very lucky). The most common price was between £40 and £70, with nearly 80 per cent coming in this range. In South Wales, by contrast, nearly half of the sessions (253 of the 523: 48 per cent) involved only masturbation and the average price was just £5. Moreover, this service was only provided for casual clients.

A further 25 of the sessions in London involved oral sex. The average charge for this service to casual punters was £38, with a range from £30 to £75. For regular punters charges ranged from £45 to £95, with 80 per cent coming between £50 and £70. In this case, the regular punters seem to be paying a premium. In South Wales, 119 sessions (23 per cent) involved oral sex and the price was no different from that of manual relief at about £5. The service was rather more commonly provided to casual punters, though the price does not, in this case, vary.

Eight of the London sessions involved some sort of SM activity and the average charge for this service was £57. Only one session involving a casual punter was recorded, so comparisons are not possible. In Cardiff, there was no SM activity as such, although corporal punishment, usually spanking, accounted for eight sessions, all with regular punters, where the average charge was between £20 and £25.

In London, a further seven sessions were reported in which no sexual contact took place. These ranged from simply talking to punters to 'groping'. Some punters were apparently satisfied with 'just looking' and there was some dressing up in fantasy costumes. These were not mentioned in South Wales.

In London, only four of the sessions in the previous week had involved anal intercourse. Two of these were with regular punters and two with casual. The average charge for the casual partners was £75, for the regulars, £60. By contrast, in South Wales, 85 per cent of the sessions with regular punters involved anal intercourse, for which the average charge was between £15 and £20. Even with casual punters, 10 per cent of sessions involved anal intercourse and the charges were the same.

Condoms

In London, 42 of the respondents had used a condom at least once, and 20 were carrying some at the time of interview. Twenty-five said that they always carried condoms while working and 13 that they sometimes did so. In South Wales, 31 (38 per cent) of the participants claimed to be carrying condoms when interviewed, but only 17 (21 per cent) always carried them while working, while another 53 (64 per cent) sometimes did so. Such figures need to be treated sensibly. The assumption that the workers should always be doing so depends on an assumption that fucking is to be a part of the repertoire. This need not be so. If a worker does not do anal intercourse, the need for condoms is less salient.

More interesting is the finding that, on the last occasion that anal intercourse occurred with a punter, the worker provided the condom in 57 (70 per cent) cases, while the punter did so in only eight (10 per cent). The most commonly cited source of supply for condoms was a machine (58 mentions) and following in descending order of popularity: an outreach worker (19), the STD clinic (17), the chemist (13), the family planning clinic (8) and, once an old favourite, the barber (2).

A total of 30 respondents reported having had anal intercourse without a condom for a number of reasons. Four had been threatened with physical violence, four reported that they were frightened of losing the punter if they refused and eight were offered more cash to provide this service. Disconcertingly, 14 reported having been raped. On the other hand, 37 of the respondents reported having refused to have anal intercourse because a condom was not available.

We may summarize the findings on condom use as follows. Condom use is more common in London than in South Wales. Overall, and including all categories of paying and non-paying partners, a condom was used in only 20 per cent of sessions involving anal intercourse in South Wales. In London, by contrast, the rate was 77 per cent. Within this difference general patterns emerge. Condom use is less common with non-paying partners than with punters in both sites. In South Wales, condoms are used in 31 per cent of sessions with punters and in only 7 per cent of sessions with non-paying partners. In London, the figures are 72 per cent with non-paying and 82 per cent with paying partners.

Condom use is more common with casual than with regular partners in both sites. In South Wales, condoms are used in 13 per cent of sessions with regular partners and 27 per cent of sessions with casual punters. In London, the figures are 80 per cent with regulars and 85 per cent with casuals. Condoms are used less often for receptive than for insertive anal intercourse, insertive anal intercourse is less common with paying than non-paying partners and, overall, condoms are used more often with casual non-paying partners than with regulars.

The pattern of practices with different types of partner points to a number of important conclusions. First, the strong pattern between the sites no doubt reflects both the differences in sero-prevalence in the two areas as well as the greater level of HIV prevention initiatives for gay and bisexual men in the capital. While it is always risky to categorize levels of risk as 'high' or 'alarming', it must be said that the level of unprotected intercourse in South Wales is higher than an objective assessment of safety would recommend.

Second, while it seems to be the case that there is a group who do not engage in anal intercourse for a set of coherent reasons, it is not the case that the group which do engage in it do so because they are stupid and feckless or that they deny their susceptibility to HIV infection. Because anal intercourse is patterned by relationship, it indicates that decisions are being made at the level of the encounter or of the relationship. While it may be the case that these decisions are unwise, even in some cases foolhardy, the fact that they are decisions needs to be taken into account when health promotion programmes are considered. Rather than seek to isolate and correct the deficiencies that lead individuals to engage in 'unsafe' behaviour, the process of decision-making needs to be identified, recognized and encouraged.

Health

The male working-class youth culture to which many of the boys belong, does not leave much space for the discussion of sexuality, or mental or physical health. There is little evidence from fieldwork observations that boys were very concerned about their health in general or HIV in particular. We specifically asked the London group about their general health.

The majority of these young men reported that, in general, their health at the time of interview was good, though in some cases their expectations were low. A number of those reporting problems mentioned the effects of drink or drugs. Nineteen reports of serious health problems were given. The majority of these were chest problems, most commonly asthma, but also recent episodes of bronchitis. The next most common group was drug related ranging from 'a fucked-up liver', to the more usual problems with teeth and gums. There were also two reports of serious psychological problems. Minor problems at the time of interview showed a similar pattern, though skin problems, including acne, psoriasis and eczema were common.

When asked about their current emotional state, there was an almost exactly equal division into positive and negative comments. Positive comments rarely went beyond equability, whereas negative comments sometimes revealed, even in the artificial context of the interview, depths of desperation and unhappiness.

> Terrible. Not happy. Not sure why. Tiredness, not in a steady relationship – would like to be. Lack of finance – money doesn't cure it but it helps.

> Bored, bit lonely, pissed off with my life, seems to be a pattern, I want to break it and do something different. Get up, go out, do this, do that, go to bed, get up ect. . . .

> I've been doing a lot of gear. Been down getting drugs all the time. Worry that I will end up doing punters all my life and will never get off smack. My flat's falling to pieces.

Conclusions

Our research has shown that complex patterns of personal and social support exist among street workers in the cities studied. In general, these are articulated around core groups of current workers and ex-workers together with a small number of clients or other, older men. It is important to be clear that these are generally supportive networks and not based on control or exploitation. Policies which have the effect of disrupting or destroying these networks, either through direct interference by police or others, or through the disruption of venues where they meet, should be avoided as being inimical to the development of a positive sex-work culture within which safer sex can be promoted and maintained. Indeed, existing social networks should be regarded by those charged with health promotion as the prime vector of intervention and the main means by which HIV education can be given both credibility and functional relevance.

Since the majority of those engaged in off-street work are integrated into the gay community, this appears the most appropriate means of intervention for this group of workers. Gay community development has been shown to result in increased levels of safer sexual practice (Kippax *et al.*, 1993). Central to such programmes is the recognition of the diversity of the community, both as a target and as a mode of delivery for sexual health promotion. Sex workers form a part of that community, yet this is routinely denied or ignored by its opinion leaders. There is a range of reasons for this. Many feel that the existence of organized sex work in the gay community will be regarded by those who would deny civil rights to gay men and lesbians as further reason to diminish their precarious freedom under the law. Others feel that sex work has no place in the gay community since it represents a form of sexual relationship which that community seeks to eradicate. Such political considerations should not, however, be allowed to obscure the fact that sex work does take place and those involved have specific needs with respect to HIV prevention work which are not being addressed. Gay community development plans should specifically include the needs of sex workers, particularly those who work off-street.

Although there was some evidence in London that a sub-set of the street workers had developed an instrumental approach to the range of agencies set up to address their many problems, in the main, street workers were reactive and passive in their dealings with them. Since many of the young men we spoke to regarded state agencies in particular as the source of problems – over benefits, for example – rather than support or help, such an attitude is understandable. Some agencies had managed, however, to establish good relations with and reputations among this group of young men.

Along with the vast majority of those we interviewed – both professionals and actual and potential clients – we were most impressed by the scope and relevance of the service provided by the Streetwise charity. Such a project is, we believe, essential in London, where the size and complexity of the street scene make such a concentration and targeting of services both necessary and cost-effective. In other metropolitan areas, such specifically targeted services will also be appropriate.

Nevertheless, such targeted provision is both expensive and complex to establish and maintain. It seems more feasible in many cases to consider other means by which young street workers can be encouraged to meet, discuss options and choices available to them and to develop their skills and strategies. Outreach work is one means (see below), but the creation of other spaces where such discussions can be enabled should be considered. This may mean no more than taking over a room in a pub for a night or the provision of more extended facilities and back-up. In other cases a telephone helpline might be more appropriate. None of these need be expensive or time-consuming interventions.

Its nature ensures that a number of individuals will drift in and out of street work over time. Where there exists a large sex-work scene, outreach is necessary both to contact new clients and to become aware of new problems of existing ones. In centres where no such large numbers are working, outreach may be the only way in which this client group can be contacted. Since the fieldwork for this project was carried out, Streetwise has piloted a successful programme of peer education with its clients (Gibson and Aggleton, 1992; Gibson, 1992). The programme met with some considerable success, yet it remains unclear whether support for it will continue.

Specific HIV Services

We have strongly argued above that HIV is one among many concerns of this group and that the risk of HIV transmission to and from members can be reduced by measures which contribute to their more general well-being and self-confidence. Nevertheless, specific services will continue to be required. At a more basic level, information about HIV, its means of transmission and safer sexual strategies, remains important for new recruits to the industry and for existing members.

Because of the reactive relationship of most street workers to health care provision, it seems inevitable that traditional means of health care delivery will need to be reassessed if efficient and effective provision is to be made. Similar problems surround the provision of care for HIV positive street workers. It is a ridiculous situation when young men may feel it necessary to become HIV positive in order to become eligible for state benefits previously denied to them. Although we have found no direct evidence to confirm that individuals have deliberately become positive in order to gain access to such benefits, the choice was one of which our respondents were well aware.

Acknowledgements .

In Cardiff, discussions were held with workers at the HIV Clinic and the HIV/ AIDS Trust (Cardiff), as well as with two owners of gay pubs in the city. In London, we are grateful to the following for their time and the sharing of their expertise:

Streetwise: Tony Whitehead, Barbara Gibson, Afame Offiah, Colin, Mark Kjeldsen, Robert, Steven; The Basement Project: Steven Clarke; Barnardo's Streets of London Project: Brendan O'Mahony; London Connection: Fazal Mahmood; Hackney Outreach: Graham Reed; Hungerford Drug Project: Christopher Piercy; Lorne House: Bill Baker; Community Liaison Team, Westminster Hospital: Dr Deborah Mincham; Salvation Army Faith House: Keith Christian; CLASH (Central London Action on Street Health): Marcus Rose and Martin Calleja; Piccadilly Advice Centre: Carlo Kampora and four others; S.A.U.C.E.: Terry Blair; Wharf Side Clinic, St Mary's Hospital: Dr David Tomlinson. We are also grateful to the Department of Health who provided the funding for this study.

References

BUTTS, W.M. (1947) 'Boy prostitutes of the metropolis', *Journal of Clinical Psychopathology*, **8**, pp. 673–81.

CHIASSON, M.A., LIFSON, A.R., STONEBURNER, R.L., EWING, W. *et al.* (1988) 'HIV seroprevalence in male and female prostitutes in New York City', paper presented at the IVth International Conference on AIDS, Stockholm.

COUTINHO, R.A., VAN ANDEL, R.L.M., RIJSDIJK, T.J. (1988) 'Role of male prostitutes in the spread of sexually transmitted diseases and human immunodeficiency virus', *Genitourinary Medicine*, **64**, pp. 207–8.

DAVIES, P.M. and PROJECT SIGMA (1992) 'On relapse: recidivism, or rational response?', in P. AGGLETON, P.M. DAVIES and G. HART (Eds) *AIDS: Rights, Risk and Reason*, London: Falmer Press.

DAVIES, P.M. and SIMPSON, P. (1990) 'On male homosexual prostitution and HIV', in P. AGGLETON, P.M. DAVIES and G. HART (Eds) *AIDS: Individual, Cultural and Policy Dimensions*, London: Falmer Press.

DAVIES, P.M. and WEATHERBURN, P. (1991) 'Towards a general model of sexual negotiation', in P. AGGLETON, P.M. DAVIES and G. HART (Eds) *AIDS: Responses, Interventions and Care*, London: Falmer Press.

DAVIES, P.M., HICKSON, F.C.I., WEATHERBURN, P. and HUNT, A.J. (1993) *Sex, Gay Men and AIDS*, London: Taylor & Francis.

ELIFSON, K.W., BOLES, J., SWEAT, M., DARROW, W.W. *et al.* (1988) 'Seroprevalence of human immunodeficiency virus among male prostitutes', *New England Journal of Medicine*, **321**, pp. 832–3.

GIBSON, B. (1992) 'HIV/AIDS health promotion with street based men who have sex with men', in P. AGGLETON and I. WARWICK (Eds) *Young People, Homelessness and AIDS*, London: Health Education Authority.

GIBSON, B. and AGGLETON, P. (1992) 'Young homeless men selling sex in central London: identifying their HIV/AIDS education needs', poster Presentation at the VIII International Conference on AIDS (PoD 5042), Amsterdam.

HARRIS, M. (1973) *The Dilly Boys*, London: Croom Helm.

HICKSON, F.C.I., WEATHERBURN, P., HOWS, J. and DAVIES, P.M. (1994) 'Selling safer sex: male masseurs and escorts in the UK', in P. AGGLETON, P.M. DAVIES and G. HART (Eds) *AIDS: Foundations For The Future*, London: Taylor & Francis.

HUMPHREYS, L. (1970) *Tearoom Trade, A Study of Homosexual Encounters in Public Spaces*, Chicago: Aldine.

KIPPAX, S., CONNELL, R.W., DOWSETT, G.W. and CRAWFORD, J. (1993) *Sustaining Safer Sex: Gay Communities Respond to AIDS*, London: Falmer Press.

KOOISTRA, O. and HAZENKAMP, J.L. (1992) 'Streetwise: survival of boys in prostitution', paper presented at the 2nd Conference on Homosexuality and HIV, Amsterdam.

LLOYD, R. (1979) *Playland: A Study of Human Exploitation*, London: Quartet.

McMULLEN, R. (1988) 'Youth prostitution: a balance of power', *Journal of Adolescence*, **10**, pp. 33–43.

MAROTTA, T., WALDORF, D. and MURPHY, S. (1988) 'Males doing sex-work in the San Francisco Bay Area: a typology and description', unpublished paper, Institute for Scientific Analysis, San Francisco.

REISS, A.J. (1961) 'The social integration of queers and peers', *Social Problems*, **9**, pp. 102–19.

ROBINSON, T.J. and DAVIES, P.M. (1991) 'London's homosexual male prostitutes: power, peer groups and HIV', in P. AGGLETON, P.M. DAVIES and

G. HART (Eds) *AIDS: Responses, Interventions and Care*, London: Falmer Press.

TIRELLI, U., VACCHER, E., BULLIAN, P., SARACCHINI, S. *et al.* (1988) 'HIV-1 seroprevalence in male prostitutes in northeast Italy', *Journal of the Acquired Immunodeficiency Syndromes*, 1, pp. 414–17.

WEST, D.J. with B. DE VILLIERS (1992) *Male Prostitution*, London: Duckworth.

WHYTE, W. (1943) *Street Corner Society, The Social Structure of an Italian Slum*, Chicago: University of Chicago Press.

Chapter 2

Sex for Money between Men and Boys in the Netherlands: Implications for HIV Prevention

Wim Zuilhof

In 1989, organized efforts resulted in the setting up of an HIV prevention programme aimed at boys in sex work in the Netherlands.[1] This rather late start was due to two factors: first, the limited visibility of sex work involving young men, second, the absence of advocates for this group within the AIDS organizations at the time. We owe it to a few former field-workers[2] that HIV prevention for boys in sex work did not in fact begin much later.[3]

Although no specific HIV prevalence studies have taken place among boys in sex work or their clients, it can be assumed that both are at heightened risk of infection. By October 1996, 4200 people had been diagnosed with AIDS in the Netherlands. Of these, 71.5 per cent were gay or bisexual men, 10.5 per cent injecting drug users and 1 per cent gay or bisexual drug users. A recent Amsterdam cohort study of 400 gay men under 30 years of age found that 6 per cent were HIV positive, an increase of 1 per cent compared to the year before (Public Health Department Amsterdam, 1996). Seroprevalence among older gay men is higher (estimates vary from 1 in 7 men who have sex with men in the built-up areas of Western Holland, to 1 in 15 in other parts of the country). In 1987, 5.2 per cent of homosexual men taking part in a Dutch cohort study reported having paid for sex at some time in the past, and 6.5 per cent had received payment (de Graaf *et al.*, 1994a). Considering these figures and acknowledging the relatively high frequency of sexual contacts with boys in sex work, the chance of one or both partners being HIV positive is quite high.

Forty per cent of the young men who took part in the Amsterdam cohort study had had one or more acts of unprotected anal sex in the previous six-month period (Public Health Department Amsterdam, 1996). In 1990 and 1991, 27 male sex workers were interviewed extensively about their experience of sex with clients. Two groups of boys in sex work appeared to be particularly vulnerable. First, there were those with a gay identity who allowed their sexual feelings to come out during paid contacts. They were more likely to consent to receptive anal intercourse, especially when they worked in more private settings where contact can be more intimate. Second, there were boys who were heavily addicted to drugs and who had less control over the nature of paid encounters when in need of money to buy drugs (de Graaf *et al.*, 1994a).

Fluidity and Change

The social fabric of boys in sex work in the Netherlands is constantly changing. Until the early 1970s, organized forms were virtually non-existent. Young men met their clients in public places (most usually railway stations, parks and squares) and to a lesser extent in gay bars (van der Poel, 1991). In the 1970s, however, organized sex work came into being because of a liberalization of legislation when the age of consent for homosexual behaviour was lowered from 21 to 16 years. At the same time, government policy began to allow (with certain restrictions) organized sex work as a business, while keeping it formally illegal. In this climate boys' clubs and private houses where sex could be paid for came into being. Because of Amsterdam's growing reputation as centre for youth and gay culture, and as a sanctuary for (soft) drug use, the population of boys in sex work became more international.

More recent changes have been brought about by increasing sexual tolerance, changing government policies on sex work, the appearance of HIV, internationalization and multi-culturalization, and changes due to drug use.

Sexual Tolerance

Dutch society is relatively tolerant about sex and sexuality compared to most other countries. Although sex work is not an everyday issue for the majority of people, in sexually liberal circles there are fewer taboos about it, on the part of both boys and clients, than there were in the past. Both male and female sex workers frequently appear in the media using their real names. On the Amsterdam gay scene, a good-looking boy with expensive clothing, equipped with a mobile phone and earning his money as an escort is seen as a welcome guest. Among the older generation of emancipated gay men, paying for sex seems to be less of a taboo. The Gay Business Association, of which most Amsterdam gay bars, bookshops and non-profit organizations are members, now includes a number of escort services and brothels. One of the most popular gay monthly magazines is owned by the proprietors of two boys' sex work businesses. In these and other magazines, frequent interviews with boys in sex work are published in which the job is described as being something quite normal.

There is, however, another side to the coin. As a result of greater sexual openness, sexual abuse is more visible and has been discussed extensively in the media. The resulting public outrage has reduced tolerance towards paedophiles, and threatens to affect the climate surrounding boys in sex work.

Government Policy

Tolerance of sex work and the political acceptance of homosexuality have made it possible for organized forms of boys' sex work to develop in the Netherlands. For years now, a change of the legislation has been discussed that would legalize sex work businesses such as brothels and escort services. Policy-makers in large cities urge this legalisation in order to control and regulate working conditions, undertake HIV prevention, treat STDs and collect taxes. Because a work permit would then become compulsory, many boys and women from non-EC countries would lose their jobs. Such an amendment would have far-reaching consequences and has therefore undergone a number of modifications and postponements. Those looking after the interests of sex workers, and proprietors who initially welcomed the amendment, now look on it with mixed feelings. Not without reason, the most often expressed fear is the emergence of a considerable illegal underground network that would be difficult to influence or control.

Nevertheless the amendment is likely to become law and, in preparation for this, a number of proprietors have joined together to form an association of 'Relax Businesses'. This association was one of the organizations that initiated moves towards a hallmark for brothels to promote self-regulation by owners, and to improve the position of boys and women working in such clubs (van Mens, 1995). In the last few years, anticipating the future law amendment, local governments have brought in stringent policies aimed at the boys' sex work sector. Increasing rigorous action towards boys with illegal status has resulted in the virtual disappearance of Czech boys from Amsterdam brothels. This policy change was probably also influenced by media reporting of police statements in the US and the UK suggesting permissiveness about paedophilia in the Netherlands and describing the part Amsterdam plays in international paedophilia networks (McMullen, 1987). A parliamentary inquiry into the criminal investigation policy of the police and Ministry of Justice in Holland, and the shockwaves throughout Western Europe after the Dutroux case in 1996, have stimulated the demand for a more forceful policy of checking boys' ages and motivations.

HIV and its Consequences

HIV seems to have had relatively little effect on the number of boys and clients. There is, however, a taboo about being HIV seropositive. Clients and boys who are seropositive generally conceal their status. To be open about this would make it impossible to work in a club. The few boys who are open have an enormous impact on risk awareness among other boys and clients. Formally, both clubs and escort services have safe sex policies. In unorganized forms of sex work safe sex also tends to be the norm. The advent of HIV also seems to have intensified the involvement of (health) policy-makers in boys' sex work, and both national and local authorities have started HIV prevention programmes for boys in sex work.

Internationalization and Cultural Diversity

Today, not only can a wider diversity of sex work be distinguished, but the populations of boys in the business have become more diverse. Thirty years ago only a distinction between straight and gay boys seemed relevant (van der Poel, 1991). In Amsterdam, boys from at least 20 different countries are involved in commercial sex (Zuilhof, 1994). These include those from West European, Latin American, Islamic and East European backgrounds. Although internationalization is a particularly strong feature of Amsterdam, it is also true in other cities. In 1993/94, van Gelder (1995) identified at least eight nationalities among boys involved in street sex work in The Hague.

Boys from Turkey, Morocco, Surinam and the Dutch Antilles generally come from families who emigrated to Holland in the last 25 years. Many German boys have been attracted by the greater tolerance towards drugs in Amsterdam. Romanian, Polish and Czech boys came for economic or political reasons. The remaining West European, South and North American boys are often seeking the greater sexual tolerance of the Netherlands.

Drug-related Changes

The rise in the number of men with drug use problems in the 1970s and 1980s has had consequences for boys' sex work in public places. For many such men, sex work became a way of financing continued drug use (de Graaf *et al.*, 1994b). While shooting and smoking heroin was popular initially, smoking small balls of cooked cocaine has become the most problematic kind of drug use among boys today. The amount of drugs used, and the ways they are used, make it difficult for users to participate in other (non-street-based) forms of boys' sex work.

However, different drugs and different kinds of drug use have become commonplace in other sex work scenes. In particular, smoking cannabis, taking ecstasy and sniffing cocaine is quite common among boys working in clubs and as escorts (as well as more generally on the Amsterdam gay scene). Consumption takes place prior to, during or after work. Sometimes clients urge boys to use drugs. These boys seem less dependent and know well how to use them. Drugs can come in handy for enhancing a sense of personal well-being during sex, and can intensify the act.

Present Forms

In Public Places

In Amsterdam, Rotterdam, The Hague and Groningen, there is a fair amount of boys' sex work in public places. In Amsterdam, two main forms can be distinguished: in public places in and around Amsterdam Central Station; and in semi-public places, in three neighbouring bars in a small back street in the city centre. Sometimes bar staff may play an active part in making contacts. They inform the clients about the reliability of boys and vice versa. The two populations of boys overlap extensively. In recent years more and more Romanian boys have been found in both contexts. Between August 1995 and

August 1996, for example, field-workers from one project made contact with 182 Romanian boys in these locations (Ramaekers, 1996). West European boys can also be found here, especially those with problematic drug use, and also Moroccan and Turkish boys.

Most public contacts in The Hague are made in the city park next to the Central Station. The majority of the boys who work here come from minority ethnic groups. In one year, 169 different boys were seen by one project (van Gelder, 1995). In Rotterdam, boys usually work to one side of an office block near the Central Station. In a small parking place in the old city centre of Groningen, 75 boys were counted in 1995, mostly of Dutch origin (de Boer, 1995). In all cities, sexual activities take place in various locations: in cars, in porn cinemas, at home, in hotel rooms and in parks.

In contrast to their female counterparts, boys working in the above-mentioned places do not wear explicit sexy outfits, nor do they emphasize their sexual readiness. They attract potential clients by wearing casual, street clothing, while presenting themselves as boyish types, neither feminine nor super-macho. Since it is not unusual to see boys hanging around somewhere, they hardly catch the eye of outsiders. Most contacts are made between afternoon and early morning the next day. The usual price is about 50 guilders, but much less is not unknown. In general, boys have only a few clients a day. Those who work these circuits tend to be between 16, the age of consent, and 30 years old.

In Amsterdam from time to time it is possible to see more 'organized' forms of sex work. Boys under the age of 16 may 'work' for a man who arranges a rendezvous with clients he has recruited beforehand. Aware of course that he is performing an illegal act, one of his main preoccupations is to keep the boys out of sight of the police and the judiciary. In other cities boys' sex work is not completely absent from the streets. For instance, in a number of cruising sites one can sometimes find a small number of boys offering sex for money.

Private Houses

Sometimes boys work in ordinary houses. The person who manages such a house, often the official dweller, often shuns the assistance of health organizations. For decades, a private house of this kind has been operating in Amsterdam and, through its increasingly open publicity, has been presenting itself more and more as a club. Because of the cosiness, the privacy and a good nose for boys, this house has been able to maintain itself up to the present day despite recent problems with the judiciary.

Clubs

Clubs, the standard name for brothels, are situated mainly in the three big cities. A few others are scattered throughout the country. Normally these venues have a bar and a few rooms. In the bar, boys and clients meet one another. The client can quietly pick a boy. He is expected to take some refreshments. Often there will be one or more video monitors in the bar showing gay porn videos. When the client has made his choice, he goes with the boy to one of the rooms. Sometimes you can also watch porn videos in these rooms. There are special rooms with Jacuzzis and a number of clubs have an SM room. The client pays a standard rate per hour for the room, ranging between 150 and 250 guilders, per club. Usually these clubs are open from the afternoon until early in the morning. Ten to 40 boys may work in one club, generally between 18 and 25 years old. Depending on the club, boys work in shifts or whenever they want to. They are selected carefully, but the criteria vary from club to club. One of the Amsterdam clubs seems to have a preference for a wide variety of ethnic origins, nice bodies and healthy, middle-class looks. Another club selects boys from a limited number of nationalities, with a lower-class background and a 'shabbier' appearance.

Escort Services

Escort services are scattered throughout the whole country. They arrange, by telephone, meetings between the client and one of the boys who work for the service. Sometimes these services are linked to clubs. When this is the case, one of the boys who usually works in the club is sent to the client's address as an escort. A client telephones the service with a request for a specific type of boy and/or a certain sex technique. When the client accepts an offer, the boy that has been described to him is contacted by the service. Then the client is phoned back to settle the time and place. This return call also checks if the client is serious. When the meeting has ended, the escort telephones the escort service to indicate that he is available again. When the meeting lasts longer than has been agreed, the escort informs the service by telephone. That way the service is able to keep track of the money that is to be settled between the escort and the service, and is also able to ensure the escort's safety. Generally speaking the client pays about 200 guilders an hour. For clients who desire an escort for a longer period of time (a night, a day, or a number of days), a reduced rate is often applicable.

Compared to other types of boys' sex work, special selection criteria apply. A handsome 30-year-old man is perfectly able to work as an escort, particularly when he possesses the specialities that are required by the client. The number of boys who work in this manner is unknown. In view of the recent increase in the number of escort services that are not attached to a club, the number of boys is very likely on the increase.

Interconnected or Separate Circuits?

Because of this diversity, a number of sex work circuits have developed which are only partly linked. Contacts between boys and the owners of different circuits do exist. The latter sometimes round up new boys from bars and streets for their clubs. Other club owners do not want to have anything to do with these kinds of boys. In fact only a small number of boys actually work across the different forms, and many remain exclusively tied to one or another, due either to personal circumstances or choice. Among boys who work for independently organized escort services, or those who acquire clients by telephone, many are unfamiliar with other forms of sex work, not too surprisingly because the client populations are also virtually distinct.

Backgrounds and Self-identification

Diversity among boys is determined not only by cultural and ethnic differences but by individual backgrounds and the age at which the boys first came to be involved in sex work. There are considerable differences between boys with regard to entry into sex work, the circumstances in which sex work occurs, how their involvement in sex work is understood, their lifestyles, social positions and sexual identities.

Youth and Social Background

In 1986 van de Lagemaat interviewed 62, predominantly Dutch, boys who worked on the street and in clubs in Amsterdam. Twenty-two of them came from working-class families, 28 of them had a middle-class background, and 12 had various social backgrounds (van de Lagemaat, 1989). Quite a number of the native Dutch boys who work on the streets and in clubs have spent a part of their youth in institutions – 35 per cent according to this same study, and 36 per cent according to de Boer (1995). On average these boys have relatively low levels of education. Many of them had difficult experiences when young (de Boer, 1995: 60 per cent) and/or ran away from home (van de Lagemaat, 1989: 34 per cent). On the whole, Romanian boys tend to be reasonably well educated (Korf, Nabben and Schreuders, 1996) while Moroccan boys who work on the streets are likely to have had relatively little education.

Such details are lacking for boys who work as an escort or independently by telephone. Field-workers have the impression that more boys among this group have had a higher education and a more average family background. The same applies to boys working in clubs.

Sexual Identity

It is often assumed that most boys who work on the streets are heterosexual, but in reality a considerable number of them have a homosexual preference. In contrast, many boys who call themselves heterosexual work for escort services and in clubs (van de Lagemaat, 1989; de Boer, 1995). Quite a number of boys say they are not sure whether they like men, women or both. As one young man I talked to put it,

> I don't fancy men . . . Are you crazy? I fuck with every chick I can lay my hands on. I don't do much with clients . . . don't have to, they still want me. Only Jacques. He's really great. You know him? I think he's really sexy! He's different. He's really the most beautiful man I know. I was his boyfriend and we still shag once in a while. I'll do everything for him. I feel we belong together. That's why I continue to work in his club. (18 years old)

Field-workers notice that some boys who started receiving money for sex at an early age seem later to be quite confused by it. This might be a result of, on the one hand, unpleasant, painful experiences and, on the other hand, warm, affectionate and sometimes lustful encounters.

Acquaintance with Sex Work

A number of West European boys who work on the streets and in clubs have been sexually abused in their youth. To them, becoming involved in male sex work seemed to be a logical next step. As a 21-year-old man described things,

> I was sexually abused by both my mum and dad. And the institution . . . something was always going on there. When I was eleven I discovered I could earn money for sex. Well, no big deal. I was used to it . . . so . . . I have worked almost everywhere. (21 years old)

Others became involved more unexpectedly: walking the streets they had met men who took care of them, providing money and shelter in exchange for sex.

> I didn't come here for that, but what can you do? I had run out of money. At first I couldn't believe that such men existed. Other guys from my country already did it and so they took me to the bars. A man winked at me and he bought me a beer. So I went along with him. I didn't do anything. He sucked my cock. He acted just like a woman. It was simple really. (22 years old, Romanian)

Boys who still lived at home and had other things to do during the day, discovered for themselves or through older friends a good way of earning extra money. Sometimes they noticed advertisements by clubs. An interview with the club's proprietor is arranged and if the boy is to his liking he can then start working.

Often in their twenties and living on their own, other boys join escort services as the result of a more or less well considered choice. Earning good money through sex with other men is like taking part in a glamorous world where they hope to meet rich men and be admired. It is often experienced as a next step in their (homo)sexual development. They assume the status and identity of a 'nice piece of ass' on the gay scene, and are much respected in the gay circles they move in.

In general, boys are not forced into sex work to the same extent that women are, but cases of compulsion have been reported such as in Rotterdam where, in 1995, two private houses were closed down by the police. Boys under the age of 16 had been traded and forced to have sex with clients (Regiopolitie Rotterdam en Rijnmond, 1995). On the whole, though, even East European boys work voluntarily in sex work. Czech boys who a number of years ago were brought to Holland by a club owner, were openly recruited for this work in the Czech Republic.

Sex Work and Personal Life

Many boys leave sex work soon after their first paid contacts. The social circumstances that led them to sex work may turn out to be only temporary, or their experiences may not match their expectations.

> I have a craze for somewhat older men and found out they sometimes thought I was a hooker. At first to earn some money for good sex wasn't a bad idea. That's why I applied to work at a club. But it just didn't work for me. I sat there waiting most of the time, while only a few clients came round. I didn't really get on with the other guys. The clients I got were simply disgusting. I hardly earned more than in the supermarket. I tried to get a job in another club, but they did not want me. I now work for an escort service. They sent me to one client, but since then no calls. I'm probably no good at it. I'm hardly interested any more. (24 years old)

For boys who pursue a career in sex work, the relevance of their work is much influenced by the quality and the accessibility of other 'social worlds'. Boys with meaningful social lives who perhaps work secretly a couple of nights a week, and boys who work openly as full-time escorts, but who are known to do such by their gay friends, tend to be less emotionally involved. Their more extensive personal social world gives them the opportunity to put their work into proper perspective and to leave it when they want to.

For a number of other boys who work on the streets and in clubs, the world of sex work assumes an important place in their lives, and they find a 'social shelter' there.

> Their self-confidence and self-esteem can be strongly enhanced by this. There they find a refuge where they can (temporarily) escape prescribed roles with regard to sexual identity and manliness. These functions can outstrip the most obvious factor, money in exchange for sex, of its importance. (van de Lagemaat, 1989, p. 232)

The sex boys have with their clients is seen as part of the deal, and as nothing unusual or extraordinary. They are able to experiment with their homosexuality without permanently identifying themselves with a particular sexual preference.

Apart from the psychological and sexual satisfaction, boys often find themselves a sense of belonging in the bar or the club, where they share a lot together. They may sleep in the club, share accommodation, or have one or more fixed sleeping-addresses with clients. Their commitment to the club gives them a certain independence from social security. Their secret world has its own social workers: sugar daddies and clients who, in their social and sexual interaction with the boys, are eager to take on the role of an (informal) social worker. If the boys go through a rough time, they are patched up by personal attention, free clothing, advice, money and shelter. Many boys participate in this private social scene for as long as possible. If their earnings fall, they fill the gap by working at the bar, doing maintenance jobs for clients or owners, or with small crimes. Some of them manage to find their own accommodation and get unemployment benefit or a job outside. Often, however, having no permanent address and not being able to account for their earnings, it is difficult to accomplish all this without outside help. A smooth return to the 'ordinary' world is impossible for many of these boys:

> you learned a great deal in prostitution, but you lack the education and working experience that is asked for. There is a 'gap' in your career history which you don't want to talk about, but at the same time you have to give some kind of explanation. It is hard to go along with a boss who treats you like a little boy. The transition to an existence on benefit or minimum wages is considerable. (van de Lagemaat, 1989, p. 232)

In recent years, and for an increasing number of boys who work in more public places, sex work has been related to problematic drug use. The need for drugs can become so demanding that everything else becomes irrelevant. The more the lifestyle of these boys becomes dominated by drug dependency, the more marginal they become on the sex work scene. More 'established' boys who look better, who are not addicted, or who are in better control of their addiction and therefore more successful in getting clients, withdraw from them. So too do former sugar daddies. Because of this exclusion, they become more and more dependent on a decreasing and unstable social network (van Gelder, 1995).

'Types' of Boys

A much used classification of 'types' of boys in sex work is offered by van der Poel (1991). She classifies boys working in Amsterdam in four groups: (1) rough trade or boys who pretend to be sex workers but use this cover as a means to other ends such as blackmail, robbery and gay bashing; (2) street hustlers or boys characterized by their attempts at survival on a day-to-day basis, having several sources of income, one of which is sex work; (3) part-time sex workers or boys who almost by accident enter into sex work; and (4) professional sex workers or boys who consider themselves committed to their work as a career, and for whom sex work has been their only or a very important regular source of income for years. This classification was, however, derived from data collected from interviews with boys between 1984 and 1986. It is highly questionable whether this typology is still adequate. Different cultural backgrounds (for example Romanian and Moroccan) imply a different style of making contact from that employed by the Dutch boys on whom the classification was based. Moreover, van der Poel's claim that professional male sex workers are an accepted part of the boys' sex work scene, and her claim that these professionals form the core of male sex work, has been altered by recent developments.

Boys who, in addition to other work or study, sell themselves as escorts or in a club a few nights a week, but who do not want to become involved with their colleagues at a personal level, are no longer an exception. They see their clients as the buyers of fantasy. They wrap up a virtually standard element, an orgasm acquired by means of a certain desired technique, in a 'one of a kind' experience.

> I have a client who likes to imagine me as a doctor. I come in, ask how he is. He then usually tells me about some sort physical complaint. I suggest I have a look while I'm here anyway. I start examining him and leave the sex for a little later. This job makes me a bit warm, and so I take off my shirt. Meanwhile he has taken off almost all his clothes. I compliment him on his body, and start to caress him. It is not until half an hour later that I start touching his cock. When he comes I've only used my voice and hands and I have got hardly out of my clothes. (28 years old, escort.)

Such boys simply play their part in the desired story which, as soon as they leave the hotel room or the house, they put back in their imaginary tool box.

Of course they try to make good money, but they respect their client and stick to the deal.

> If I have agreed with a client on one hour I'll bear that in mind. But if I'm there with him in the bath, nice and cosy and he enjoys the calm foreplay, I don't want to rush things. After 50 minutes I will give him the choice: finish the job quickly or pay for another hour. It would of course be really nice if he had enough money and I could manage to persuade him for an extra hour. But if he sticks to an hour, I will try to bring him off within the agreed time. A satisfied client shouldn't feel robbed, because he won't come back again. (23 years old, club worker)

Unfortunately for many boys currently working, neither their clients, the sexual activities nor the environment (be it physical, emotional, legal or otherwise) are sources of inspiration for professionalization. Frequently clients are regarded as their friends, lovers, social workers, or providers of sleeping accommodation. At times, sex with them can be pure lust, but it can also be a bad exchange, giving much more than one gets, or purely a cry for support or attention. Many boys see their sex work environment more like a home than a working-place. When and if the ban on brothels is lifted, these relations and interactions may move to the unregulated circuits.

Clients

In the Netherlands, as anywhere else, relatively little is known about clients. What we do know derives from small numbers of interviews with clients (van der Poel, 1991; de Graaf *et al.*, 1994a) boys' descriptions of clients to fieldworkers (van Gelder, 1994), or sex premises' owners' descriptions, and the accounts given to field-workers by a few frank clients themselves. The variety seems to be immense. Generally, the various forms of sex work attract their own groups of clients. The boys who work the streets attract both 'sugar daddies' and 'bargain hunters', who aim for sex for the lowest possible rate and therefore sometimes wait for hours until a drug-addicted boy offers himself for a minimum price. Although working- and lower middle-class clients generally use the (cheaper) public forms of sex work, the latter also attracts some better-off clients who prefer the kinds of boys who work there and the atmosphere that goes with it.

> Look, I really go for those guys. They're real, they're not like these fruits! A number of them I know very well, they're my friends. Sometimes I sleep with three of them at the same time. I mean, what else can you do? There is no one else they can turn to. (48 years old)

Clients who visit clubs know that they are likely to spend a lot of money. The bill can run up quickly when paying 200 guilders per hour for a room and expensive drinks. Clients who visit the clubs have a wide variety of ages, sexual identities, nationalities and cultural backgrounds. Their motives for visiting a boys' club are similarly diverse. One can find the 'sober' clients who just want sex for an hour with a particular type of boy, but also the 'fanatics' who want to fall in love. The clients serviced by escorts are partly comparable, with a higher percentage of older men who do not go out so much any more, and celebrities who are still closeted.

HIV: a Well-kept Secret

In some circuits, awareness of HIV is still very low. Younger boys particularly, and boys of Moroccan and Romanian origin, tend to be badly informed about HIV, especially at the beginning of their careers. In the world of boys' sex work, there is no place for HIV infected men. Many infected boys and clients therefore keep quiet about their seropositivity. Boys and clients who do not look well are automatically seen as being HIV infected. When it is finally known that a client or boy is HIV positive he will be shunned. Seropositive boys who are still working in a club will be thrown out, and their former sex partners become terrified. Boys who are known to be HIV positive gradually disappear from the scene. If they refuse to leave, there will always be a 'friendly' colleague informing potential clients about the boy's status. In contrast, when a field-worker tells a boy that some of the clients at the club are likely to be HIV positive, it is not unusual for the boy not to listen. Romanian boys, coming from a culture where all deviant or seriously ill individuals have until recently been 'put away', may even believe that Dutch society will have removed HIV infected people from daily life (Zuilhof and Ramaekers, forthcoming).

Implications for HIV Prevention

Until 1989, it was often assumed that boys and their clients would be reached by the use of large-scale national public information campaigns. However, the varying backgrounds of boys, and the relative seclusion of boys in sex work, make such an effect improbable. Their circumstances require small-scale or even individual face-to-face HIV prevention initiatives.

Supportive Environment

Both boys' and clients' preventive actions are partly influenced by their environment. In a sex work circuit, where risks for HIV may be denied or trivialized, safe sex is far from a matter of course. Bar or club owners therefore have an important role to play. They decide whether or not suitable condoms and lubricants will be available, whether or not boys will begin work only after being fully informed about health risks, and whether or not clients should understand there is a safe sex policy. HIV prevention aimed at boys in clubs depends, therefore, very much on club owners.

The norms and attitudes about sex with clients that boys share are also an important part in this generally (un)supportive environment. Field-workers working with drug users, youth agencies and municipal health services have an important role to play in creating supportive environments. In the past they have set up distribution systems of suitable condoms and lubricants as well as leaflets and posters. Another contribution that field-workers can make to this supportive environment is to provide individual face-to-face contact and group activities. For boys who work on the streets, such a supportive environment is not a matter of course. For these boys, field-workers and drop-in centres linked to their organizations play a more important role.

How to Address Boys?

Most boys are particularly sensitive to moral rejection. The only way in which contact can be made is through showing respect for their choice of lifestyle, of which paid sex is an essential part. The variety of boys, and their varying motivations and attitudes with regard to sex work, make a standard approach impossible. Adequate HIV prevention starts with an understanding of unsafe sex. A number of boys have unprotected sex particularly with special partners, male or female, and the distinction between clients and other partners can be rather vague. Therefore the field-worker needs to discuss, whenever possible, all sex contacts, paid and unpaid. Sex work needs to be viewed as work to which rules of safety should apply. For less privileged boys, choosing safe sex is hardly an option. Housing, drugs and the need for affection may have a higher priority for them. In the short term, fulfilling these needs may be the most effective way to motivate them to have safe sex. Letting them organize their own activities, make their own leaflets and so on, may prove most effective in the long run. That way, boys learn to develop other personal qualities. It helps set them on their own feet, makes them less of a victim, enhances self-respect and thus makes practising safe sex an option.

Like many other gay men, boys with strong sexual feelings for particular men may be tempted to have sex unsafely. Effective HIV prevention should acknowledge the complexity of this kind of situation and seek to address clients' sexual behaviour too.

Who's the Messenger?

Knowledge of HIV and the attendant risks is not sufficient to change individual sexual behaviour. Such a change requires boys to adjust their own attitudes and to learn new behavioural skills. It is impossible for one person to influence all these aspects optimally. It is often stated that peer education is most suitable in this case. However, reality is more complicated: when it comes to factual information on HIV, boys are generally highly sensitive to the status of the counsellor. Another boy or peer is usually not felt to be as credible as an information source. A professional health-worker, especially a doctor, will often get a more attentive ear. For other skills, like attitudes towards clients and HIV risks, or skills to keep sex contacts safe, peer education works and boys are particularly able to learn from each other.

Peer education can be facilitated through group meetings arranged by field-workers. By arranging these meetings in a calm and familiar setting, boys can be encouraged to talk about subjects they rarely discuss elsewhere. In Holland, peer education on a daily basis for boy sex workers has never worked out. Differences between boys, their mobility and their unplanned lifestyles make this impossible.

What to Talk about

In individual counselling, the field-worker can address individual risk determinants. The personal and sensitive nature of these makes it hard to discuss them in group meetings. Through such counselling, boys can become more open about, for example, homosexual feelings, their fear of being HIV positive, or their choice to have unprotected sex with certain partners. In Amsterdam, these counselling sessions take place at a drop-in centre, in clubs, on the streets, or in bars and coffee shops.

Meetings need to be organized to meet the needs of different groups, for example, gatherings for German drug users, Romanian boys or newcomers in clubs. An emphasis on safe sex rules and HIV risk is central, but also information about certain job skills can be exchanged. For certain themes like SM practices, special group sessions are organized. Recently STD prevention and treatment have become more important in outreach work. Boys are often anxious about catching an STD, since it means not being able to work for a number of days and the STD may have been passed on to clients who in turn may inform other (potential) clients.

A double message needs to be conveyed about STDs: first, most STDs are not entirely avoidable, so if you have symptoms get a check-up and possible treatment; second, by practising safe sex you can reduce the possibility of catching an STD.

Future Directions

In the Western world, HIV prevention seems to have entered a new phase with the advent of combination therapies for HIV. Although it is premature to predict the future, the threat of HIV seems to be changing. For prevention, this can have both positive and negative consequences. For example, some less privileged boys in sex work are highly susceptible to sensational media with superficial and oversimplified headlines. Already there are boys who think that HIV is curable. Continuing to provide accurate information is therefore one of the greatest challenges for the coming years. Thinking about and having regular HIV tests will be more pressing as a result of new treatment options. Some new medications will be unsuitable for many boy sex workers because of the stringent conditions of use and the tightly required regularity in eating and sleeping habits. In the coming years, field-workers will have a difficult task giving good advice in coping with these new situations.

Notes

1 'Boys' is the best translation of the Dutch word 'jongens'. The term is not restricted to teenagers, but also includes men in their twenties. In certain gay circles, the term is also used to describe men of an undefined age who want to be addressed as young.
2 I use the term 'field-workers' to describe outreach workers from different backgrounds and disciplines including care, prevention and social work.
3 In Holland, sex between men involving some kind of reward is quite frequent. In popular speech most of these contacts are called 'prostitution', often with a negative connotation. The term 'boys' sex work' will be used in this chapter to describe situations in which young men have sex with men with whom, prior to sexual interaction, some sort of material reward has been agreed upon by both parties. A situation in which a man rewards the sexual act with (expensive) presents is not regarded as prostitution so long as the boy, prior to the act, does not claim any form of compensation. Moreover, when a client takes a boy away from the job by providing him with accommodation and money so that the latter stops having sex on a reward basis, we are no longer dealing with sex work. This chapter therefore works with a definition of sex work which emphasizes that some reward is more or less agreed beforehand (though paid afterwards) and is an essential and definite part of the act. The actual terms 'sex worker' and 'sex work' are rarely used in the Netherlands.

   Transgender sex work can be categorized partly as boys' sex work but will not be discussed in this chapter. In the Netherlands transgender contacts mainly take place through female sex work circuits that are separated from circuits of boys' sex work.

References

DE BOER, S. (1995) *Het Land der Klinkers*, Groningen: Municipal Health Service.

VAN GELDER, P. (1994) ' "Bisnis", mannelijkheid en seks', *Etnofoor*, **2**, pp. 42–58.

VAN GELDER, P. (1995) *Tussen 'bisnis' en taboe*, Amsterdam: het Spinhuis.

DE GRAAF, R., VANWESENBEECK, I., VAN ZESSEN, G., STRAVER, C.J. and VISSER, J.H. (1994a) 'Homosexual prostitution and the potential spread of HIV in the Netherlands', *Journal of the Acquired Immune Deficiency Syndromes*, **7**, pp. 526–9.

DE GRAAF, R., VANWESENBEECK, I., VAN ZESSEN, G., STRAVER, C.J. and VISSER, J.H. (1994b) 'Male prostitutes and safe sex: different settings, different risks', *AIDS Care*, **6**, pp. 277–88.

KORF, D.J., NABBEN, T. and SCHREUDERS, M. (1996) *Roemeense trekvogels, nieuwkomers in de jongensprostitutie*, Amsterdam: Thesis Publishers.

VAN DE LAGEMAAT, G. (1989) 'Jongensprostitutie, een carriere van betekenis', *Jeugd en samenleving*, **19**, pp. 211–33.

McMULLEN, R.J. (1987) 'Youth prostitution: a balance of power', *Journal of Adolescence*, **10**, pp. 57–69.

VAN MENS, L. (1995) 'Erotikeur', *SOA bulletin*, **4**, pp. 22–3.

VAN DER POEL, S.C. (1991) *In de bisnis, professionele jongensprostitutie in Amsterdam*, Arnhem: Gouda Quint bv.

PUBLIC HEALTH DEPARTMENT AMSTERDAM (1996), Press Report, 'Many HIV-infections among homosexual boys', Amsterdam.

RAMAEKERS, S. (1996) *Eindevaluatie project AIDS preventie bij Oost-Europese jongens in de prostitutie*, Amsterdam: AMOC.

REGIOPOLITIE ROTTERDAMEN RIJNMOND (1995) *Eindrapportage onderzoek naar handel in kinderen en sexuele exploitatie van kinderen*, Rotterdam: RRR.

ZUILHOF, W. (1994) 'Boys in prostitution and prevention on aids', working document from European Expert Meeting on 'How to reach youth in the outside school setting', Utrecht: Dutch Centre for Health Promotion and Health Education.

ZUILHOF, W. and RAMAEKERS, S. (forthcoming) 'HIV en soa preventie voor Roemeense Jongens in de prostitutie'.

Chapter 3

Travestis and *Gigolos*: Male Sex Work and HIV Prevention in France

Lindinalva Laurindo da Silva
Translated by Peter Aggleton

This chapter examines some aspects of male sex work in the Paris region of France. It focuses on those kinds of sex work practised by *travestis* and *garçons* who sell sex exclusively to other men and occasionally to couples and/or women.[1] The aim is to understand the context in which male sex work takes place and the opportunities for HIV prevention that present themselves. Male sex work in France has been very little studied from a sociological point of view. While mentioned in nineteenth-century works on public health, morality and social administration, as well as in medico-legal studies of indecent assaults, it was only from the 1970s that publications focusing exclusively on male sex work began to appear.[2]

With the advent of AIDS, questions of male and female sex work were given new impetus, and a number of different studies have been carried out focusing on women and/or men providing sexual services. Among these studies, those by Ingold and Toussirt (1993) carried out in Paris, and that of Welzer-Lang, Barbosa and Mathieu (1994) in Lyons, address issues of sex work generally. Ingold and Toussirt's work focuses on drug-using sex workers, with sex work being seen primarily as a means of obtaining both licit and illicit drugs. Welzer-Lang, Barbosa and Mathieu (1994), on the other hand, examine changes in sexual identity and social-sexual interaction in the sex work context. The *travesti* or transgendered sex worker is the focus of these changes. Very few studies, however, examine the sex work practices of the many men providing sexual services who are not *travestis*. For Welzer-Lang, for whom prostitution is best characterized by a blurring of identity categories, 'there is no clear break but a continuum between *tapins*,[3] hormone using *travestis*, and transsexuals awaiting surgery' (*ibid.*, p. 26).

In contrast, we regard *travestis* and *garçons* as two very distinct categories of sex worker.[4] They are situated at opposite poles with respect to femininity and masculinity: in their sex work practice, *travestis* affirm their femininity, while *garçons* affirm their virility. If there is a tendency for *travestis* to see themselves as 'homosexual' in some way, *garçons* do not always know themselves as such. Often, the latter describe themselves as *gigolos*,[5] a term which suggests that for payment they will have sex with, or spend time with, either women or men. As well as being situated at opposite poles in relation to femininity and masculinity, *travestis* and *gigolos* differ in the places where they practise sex work, in the way they do it, in their clientele, and in the ways in which payment for sexual services takes place.

All HIV prevention messages need to be adapted to the social characteristics of the group concerned. In order to respond to the question (how should we undertake HIV prevention with male sex workers?) we must first identify how a particular kind of sex work is organized and how it takes place. Using a qualitative approach, we have carried out analyses of different sex work careers and different types of sex work in order to better understand the relationship between sex work practices and HIV-related understandings and risk. We have also tried to find out how different factors affect HIV risk perception, such as the client's appearance (good-looking or dirty), the type of services asked for and the kind of social interaction that takes place between a sex worker and client.

Method

The issues and themes we explore here come from an action research project carried out in Paris. This involved us working together with male sex workers to undertake HIV prevention.[6] The work occurred in two phases. The first involved a group research project conducted between 1990 and 1992 on male sex work and HIV prevention. The team consisted of sex workers, ex-sex workers, social workers, members of local authority and non-governmental groups, as well as the researchers themselves. The second phase of the study involved inquiry among sex workers in their place of work. The aim here was to learn more about the opportunities and constraints on HIV prevention in the sex work context. This chapter draws heavily upon information collected during the second phase.

Before fieldwork commenced, data collection procedures were discussed collectively. Additionally, a decision had to be reached whether to pay sex workers who were interviewed in their place of work; it was suspected, for example, that in the absence of such payment some might refuse to participate.[7] This procedure, however, was not without problems. It can be asked if, as a result of making such payment, the project might run the risk of focusing only on those actively involved in sex work. Moreover, generally speaking, researchers do not remunerate informants, since the aim of most studies is to solicit information rather than a service.[8] After much discussion, it was agreed that every sex worker agreeing to participate in the study should be offered 200 francs as remuneration. Seventy-one interviews were carried out between June 1990 and September 1991: 14 *travestis*, 53 *garçons* (of whom 43 were interviewed face to face and 10 by telephone), and 4 clients.[9] The 67 workers interviewed were contacted in the following ways: 8 through organizations providing social support to sex workers, 49 in their place of sex work or through contact with other sex workers, and 10 via Minitel. The four clients were contacted through one member of the research team. They were interviewed either in cafés or their homes.

Interviews with sex workers were generally carried out close to the context in which they worked, most usually in a car or café. Some *travestis*, however, were interviewed in their own homes. Interviews were semistructured in design and tape-recorded. They focused on entry into sex work, ways of meeting clients and places in which this could occur, the kinds of negotiation that preceded sex, social and emotional life, future hopes and aspirations, perceptions of HIV infection, responses to previous and ongoing prevention campaigns, access to health care, and the relationship between sex work and drug use.

In order to interpret the information obtained, a thematic analysis was carried out. Interview coding allowed us to identify a number of key messages in the body of the information collected. Once the coding had been carried out, a re-analysis of each interview was conducted in order to trace the individual history of each informant. This double reading of the interview data enabled us to identify a number of recurrent themes pertaining to male sex work, which are discussed below.

Entry into and Settling into Sex Work

Becoming a Sex Worker

Sex work is like a journey in many ways and constitutes a career as defined by Becker (1985). In order to become a sex worker, the individual needs to pass through several stages: first, occasional, sometimes difficult, experiences; second, experiencing pleasure or reward as a result of providing sexual services; third, becoming accustomed to sex work; and finally, giving up sex work. While entry into sex work can occur in a variety of ways and at different stages in life, the majority of respondents in this study began to sell sex between the ages of 12 and 17. For both *garçons* and *travesti*, the major reason given to explain their entry into sex work was easy money. But when questioned more deeply, other reasons emerged: sometimes there were emotional reasons, and sometimes entry into sex work coincided with a desire to have sex with other men. Most usually when the young men interviewed entered sex work, they practised it only occasionally, and only later did it become a more regular activity for a large number of informants.

On the whole, the *travestis* interviewed reported becoming sex workers as a result of individual choice, often linked to their desire to live as a woman.[10] Once a decision had been made to cross-dress, few employment opportunities exist other than in sex work or in shows. It is relatively rare, though, for a *travesti*, through her own talent, to become a real professional in the artistic world. Some *travestis* began their career in sex work as *garçons*, and relatively rare are those who dress as women only in a sex work context.

In contrast to *travestis* who, generally speaking, identify as homosexual, *garçons* often do not identify as homosexual and may see themselves as bisexual or heterosexual.[11] In response to the demands of the sexual market, these *garçons* adopt a manly and youthful appearance. Many were initiated into sex work through friends who were already sex workers, but others took the initiative themselves. As a result of our research, we can identify three principal ways in which *garçons* entered sex work:

First there are those who become involved in sex work in order to obtain occasional pocket money. They most usually begin such work in recreational settings such as swimming pools, cinemas or fairgrounds. This coincides generally with their discovery of their homosexuality. They feel happy, they like to receive presents from the men they meet, and little by little they become sex workers. Second are those who are escaping from difficult family circumstances, searching for a better life with more freedom and less stress. On leaving their families, direct entry into sex work is not inevitable. Sometimes these young men find a little work. Gradually, however, they begin to realize that by selling sexual services they can earn much more each month than otherwise. This may lead to them leaving other employment in order to devote themselves full-time to this more lucrative activity. Finally, a minority begin sex work in order to obtain drugs such as heroin and cocaine. Among our informants, four explained their involvement in sex work in these terms.

Settling into Sex Work

Finding a place in the sexual market-place is central to self-definition as a prostitute. This is usually marked by movement from the occasional to regular sale of sexual services.[12] Gaining a niche in the sex market was accomplished through getting to know well those who were already sex workers, but it could also occur more forcibly. And when it comes for standing up for their rights, *garçons* and *travestis* use male power in order to defend their territory and place.[13] Because pimping is unknown in male sex work in France, for most of the time workers have to defend themselves in order to maintain their market position. This is especially the case for *travestis*, who work for the majority of their time in a fixed public place.

Among *travestis*, placement in the sex work scene (including where you work) is influenced by a number of factors, of which nationality is the most important. Different groups of *travestis* arise as a result of both affinity and patronage by older friends, as is shown in the following quotation:

> Where I work there are only French [*travestis*] ... but 100 metres away there are Colombians. Really it's a bit like seeds that have fallen in the Bois de Boulogne, they take over, they take over, they spread, they nibble away at a 100 metres [space], 100 metres and then they take over an entire area. If a new [*travesti*] arrives, I see her off.

When you are involved in sex work, you develop a double personality. You become like an animal . . . that's what happens . . . it's like a bitch looking after her puppies, like an eagle guarding its eggs. You're like an animal . . . that's what happens. It's human nature, it's the strongest who win in life. (45 years old, French)

Territorial rules are generally implicit. They are, however, imposed and respected by all. This is true both for *travestis* and for *garçons*. In the case of *gigolos*, sex work locations are not as fixed as they are for *travestis*. In certain areas of the city, *gigolos* work in a fixed location, but for the majority of the time they move around between the main railway stations and certain neighbourhoods, between gay bars, gay cinemas and sex shops. They can also be contacted by telephone and may receive clients at home. For *gigolos*, one of the main means of ensuring success in the sex market is constantly to move around.

Not resting in the same place allows you to avoid being labelled as a sex worker.[14] It also means that you do not have to constantly meet the same clients. This is useful because the latter are usually looking for new faces. But this tactic only works for those who are young or at the start of their sex work career, or those who after many years' involvement in sex work still preserve a good-looking appearance. When you are older than 30 or at the end of your career in sex work, it is more difficult to find clients and there is less possibility of going to bars or other places frequented by men in the medium to higher socio-economic class who may be willing to pay. At this point in their careers, *gigolos* may return to work in places such as railway stations, where all types of sex workers can be found: those beginning their sex work careers, those selling sexual services in order to buy drugs, and those who are just cruising. Because stations are closed spaces in which a multitude of people can be found, and since there are many possible reasons for being there, they permit everyone to keep their anonymity. As one sex worker put it:

In the stations it's a fantasy world, and that excites me. They are places of movement, places of anonymity, that's what crowded places are. The toilets . . . sometimes they are good places to go for a quick one, the people who go there don't look obvious, in fact for the majority of the time they look quite the opposite. There are married men who do it, who want to have quick sex without speaking. In the stations it's often like that, there is a client who's there, he says 'I'll give you this if you do that for me.' That sort of thing goes on in the [booking] halls and then you go to the toilets and you masturbate each other, that sort of thing. They show you the money to get you excited in order to . . . even if you're not a prostitute you could become one because the money gives you ideas . . . (38 years old, French)

Relationships with Clients

From the start of this study, male sex work was seen as a relationship involving two principal parties, the sex worker and the client. Essentially, sex workers are service providers who respond to the various needs of clients who are seeking a wide range of sexual services.[15] The relationship between the sex worker and the client is negotiated in accordance with relatively clear rules of sexual exchange.

Travestis

For the most part, the clients of *travestis* are men who see themselves as heterosexual. Negotiation is generally carried out in the street in order to establish the fee and the service required. Payment is made in advance. As a rule, *travestis* never trust their clients because there is always the possibility that they may leave without paying. The services that are asked for include fellatio, touching and feeling the breasts, and masturbation; but all *travestis* practice insertive and receptive anal sex. All of those interviewed had experience of clients who asked for SM and scat. For these practices, the price asked is much higher. The majority refused to provide this kind of sexual service. *Travestis* service their clients either in their own homes or in rented rooms, or occasionally in alleyways. They also provide sexual services in cars or in the woods. Only rarely will they visit a client. The relationship between a *travesti* and a client is generally governed by strict rules established in advance and does not continue beyond the agreed time, usually 15 to 20 minutes. For them, the central principle is to provide the service as quickly as possible while giving the least away.

    Travestis occasionally receive gifts from regular clients, sometimes a rose or a box of chocolates. Clients often use their services regularly, perhaps once a week or a couple of times each month. In general, the relationship between *travesti* and client is confined to the duration of the sexual service provided. *Travestis* generally do not permit clients to show them affection or intimacy, nor do they spend the night with clients. According to them, someone looking for a *travesti* is seeking a sexual service, nothing more. A good sex worker will not go beyond the provision of this service, for to do more than this is not proper. This principle is strictly adhered to by *travestis* of French origin, who often criticize newer *travestis*, especially foreigners:

> A French prostitute . . . she sucks him off and that's it. She doesn't give favours to her clients or let them fondle her. She certainly doesn't lie on the grass with them. No, no. A real prostitute sucks them off for 100 francs, she lets them touch her breasts a little and that's all. That's where it stops. There is no relationship. A client is a client, he stays a client. (45 years old, French)

Nevertheless, certain *travestis* do not respect this principle and may search for something more than money, such as an emotional relationship with a client:

> A client, they have it off and then that's it. Off they go, it's just sex, just 'coming', and off they go. I like to have someone who will be with me. Last Saturday, for example, I met someone ... he said to me 'How much do you want?' I said 200 francs. He said 'Can I stay for a little while?' I said, 'Well, 500 francs then.' He said to me 'I can't, I've only got 300 francs.' I saw that he was an honest man and now he is here I have money that I share with him. He has no work. He is looking for a job and I invite him. It's normal. He needs to eat. I am like that. (40 years old, French)

While an emotional attachment can sometimes arise between a *travesti* and a client, among themselves *travestis* tend to say that when a man stays with them it's because it's in his material interest to do so. In this respect, *travestis* tend to differ from *gigolos*, who will stay with their clients whenever it is to their (the *gigolo*'s) material benefit to do so.

Gigolos

The clients of *gigolos* are composed principally of gay and bisexual men. When we began talking with *garçons* about their sexual practices, the majority stated that they played the insertive role and refused to be penetrated. For some of them, this refusal of penetration is a way of preserving a part of the self:

> I make excuses ... I've never been taken. It's the only thing I've managed to get away with, not because I'm ashamed of being fucked, but because it's the last scrap of dignity I've got. (34 years old, French)

By affirming that they only engage in insertive sex, these young men seem less concerned with avoiding being labelled homosexual than with finding a way of ensuring that their virility is not called into question.[16] This is equally true for those who define themselves as gay or homosexual and for those who see themselves as heterosexual. This tendency can be seen among *garçons* of all nationalities, but is particularly strong among those of Algerian origin, where the desire to protect their manhood prohibits fellatio. Algerian informants said that they only practised insertive sex and never touched the penis of their client, nor let him touch theirs.

Overall, based on the accounts given, it would seem that, as for the *travestis*, the majority of *garçons* respond to a varied list of requests: the services demanded most are oral sex by the client, masturbation, oral sex on the client and insertive sex.[17] Once the price is fixed, *garçons* usually go to the client's place or to a hotel, which may be anything from a hotel where there are rooms by the hour, to a three-star hotel. Alternatively they may have sex quickly in building entrances near the place of work. When they are working on the street or in stations, time is of the essence. Things must happen quickly and then they must get rid of the client, and in these circumstances the service provided is rarely anything more than fellatio or masturbation.

The pattern of interaction between *gigolo* and client is extremely variable. Some clients, for example, simply want to have a conversation or to go for a drink. Also, money is not the only way of making payment: other forms of recompense include invitations to clubs or restaurants, presents, holidays, or the opportunity to sleep with a client in an expensive hotel. In this form of exchange, time and price are very malleable, and the principles governing sexual exchange are neither fixed nor absolute. The actual 'act of prostitution' becomes blurred: touching, a conversation, a beer – it is difficult to decide when the sex work encounter begins and ends.

> I have three clients who spoil me terribly. They buy me things – trousers, trainers, jackets. Sometimes they give me money or we go out together, or we go and have a drink and then they give me money. Maybe they give me 300 francs or 200 francs. These are men of 50 or 40 years old. Those are not like the others. They are not clients any more. (19 years old, Turkish)

This heterogeneity in the modality of sexual exchange makes it difficult for some *gigolos* to establish clear boundaries around sex work. It can cause both sex worker and client to enter a realm where roles and identities become blurred, and where it is hard to know whether their relationship is one of sex work or not. The client can become a lover who gives money regularly, or sometimes a friend:

> I have clients who help me all the time, they don't just help me because . . . I make love with them, they give me money also . . . and then we become friends . . . they're not just queers . . . they help me when I'm in difficulty. (28 years old, Algerian)

It is difficult to analyze these kinds of interaction simply in terms of market relations. What characterizes them, however, is that nothing is given away in sexual or emotional exchange. We can see here the tension of reciprocity described by Mauss (1974) in his theory of the gift relationship. According to Mauss, these types of exchange appear to have a voluntary basis when in fact they are obligatory. In the case of *garçons*, they do not demand remuneration for their company, but without fail they get it in the form of gifts of one kind or another. This is most likely to occur if the *gigolo* is young or good-looking.

The sexual and emotional rapport that exists between a *gigolo* and his client can sometimes lead to them living together, perhaps as a couple. This type of relationship often runs into difficulty after a few months. The break-up is usually attributable equally to one or the other, but often the *gigolo* claims that he has been dropped, perhaps in order to gain sympathy. In reality, for most of the time the relationship has been socio-culturally unequal, and mutual suspicion does not completely disappear. As a result, sex cannot make up for differences of age or social background.

If there is a golden rule adhered to by *gigolo*s, it is to never trust a client. Here, they share something in common with *travestis. Gigolos* say that clients often promise many things at the start, but then as they become older, clients lose interest in them.

> Before, I was with a guy that . . . it was like he was my wife . . . I was young, about 19 years old. At that age you have golden balls, as long as you are young and can get a good hard-on, that's all the queers want. By the time I was 23 or 24, that was all over, and when you get old they prefer younger men. That's what queers are like. What is a queer? It's a guy who buys you with his money, and then when he sees that you are too old, he chucks you out. He takes someone younger. Why? It's money, it's the game. It's the way things are. That's how it is. (28 years old, Algerian)

The *garçon* who explained this, though no more than 28 years old at the time, already feels used by his life in sex work. In the course of the fieldwork, however, we also met *garçons* of the same age who had met 'good clients' and who were receiving plenty of money. The previous young man, however, was dependent on heroin, which had damaged his appearance and made it difficult for him to maintain an erection. He did not appeal to clients looking for a beautiful face and a beautiful body. If a *gigolo* wants to remain in sex work for a long time, he needs to make sure he remains young and good-looking.

If clients tend to look for younger men, there is a tendency for *gigolos* to search out those who are older. By choosing carefully the contexts in which they work, *gigolos* were able to exert some influence over the clients they were likely to meet.

> I go to the Gare du Nord because I'm trying to find older men. I often look for men who are 40 or 50, who can show me affection, who are going to be OK with me, you know what I mean? I don't go to other places like the Tuileries, for example. (21 years old, French)

In a similar way, some *gigolos* who sell sex only occasionally may be trying to find an emotional relationship, or perhaps love.

> When you're on the scene and you fall in love with someone, some-one you want to stay with and he doesn't want you when you've had

some good times together, and it's not exactly clear why, then you begin to feel really upset . . . and it's terrible because it doesn't lead to suicide exactly . . . but almost . . . you get really depressed, you cry, it hurts a lot . . . yes it's happened very often to me. Yes, it's true. If I were honest, there are clients that I would have wanted to see again, but they always want someone new. (22 years old, French)

This *garçon* never set a fixed price in his negotiations with clients. By doing so, he was able to get more money by putting himself in an advantageous position emotionally, with the hope that things might become more permanent. But he often ended up trapped by his own strategy, because when the desired outcome is not realized, he feels deceived and hurt. There exists a fundamental rule for many clients: do not become attached to a *gigolo*, always try to find someone new. The main advantage of buying sex from the point of view of the client is that by paying there is no commitment, either of body or heart.

Between us, I'm not a *micheton*.[18] When they come to sleep at my home, it's not just a help for them, it's a pleasure for me. But having said that, and not being sentimental about it, none of the *garçons* sleep with me. They can sleep fine on the seats six feet away from me. When we have finished, we can smoke a last cigarette together, but I don't like to have someone sleeping beside me, handsome as he may be, because I haven't believed in love affairs these past 25 years. I don't want to fall in love with someone and I don't want all that comes with a loving relationship. (client, 52 years old)

In the complexity of sex work, this kind of self-protection is no guard against one of the partners running the emotional risk. In every encounter, each person needs to protect himself against this possibility. In one sense, therefore, emotional risks are professional risks: money is the third party protecting the sex worker and client from this possibility. These risks exist equally for clients and *garçons*; the latter perhaps can protect themselves less because they are linked to clients through a material dependency. Some *gigolos* claim, however, that they have left a relationship with a client because they need their independence and to be constrained in this way is an interference with their life as sex workers.

Often, *gigolos* state that in their work they have to be 'professional'. One becomes professional with experience. A professional is 'someone who is not going to be "had" by his client' and, in order to avoid this, you must know the rules of the game. The real professional never mixes emotional life with his life as a *gigolo*. The more advanced they are in their sex work career, the more *garçons* adopt this purely professional logic within relationships, being limited to the practices of relatively short-term duration agreed in advance so as to avoid this kind of emotional confusion.

Becoming an Occasional Sex Worker and Leaving Sex Work

In general, *travestis* can continue to sell sex until the age of 45 or more. The majority of *gigolos* sell sex less often when they reach their early thirties, either because they have become tired of doing so or because they cannot find clients. They may return to sex work areas from time to time in order to get money when they need it, or maybe because of the enjoyment of going back.

Certain *gigolos* at the end of their careers in sex work may be successful in prolonging a relationship with a client who regularly provides for them while they continue to sell sexual services occasionally to others.

> He's married. He's a grandfather and lives in the countryside. He's very well known. He comes up once a month to Paris in order to see me. He pays the rent, he pays for the telephone, he gives me 4000 francs a month, jewellery, things like that. He's good luck for me, there's an emotional relationship between us of course. If there wasn't, things wouldn't have lasted for three years. He says to me 'You've given me a lot, before I was withdrawn, before I felt bad about myself, I was hung up, but you've given me a lot.' And every day for three years he has rung me at midday. He has taken me to Turkey, he's taken me to Egypt. I love him a lot and if we ever broke up, it would make me very upset because in three years a bond has been created. He's the father I never had, he's the father I never had and so . . . if one day he said to me 'I haven't got any money', I would accept him as before, because for three years he's given me a lot. If he said to me tomorrow 'I haven't got a centime, can I come and eat with you?', I would say to him 'Of course, eat, sleep, drink!' (30 years old, Tunisian)

This *garçon* sells sexual services occasionally and is kept by the man whom he treats as a father. For the *garçon* concerned, this client is no longer a client, and certainly for the latter, his friend is no longer a *gigolo*. It is fair to say, however, that these types of relationship were not very frequent among the young men interviewed, as we found only two of them.

It seems that at the end of their careers some *gigolos* are able to disengage from sex work relatively easily. while others when they leave are completely de-socialized. A dozen *gigolos* said they were saving money for when they finally left sex work. Of these, two said they had bought a house. Of the 13 informants who could be considered to have reached the end of their sex work careers, three had found other work and six were receiving social security. The latter sold sex occasionally wherever they could, and with whatever clients they could find. They had little say over the choice of client, over the services provided, or over what they would receive by way of payment. Five of them were heroin users and three were reduced to begging in order to survive.

Sex Workers and AIDS

In 1992, when our study commenced, AIDS was already a real issue for sex workers, and condoms were familiar to a large number of the men involved. The *gigolos* and *travestis* who had been involved in sex work before the advent of AIDS, all spoke of the changes that had come about: neither clients nor sex workers dared go so far as they used to when it came to sex.

According to informants, it was rare nowadays for someone to have sex without using a condom. The majority of clients, both of *travestis* and *gigolos*, are happy to use condoms for penetrative sex. Moreover, some clients encourage younger *garçons* to use condoms. However, AIDS is not a subject to be talked about, either between sex workers or between client and sex worker. Instead, it remains a taboo subject, but one implicit in most situations and relationships.

> It's a subject which everyone avoids talking about . . . speaking about it. It breaks your spirit to do so. (27 years old, Algerian)

Among the 14 *travestis*, 10 said they had taken an HIV test at least once. None stated that they were either seropositive or had AIDS. Among the 43 *gigolos* interviewed face to face, 29 said they were seronegative, of whom 20 regularly had an HIV antibody test or gave blood in order to find out their serostatus, and of whom nine said they had never had a test. Among the others, three had been diagnosed with AIDS and seven were HIV seropositive. The remaining four did not answer the question.

If *travestis* think that AIDS is an illness of 'others' and danger lies in the client, in the eyes of *gigolos*, AIDS is an illness that can affect anyone, including themselves. A few *garçons* adopted a fatalistic attitude, taking the view that whether or not you protected yourself, you could always become infected. Others, however, played down the risk:

> AIDS . . . I don't give a fuck [about it]. I tell you honestly, the day I die, I will die of a natural illness or some other thing. I don't give a fuck. You know, I'm going to tell you something when people speak about that, it does my head in . . . I don't want to hear about it. Anyway, I might have AIDS already, and I tell you I have sex without a condom. I don't use them. (34 years old, French)

When sex workers find themselves under social pressure or when they are at the end of their sex work career, AIDS is seen as just another risk. To get AIDS is just bad luck and therefore not to be taken seriously. You might just as well die of AIDS as of an overdose or through suicide, it is all the same thing.

Practices of Protection

All the *travestis* that we met stated that they used condoms in their work. The majority said that before AIDS they would protect themselves against other STDs in the same way. In this sense, AIDS has not changed anything in their use of condoms. From the client's point of view, condom use is equally normal and sometimes certain clients carry their own condoms, but there are always those who are willing to pay more for unprotected sex. So among the 14 *travestis* who said they used a condom for penetrative sex, nine said they did not do so for fellatio. In order to protect themselves here, they did not let the client ejaculate in their mouths. This was true also for *gigolos*, among whom fellatio was a much requested service, and one that was very rarely protected. Two types of arguments were used in order to justify the absence of protection: the first made reference to medical uncertainty about whether or not HIV can be transmitted through oral sex and saliva; the second took the form of what might be described as a kind of 'threshold effect'. For some sex workers, fellatio is seen as constituting a kind of 'free space' unlinked to other more dangerous practices.

While *travestis* stated that they used protection with all their clients, there were situations in which condoms might not be used. These included having sex with a friend or with a client who was somehow different from the others.

> I really think that not using condoms is like playing with death and I use them 99 per cent of the time. But one day I might meet a guy and say to myself 'He's good looking, I won't use a condom with him.' At times the flesh is weak, but of course that kind of guy could kill me, that's how it is, that's my choice [laughs] . . . for my personal desires I don't use one . . . (43 years old, French)

Through these examples, we can see the high stakes involved in HIV prevention. On the part of the client things may be similar, and protection against HIV can be particularly difficult when one is in an unusual situation with a sex worker.

> I had an orgy with a *travesti* and with another guy, a famous actor that I wanted to . . . anyway I was astonished because before being sucked the *travesti* put on a condom. You see, I had been sucked by the other guy without a condom. I was sucking with him without a condom. Well, I don't know if I'm sick, I don't know if he's sick and he let himself be sucked without a condom. Maybe he is sick, you understand? . . . It's complicated . . . and then there were moments when you don't want to think about it, you're in the middle of making love, it's great, it's wonderful, I don't want to say I have got to protect myself. (50 years old, client)

We can see here that when the partner is not a sex worker, less risk is perceived. Statements like this also suggest something of the anguish that can arise in situations that are difficult to control or when beauty, sensuality, or something similar, makes the risk of infection seem weaker. This is a complicated aspect of sexual relations, be they linked to sex work or otherwise, and is something which HIV prevention needs to take into account.

Among the *gigolos*, a small number stated that they did not use protection at all except when the client was very old or dirty. Others said they protected themselves systematically whenever they had insertive anal sex with a client. The majority did not protect themselves for fellatio and simply avoided getting semen in the mouth.[19]

Always carrying a condom was seen as a sign of professionalism. Whenever we talked with *garçons* who defined themselves as professional, they quickly took out a condom. But not all *garçons* see themselves this way and not all carry condoms with them at all times. In this kind of situation, they must rely upon the client to provide them.

> If the *micheton* hasn't got a condom, I suggest we get one. Or if I haven't got any . . . well . . . we go to the pharmacy to buy one. If there's no pharmacy . . . well . . . we arrange something else . . . once (I had a client who) came inside me. He didn't have time to get one . . . well . . . I did everything necessary . . . well . . . I know I don't have AIDS. I clean myself well inside with water afterwards. That's OK for me. (21 years old, French)

This strategy of washing after having sex is not an efficient means of preventing HIV transmission and may in fact increase the risk of infection.[20]

Prevention strategies also vary according to the situation, and a hierarchy of risk protection exists: if a condom is not available, then avoid ejaculation; if that is impossible, then clean yourself well afterwards and (maybe) have an HIV test, and so on.

> I know that I could get caught but . . . but well . . . if you take the test there's no problem. That's why a lot of young men like me go and take the test every three months . . . (21 years old, French)

In fact, taking the test, and interpreting the results, can create confusion. Among the *gigolos* interviewed, 10 stated that they regularly took an HIV antibody test as a means of prevention. This was particularly true of those who did not protect themselves systematically and who found themselves trying to adapt to both the situation and the client.

According to the *gigolos*, the majority of clients try to protect themselves against AIDS, but they sometimes find themselves in situations where cruising and sex work confuse them. Here, HIV prevention can lose its importance.

Now all the clients understand the situation . . . you forget your condoms for example, I do sometimes, I go out working without condoms. I do three clients, they all have condoms and lube, you know!
But the worst are those who haven't understood, (who) are not on
the game, those who go to places like the Tuileries and that, or who
go cruising for nothing. I went there once, I saw guys fucking without
condoms, coming without condoms, you see that sort of thing. (20
years old, French)

According to this account it seems that many men who use cruising grounds in
Paris may be at greater risk of AIDS than those who provide sexual services.
This confirms one of our hypotheses that HIV prevention activities need to be
adapted to the situation. This switching from the form(s) of interaction char-
acteristic of sex work to those typical of cruising can seriously interfere with
HIV prevention work.

In fact, a range of very diverse factors militate against the success of
prevention work. A large number of sex workers claim that they use condoms
with clients, but they do not do so with girlfriends and boyfriends, nor do they
necessarily do so with people they meet in their leisure time in clubs.
Moreover, they tend not to use protection in their relationships with women
generally. In the case of *gigolos* this was particularly clear:

Oh, that bit of plastic, no. When it's work, OK, but I'm not going to
fuck with it when I'm doing it for pleasure. Even if it's someone I
don't know very well, that I'm just beginning to get to know, I don't
use protection then . . . It's a risk that I take but it's a small risk you
see, if you like a guy . . . it's the same with a woman, hein? (32 years
old, French)

Such respondents display little understanding of there being a chain of infection, since outside the context of sex work, they see little risk. In the course of
our work, we did not meet one *garçon* who said that he used protection outside
sex work. Thus in thinking about how to promote HIV prevention in the sex
work context, we must emphasize the risk of HIV infection off the scene as
well.

Conclusion

In the course of this chapter, we have tried to describe the diversity of practices
constitutive of male sex work, as well as implications for HIV prevention. We
have shown that the majority of *travestis* sell sexual services as a result of their
decision to cross-dress, and their relationships with clients rarely go beyond
simple market exchange (money in return for sexual services). By way of
contrast, for *gigolos* it is difficult to establish clear boundaries between sex

work and other activities, and sometimes a purely market relationship is superseded by one of a more affective and emotional character. In this way, they may mix their interests with more complex kinds of interaction occurring in the context of gift relationships. Here, the selling of sexual services and HIV prevention concerns may become blurred. The majority of *gigolos* claim they use protection when they are selling sexual services, but outside this context they do not protect themselves (and their partners) consistently.

On the other hand, the status of condom use changes during the course of an individual's sex work career, as well as according to sexual practices and whether or not the person is in an emotional relationship. Consistent HIV prevention does not sit easily alongside love, physical beauty and the pursuit of personal pleasure, nor does it go well with situations of extreme social stress.

The material and emotional circumstances that some sex workers find themselves in, principally those linked to the use of drugs or likely to be found at the end of a sex work career, can increase the risk of HIV infection as well. The success of HIV prevention is also determined by the life situation of the person concerned. Few options present themselves by which male sex workers such as those interviewed in this study can lead decent lives: begging and selling sex in order to get something to eat. It is easy to understand how, in these kinds of situations, AIDS does not seem important.

The majority of the *travestis* and *gigolos*, however, stated that it was important to undertake prevention work both with sex workers and clients, and that so far the majority of prevention campaigns have not been directed towards such groups. According to them, prevention work for male sex workers must seek actively to involve the latter: sex workers are the best people to talk to other sex workers if prevention messages are to be clearly understood.[21]

On the other hand, HIV prevention discourse is changing, as findings concerning the effectiveness of new therapies become available: the advent of protease inhibitor drugs, for example, and multiple combination therapy may have important consequences both for infectivity and for the nature of prevention messages. Similarly, it is possible that HIV risk reduction practices can also evolve. The descriptions and information in this chapter relate to the years 1991–92, but we think that they remain valid today, especially in contexts where people switch from one situation to another (for example from a work relationship to an affective relationship). In order for prevention work to be effective, it is necessary to use appropriate intervention strategies. But we must anticipate changes in the way in which HIV and AIDS are socially represented if we are to carry out work that systematically enables individuals and groups to protect themselves against risk. This work, which can be both time-consuming and difficult, implies the need to change risk perceptions, particularly those associated with enjoyment and sexual pleasure, and particularly those context-specific risk perceptions linked to emotion and sexual enjoyment. Nevertheless, it seems to us that this is the way in which new prevention approaches need to be conceptualized and implemented.

Acknowledgement

I would like to thank Peter Aggleton who asked me to write this chapter and I would like to thank Yves Souteyrand and Jean Javanni for their critical reading of the text.

Notes

1 In this chapter, sex work is seen as a service involving the supply and demand of the body, generally with the purpose of a sexual and/or emotional relationship in mind. For reasons of methodology, this chapter will not examine young men who provide sexual services largely to women, and who frequent certain bars and brasseries in Paris.
2 See Weis (1985), Feschet (1986), Hennig (1978), and Schérer and Hocquenghem (1977).
3 *Tapin* ('drum-beaters') is a description given to men who provide sexual services to other men. The term is used colloquially to describe those who sell sex in the street – be they women, *garçons* or *travestis*. It is often used pejoratively by both clients and sex workers themselves.
4 See also Perlongher (1987).
5 The majority of *garçons* that we have had contact with, prefer to describe themselves as *gigolos*. In this chapter we will use the terms *gigolos* and *garçons* interchangeably to describe this type of sex worker. In other accounts, such men may be described as *tapin* (Welzer-Lang, Barbosa and Mathieu, 1994) or *garçon de passe* (Hennig, 1978). According to how they behave in places of sex work, *garçons* who see themselves as *gigolos* may be *tapin*. Colloquially, *fait le tapin* means to stay immobile at one place on the pavement or street. The *gigolo*, on the other hand, is the one who takes the initiative by going up to prospective clients in the street, asking them for a cigarette and so on, behaviour which for many people is not seen as a sign of sex work at all.
6 The project was carried out in association with APARTS (Association Pour les Appartements et les Actions de Relais Thérapeutiques et Social). It was financed by ANRS (Agence Nationale de recherches sur Sida) and AFLS (Agence Française de lutte contre le Sida). The work was conducted jointly with Sibel Bilal, and with the assistance of Maryline Rébillon and Abdalah Toufik (see da Silva and Bilal, 1992).
7 We noticed that when we called on sex workers in the context in which they worked, the majority asked to be paid for their time. A few, however, tended to refuse the payment offered. The *travestis* interviewed in Boles and Elifson's (1994) study in Atlanta (USA) were paid.
8 In some social and ethnological research, the offer of gifts to informants in exchange for information and acceptance is part of the overall style of work. Although making such a donation is not strictly comparable to the

monetary exchange that occurs between sex worker and client, it must nevertheless be recognized as a form of exchange in itself.

9 Of the 14 *travestis* interviewed, 6 were French, 3 Algerian, 3 Brazilian and 2 Argentinian. Of the 43 *garçons* interviewed face to face, 31 were French, 6 Algerian, 2 Romanian, 2 Yugoslavian, 1 Brazilian and 1 Turkish. The median age of the *garçons* was 27: the youngest was 19 and the oldest 38. Of the *travestis*, the median age was 40: the youngest was 28 and the oldest 50. The majority of interviewees had no professional qualifications, having been educated at school until the 5th or 6th grade. Among the *garçons*, we encountered one informant who was a physics teacher and who sold sex only occasionally. Another was preparing for his *baccalaureat* with a view to studying accountancy. Another had a higher technical qualification in agriculture. Yet another had completed higher level studies in information technology. Except for this last *garçon*, who was Romanian, the others were of French origin. Among the *travestis*, we interviewed one Argentinian who had studied veterinary medicine. Another Brazilian *travesti* had completed higher level studies in accountancy. Yet another Brazilian was a doctor. While it might be said that these are exceptions, they demonstrate clearly that male sex work cannot be understood simply in terms of economic need. Libidinal motivations cannot be ruled out.

10 This search for femininity can be achieved via different techniques, from the injection of silicone through to the total removal of male organs and the creation of a vagina. Those who undergo surgery in this way are called transsexuals. It is very important to distinguish between these *travestis* and those who may occasionally wear women's clothes for parties and shows, but who do not change their bodies in a permanent way.

11 Of the 53 *garçons* interviewed, 22 defined themselves as homosexual, 18 as bisexual and 13 as heterosexual.

12 Out of the 14 *travestis*, 11 sold sexual services regularly and 3 did so occasionally. Of these 3, 2 were in the latter stages of their sex work career. Of the 53 *gigolos*, 31 sold sexual services regularly with this being their principal activity, 9 did so occasionally either for money or enjoyment, and another 9 were at the end of their sex work career, rarely finding clients. Four *gigolos* considered themselves to be ex-sex workers and only sold sexual services very occasionally.

13 See da Silva (1995a).

14 See note 5, above.

15 According to informants, clients can be men of all ages, from 18 to 70 years old, but the majority are between 40 and 50 years of age.

16 See Fry (1982), Perlonguer (1987), Macrae (1990), da Silva (1995b).

17 Out of the 53 *garçons*, 27 stated that the service offered depended upon negotiation with the client but they practised mostly fellatio, masturbation and insertive sex. Eleven said that they only practised fellatio (either insertive or receptive), masturbation and insertive anal sex, 8 stated that

they only practised insertive anal sex, and 7 stated that they only allowed themselves to be fellated.

18 *Micheton* is a name used by *gigolos* to describe their clients.
19 Out of the 53 *garçons*, 10 said they used a condom for all practices, and 13 for insertive or receptive sex; 11 used a condom if the client suggested it, but if not, suggested they avoided contact with semen; 14 said they did not use a condom for fellatio. Among these, 10 avoided contact with semen and 4 only allowed themselves to be fellated by a client. Six said they did not use protection at all.
20 See Messiah *et al* (1993).
21 These suggestions have led to the creation of the PASTT (Prévention-action-Santé, pour les travestis et transsexuels) a project run by *travestis* encountered in the course of our research, in partnership with state organizations.

References

BECKER, H.S. (1985) *Outsiders*, Paris: Métailié.
BOLES, J. and ELIFSON, K. (1994) 'The social organisation of transvestite prostitution and AIDS', *Social Science and Medicine*, **39**, 1, pp. 85–93.
FESCHET, J. (1986) *Garçon pour le trottoir*, Paris: La Découverte.
FRY, P. (1982) 'Da Hierarquia a Igualdade: a construção historica da homosexualidade no Brasil', in P. FRY, *Para o Inglès ver*, Rio de Janeiro: Zahar.
HENNIG, J.L. (1978) *Garçons de Passe, enquête sur la prostitution masculine*, Paris: Hallier.
INGOLD, F.R. and TOUSSIRT, M. (1993) *Le travail sexuel, la consommation des drogues et le VIH: investigation ethnographique de la prostitution à Paris*, Paris: IREP.
MACRAE, E. (1990) *A construçâo da igualdade: identidade sexual e politica no Brasil da 'Abertura'*, Campinas: Editora da Unicamp.
MAUSS, M. (1974) 'Ensaio sobre a Dadiva. Forme et razão da troca nas sociedades arcaicas', *Sociologia e Antropologia*, **2**, pp. 37–184.
MESSIAH, A., BUCQUET, D., METTETAL, J.-F., LARROQUE, B., ROUZIOUX, C. and BRUGEAT, A. (1993) Factors correlated with homosexually-acquired HIV infection in the era of 'safe sex', *Sexually Transmitted Diseases*, **20**, pp. 51–8.
PERLONGHER, N. (1987) *O Negocio do Miché*, São Paulo: Ed. Brasiliense.
SHERER, R. and HOCQUENGHEIM, G. (1977) 'Sur la prostitution de jeunes garçons', *Recherche*, **26**, pp. 51–76.
DA SILVA, L. (1995a) 'Styles de vie homosexuel: l'exemple de São Paulo – Brésil', in R.L. MENDES (Ed.) *Un suject inclassable? Approches Sociologique, littéraire et juridique des homosexualités*, Lille: Cahier GKC.

DA SILVA, L. (1995b) 'Être un homme et une femme: ou la permanence de la personne dans l'exemple du travesti', *Journal du Sida*, **79**, pp. 30–3.

DA SILVA, L. and BILAL, S. (1992) *La prostitution masculine et la prévention du VIH à Paris. Rapport de Recherche*, Paris: APARTS – ANRS.

WEIS, J. (1985) *Arraché au trottoir – Le drame de la prostitution masculine*, Paris: Ed. Garancière.

WELZER-LANG, D., BARBOSA, O. and MATHIEU, L. (1994) *Prostitution: les uns, les unes et les autres*, Paris: Métailié.

Chapter 4

Male Sex Work and HIV/AIDS in Canada

Dan Allman and Ted Myers

Many of you will ask yourselves, or perhaps each other, how, in this era of AIDS, of a deadly fatal disease, which we all know is not primarily a gay disease, how can such things as male prostitution exist? Should they not be stamped out by the forces of law and order which must dedicate themselves to eradicating such vice in our fair land?

> Wallace [Win] Cummings, *Hustling* (Gilbert, 1986)

Unlike some deviant sub-populations which only began to be seriously scrutinized by researchers upon the advent of HIV, the study of sex work in Canada was well developed by the time HIV was identified. Though sex work as a social issue has been much discussed in Canadian academic, political and legal discourses over the last 20 years, there have been few attempts to understand the experiences of male sex workers. In this chapter we will describe findings from a recent review of male sex work and HIV/AIDS in Canada. This review examined past and present understanding of male sex work in Canada, with an emphasis on issues relating to HIV and AIDS.

Much of the pertinent literature was obtained through university and reference libraries. Other useful sources were municipal, provincial and federal archives, community-based resource centres, government libraries, public health departments and sex workers' alliances such as CORP (The Canadian Organization for the Rights of Prostitutes), Maggie's (Toronto) and SWAV (Sex Workers Alliance of Vancouver). In addition, many past and ongoing HIV behavioural and epidemiological studies of young people and injecting drug users have collected data on male sex work in tandem with other factors, and many of these studies' investigators have made their writings available to us.

While male and female sex workers share certain commonalities, there are many differences. To those who accuse us of marginalizing the female sex worker, we plead guilty – and intentionally so. We focus on male sex work because we believe that male sex work and HIV is not well understood in Canada, and that better understanding is needed. To study male sex work is not to belittle the experiences of female sex workers. Those experiences have been and are being addressed in a number of initiatives. Rather, it is to reflect the facts that the risks faced by the two populations may not be the same and that different interventions may be needed.

Because our focus is on male sex workers, we have not included socio-behavioural, epidemiological or experiential data on transgendered sex workers. This largely follows the lead of Namaste (1995) who believes that regardless of anatomy, transgendered sex workers often do not self-identify as male, that many of the issues as they relate to HIV and AIDS are distinct, and thus that the two populations should be considered separately. Finally, while many in Canada argue for a two-tier system of sex work law and policy – one that pertains to younger sex workers and another for adult sex workers – this chapter will consider both together, except where the division is warranted by specific research findings.

Canadian Prostitution Laws

Even though the United Nations passed a resolution in 1958 that prostitution should not be treated as a criminal act, Canada has always taken a criminalized approach to its control (Lowman, 1991; Achilles, 1995). Whereas in Canada prostitution is legal, many of the activities which may be associated with or related to sex work are considered illegal by the Criminal Code. These include communicating in a public place for the purpose of engaging in prostitution, keeping or being an intimate, providing directions, taking or showing someone to a common bawdy house, procuring or assisting or obtaining a person for sexual services on behalf of a third party, and living on the avails or benefiting from the prostitution of another person. One of the pitfalls of Canadian prostitution law is that, since the federal government has exclusive power over criminal matters, neither provinces nor municipalities are able to regulate sex work in any way other than that set down in the Criminal Code (Achilles, 1995).

Sex Work Research in Canada

The genesis of Canadian male sex work research can be traced to 1977 and the discovery of the body of 12-year-old shoeshine boy Emanuel Jaques behind Charlie's Angels body-rub parlour (Moyer and Carrington, 1989). At that time the Canadian media speculated whether or not he had been a sex worker. Concurrently in Vancouver, the police estimated there were about 200 male sex workers on the city's downtown streets (Forbes, 1977; Lowman, 1986). Some three years later, then federal Justice Minister, the honourable Jean Chrétien declined a tour of the area, remarking 'that he only had to look out his hotel room to see prostitutes' (*Vancouver Sun*, 1980, p. 7).

In the early 1980s, the federal government funded two large-scale research initiatives: the Committee on Sexual Offenses against Children and Youth, known as the Badgley Committee (1984); and the Special Committee on Pornography and Prostitution, known as the Fraser Committee (1985). Combined, these two studies interviewed 501 sex workers, 131 of whom were male (Lowman, 1987). As we shall see, these studies provide us with a baseline for much of our current understanding of male sex work and HIV/AIDS in Canada.

In overviewing the theoretical approaches that Canadians have applied to the study and understanding of sex work, it is important to recognize that this literature has largely attempted to describe female sex workers and their male clients. Lowman (1991) argues that no one theoretical perspective on sex work is distinctively Canadian. He believes that for the most part, the Badgley Committee worked from a social-psychological perspective which gave little specific attention to the role of the family. The Fraser Committee, on the other hand, 'developed a political economy of prostitution informed by a feminist analysis of patriarchal social relations', stressing inequalities in job opportunities and earning power as well as sexual socialization (Lowman, 1991, pp. 126–7). It is arguable that neither a social psychological perspective nor a political economy approach apply unproblematically to the study of male sex work, where special issues such as sexual orientation and community affiliation may come into play. Alternatively, dominant perspectives that have generally been used to theorize Canadian sex work need to be redefined or reapplied to consider the experiences specific to men and to women (Lowman, 1991).

In 1898, Stafford, writing in the *Canadian Journal of Medicine and Surgery*, defined both female prostitution and male same-gender sex as 'perversions' (cited in Kinsman, 1994). To some extent such practices, together with same-gender sex work, continue to be understood not simply as deviant, but as perverse. Kinsman (1994) believes that because male sex work is considered to be a sexual problem or perversion as opposed to an occupation or consensual sexual expression, we need to ask

> Who is defining sexual problems? Who is being defined? Whom are the definers silencing or opposing? It is especially important to investigate where these definitions have historically and socially come from. If we can grasp where they have come from, and how they have been put in place, we can act to challenge and transform them. (Kinsman, 1994, p. 166)

The dialectic which Kinsman extols has often been the vantage point from which many of Canada's sex worker coalitions and alliances have approached the legal inconsistencies, which some have suggested make sex work, especially male sex work, a more unsafe occupation than it necessarily need be.

Canadian Male Sex Workers – Who are they?

It is extremely difficult to estimate the size of the Canadian sex work industry. It is perhaps even more difficult to estimate the size of the male sex work industry. Definitions of male sex work vary, sex work is subject to personal shifts, and male sex workers in particular may drop in and out of the industry (Shaver, 1996). It is also hard to estimate the number of escorts and masseurs, as the individuals concerned may change names, addresses, and telephone numbers to avoid contact with police (International Conference on Prostitution and Other Sex Work, 1996).

Field studies conducted for the Federal Justice Department in the late 1980s showed that from 10 to 33 per cent of street sex workers in a number of large Canadian cities were men – 10 per cent in Vancouver, 18 per cent in Calgary, 20 per cent in Montreal, 25 per cent in Toronto and 33 per cent in Halifax (Moyer and Carrington, 1989). The Fraser Committee estimated that 25 per cent of sex workers in Canada were male. In the early 1990s it was estimated that in Toronto there were approximately 200 male workers working indoors and 150 male sex workers working on the street (Prostitutes' Safe Sex Project, 1991). It has been estimated that in Canada, men and women under 18 years of age represent between 10 to 12 per cent of individuals involved in sex work (Task Force on Children Involved in Prostitution, 1997).

How Canadian Male and Female Sex Workers Differ

There is consensus in Canadian sex work research that the careers of female sex workers tend to be longer than those of males (Lowman, 1992). 'For males, their term in the business is typically finished by the time they are in their early 20s as they are no longer competitive with the new and younger hustlers' (Fraser Committee, 1985, p. 372). It is not surprising, then, that most studies show male sex workers to be younger than females (Sasfaçon, 1985; Earls and David, 1990; Lowman, 1992).

There is controversy concerning the earnings of male sex workers. The Fraser Committee (1985) found, for example, that male sex workers can earn higher incomes because the prices they charge are higher than those of females, and pimping of male sex workers is virtually non-existent. Sansfaçon (1985) also reported that male sex workers earned more than their female counterparts. Shaver (1993), on the other hand, reported that the male sex workers earned much less than their female counterparts – between 600 and 800 dollars a week, compared to 1800 to 2000 dollars a week for females. She notes that 'the differences between female and male prostitutes regarding job hazards and earning power suggest that most of the undesirable aspects of prostitution are linked to broader social problems rather than the commercialization of sex' (Shaver, 1993, p. 167).

Earls and David (1990) reported that male sex workers in their study had been involved in sex work for an average of 5.1 years. Maggie's, The Toronto Prostitutes' Community Service Project (1994), in their study of sex workers in Toronto, found that for males, the average length of time spent in sex work was 5.2 years.

While the risks involving HIV and AIDS may be higher for male sex workers and their clients than for female sex workers, statistics regarding other forms of risk, specifically violent events, show that it is female sex workers who face the greatest dangers. For example, Statistics Canada (1997) notes that between 1991 and 1995, 63 known sex workers were murdered. Of these, only three – or less than 5 per cent – were male. The latter are also much less likely to be charged or convicted of a prostitution-related offence (Fraser Committee, 1985; Fleischman, 1989; Lowman, 1990; Gemme and Payment, 1992; Shaver, 1994; Achilles, 1995). Male sex workers are less likely to report rape, assault, or robbery, although when male sex workers are confronted with violence, it is often related in some way to homophobia (Lowman, 1992).

Male Sex Work and HIV/AIDS in Canada

The AIDS Case Reporting and Surveillance System was created by the Department of National Health and Welfare (now Health Canada) in February 1982. By the end of December 1997, 15 528 AIDS cases had been diagnosed, with 14 324 or 92.2 per cent of all cases involving adult males (Health Canada, 1998). In Canada, sex work is not a risk or demographic category that is recorded as a possible factor in terms of HIV testing or AIDS reporting and surveillance (Achilles, 1995).

Much data on male sex workers therefore derives from other sources, in particular, information on young people and injecting drug users. These two groups were identified early in the epidemic as *at risk* populations, and much of the information we have been able to gather has derived from studies of them. Though some studies exist which include male sex workers of all ages, they are very much in a minority.

Haug and Cini (1984) found that young men aged 20 to 24 made a significant contribution to the spread of gonorrhoea, while at the same time being less informed than other age cohorts. Earls and David (1989) report on 108 Canadian males recruited from several areas of a major eastern Canadian city, 55 who claimed they were actively involved in sex work, and 53 who had never had any direct experience with sex work. They found that 42 per cent of the sex workers indicated that they had ever had an STD. Ninety-two per cent of the male sex workers reported that they sought medical check-ups on a regular basis. These same authors also found that 96 per cent of their male sex worker sample were aware of the existence of AIDS, and 58 per cent indicated that they had changed their sexual practices as a result of AIDS. Bastow (1996) found that among Toronto male sex workers, 'the most common sexual activity engaged in was oral sex. The second most common was anal intercourse, 'with the sex worker giving rather than getting' (Bastow, 1996, p. 12).

Shaver and Newmeyer (1996), comparing data from 40 male sex workers collected in 1991 with comparable data from the 1991–92 Montreal site of the

National Men's Survey (Myers *et al.*, 1993) and the 1991–92 Quebec study, Entre Hommes (Godin *et al.*, 1993), found that male sex workers were more likely to have been tested for HIV than men who have sex with men recruited through gay identified venues (88 per cent compared to 61 per cent and 68 per cent) and less likely to report a seropositive result (0 per cent compared to 11 per cent and 21 per cent). Seventy-one per cent of male sex workers used condoms most or all of the time for oral sex with clients, and 45 per cent for oral sex with partners. Ninety-two per cent used condoms most or all of the time for anal sex with clients (less than 25 per cent of males provided this service), and 71 per cent with partners.[1] Male sex workers in the study spent an average of 40 minutes with each client with a mean number of 15 clients a week (Shaver, 1996).

Shaver also found that male sex workers were cautious with respect to risks related to HIV and other STDs, reporting an average of 0.77 episodes of STD over the last two years. However, 63 per cent reported no episodes in the last two years. Shaver suggests this may indicate 'that there is a small number of sex workers who are chronically infected, as opposed to a large number of sex workers who are occasionally infected' (Shaver, 1996, pp. 51–2).

Shaver and Newmeyer (1996) found that among male sex workers, consistency of condom use increased with the riskiness of sexual activity. Male sex workers were much less likely to engage in high risk activities with clients than they were with their primary partners, and were more likely to use condoms with clients, regardless of the sexual activity, than they were with their primary partners. With regard to both sexual practices and risk taking behaviour, sex workers' behaviour with partners seems to be more similar to that of gay and bisexual men in general than it is different. In addition, both groups are knowledgeable about AIDS and the risks involved, and both have made some changes in their sexual practices. Higher levels of condom use and the limitation of sexual practices with clients may well serve to differentiate work-sex from personal-sex. Clients are business – one does not have to enjoy sexual relations with them, or even see the encounter as being other than a cash for service transaction (Shaver and Newmeyer, 1996, pp. 13–14).

HIV/AIDS and the Younger Male Sex Worker

Younger male sex workers have been the subject of interest in some early Canadian research initiatives, from the work of the Badgley Committee (1984) through to the work of Visano (1987, 1991). Highcrest (1997) points to the need to differentiate between younger sex workers whose occupation is prostitution, and youth who participate in 'survival sex'. The educational and social service needs of these two groups are distinct. Sex workers may be more informed than youth participating in sex as a means of survival; for the latter, AIDS may be a relatively low level concern (Tremble, 1993).

The Badgley Committee (1984) found that 52 per cent of their male respondents indicated that they had contracted an STD, a sex-related disease or another condition since they began to actively participate in sex work. Eighty-four per cent of these had sought treatment. In addition, 66 per cent of males indicated that they had regular medical check-ups, regardless of suspected STD infection. The Committee reported that 64 per cent of males indicated that active fellatio was the most requested act, while 12 per cent reported that passive fellatio was the most requested act. Approximately 5 per cent stated that anal sex was most frequently requested and another 12 per cent said that a 'straight lay' was the most frequently requested act. In terms of the sexual acts that they were unwilling to perform, 43 per cent indicated that they would not receive anal sex. When engaged in sexual activities with clients, 12 per cent indicated that they usually used some form of protection. Eighteen per cent used condoms for oral sex, and 19 per cent for anal sex. The Committee notes: 'it is relevant in this context to recall that these findings were obtained during 1982–83 when there was a growing public awareness of the sharp increase in the reported incidence of Acquired Immune Deficiency Syndrome' (Badgley Committee, 1984, p. 1023).

Read *et al.*, (1993) report that 11 per cent of their sample of street youth who had ever sold sex were HIV positive. Ten (67 per cent of 15) youths testing HIV positive reported that they had engaged in same-gender sex work in the previous six months. Seven of those same 10 reported having had no anal sex with clients. The three who reported anal sex with clients all reported consistent condom use. It was with their regular partners that these three reported sometimes engaging in unprotected anal sex. These same authors found that males were more likely to always use condoms with female clients (68 per cent) than with male clients (54 per cent). Ten per cent of male sex workers reported that they engaged in unprotected anal sex, at least occasionally, with clients. Nearly one-third of male sex workers reported 26 or more clients per month, and 38 per cent of males involved in same-gender sex work reported practising anal sex.

Data from the Canada Youth and AIDS Study indicate that 14 per cent of 712 street youth recruited were reported sex workers with a male/female ratio of 0.8:1 (MacDonald *et al.*, 1994). Forty-five per cent of male sex workers reported having had an STD. Among these male sex workers, 63 per cent had engaged in anal intercourse. Regular condom use was associated with a lower reported STD history (36 per cent) than for those who inconsistently used condoms (61 per cent). The authors found that 52 per cent of male sex workers reported over 100 different sexual partners. In addition, 69 per cent of male sex workers reported worrying about AIDS, 60 per cent reported having engaged in anal intercourse, and 55 per cent reported that they always used a condom. More recently, Roy *et al.* (1996) have reported that six of 122 male street youth interviewed who had sex with men were HIV seropositive. All had a history of sex work and five had also injected drugs.

Injecting Drug Users, Male Sex Work and HIV/AIDS in Canada

Millson *et al.* (1991) reported that among male sex workers with same-sex clients, 61 per cent reported always using a condom compared to 15 per cent reporting that they never did so. Of males with female clients, 34 per cent reported always used a condom, while 51 per cent had never used a condom in the last six months. At the 1994 national meeting on HIV infection in injecting drug users in Canada (Laboratory Centre for Disease Control, 1994), Millson *et al.* (1994) reported on a series of repeated cross-sectional surveys of injecting drug users entering drug treatment. In 1991–92 4.0 per cent of 372 male injecting drug users reported same-sex clients in the previous six months, compared with 3.4 per cent of 380 in 1992–93, and 9.2 per cent of 414 in 1993–94. Of male injecting drug users reporting an involvement in sex work, approximately half indicated that they always used condoms with female clients (vaginal sex only), while 21.7 per cent, 12.5 per cent and 22.2 per cent, during these three periods respectively, reported that they never used condoms. For same-sex clients (and in relation to anal sex only), 40 per cent, 66.7 per cent and 76.5 per cent reported that they always used condoms (for the years 1991–92, 1992–93, and 1993–94 respectively) while 10 per cent, 0 per cent and 11.8 per cent respectively indicated that they never used condoms with male clients (Millson *et al.*, 1994).

Rekart (1993) reports on a study conducted between 1988 and 1992 of street-involved persons. HIV prevalence over five years for the entire sample (n = 825) was 6.4 per cent. The author notes that sex between men was an important risk factor. Dufour *et al.* (1995) report that 12.2 per cent of 41 male prison inmates who had engaged in sex work were HIV positive. They note that all of the HIV positive individuals were also injecting drug users. Lamothe *et al.* (1996), reporting on a study of 694 injecting drug users receiving treatment and 213 injecting drug users not receiving treatment, found that HIV seroprevalence for sex workers/injecting drug users not receiving treatment was higher than that of sex workers/injecting drug users under treatment. The seroprevalence of male sex workers/injecting drug users was also found to be higher than that of female sex workers/injecting drug users.

Baskerville, Leonard and Hotz (1994) have described an evaluation of a needle exchange programme in which 34 per cent of male injecting drug use survey respondents (which included both attenders and non-attenders of the needle exchange clinic) indicated that in the last three months they had had sex with male clients for either money, goods or drugs. Ninety-six per cent reported oral sex with a same-sex client in the three months prior to the study, while 46 per cent of men with same-sex clients reported insertive or receptive anal intercourse. Seventy-two per cent of the respondents reporting anal sex with a client in the previous three months had always used a condom, while 29 per cent reported never using a condom for anal sex with a client.

Parent *et al.* (1994) report that among 212 male injecting drug users in their Quebec City study, HIV prevalence was 28.6 per 100 for the injecting drug users who were also male sex workers, and 9.7 per 100 for injecting drug users who did not report male sex work.

Bisexual Men, Male Sex Work and HIV/AIDS

In 1996 we conducted the BISEX Survey, involving 1314 anonymous interviews with behaviourally bisexual men (defined as having had sex with a man and a woman in the previous five years) across the province of Ontario (Myers *et al.*, 1997). Men were recruited through extensive advertising in mainstream, community and alternative sources. Interviews were carried out by way of a toll-free telephone line. Respondents provided information on the sexual activities of their last safe and unsafe sexual encounters with male and female 'casual' and regular partners. In total, 20 men reported that their last casual male partner had been met through sex work.[2]

For these 20 men, the mean age was 35.9 with a range from 19 to 51. All self-identified as bisexual. Of these men, 26 per cent were married and 58 per cent were single. Six per cent reported unprotected receptive or insertive anal intercourse in the previous year with men only, 47 per cent reported unprotected vaginal or anal intercourse in the previous year with women only, 23.5 per cent reported unprotected vaginal and/or anal intercourse with both men and women, and 23.5 per cent reported only protected vaginal and/or anal intercourse with both men and women.

Twenty-seven percent of these men had ever been tested for antibodies to HIV. None reported that they were HIV seropositive. When asked what they thought their current HIV status was, all men reported that they believed that they were HIV seronegative. Men were asked how likely they thought it was that they would become infected with HIV. Twenty per cent believed it was likely and 73 per cent believed that it was unlikely.

Hidden Male Sex Work

In Canada, public concern regarding sex work is generally limited to the visible manifestations of street work, and 'all legislative attempts to control prostitution in the last 15 years have targeted only street prostitution' (Achilles, 1995, p. 1). The Bureau of Municipal Research (1983) found that only 20 per cent of all sex work was visible or on the streets of Toronto, and as little as 5 per cent in the winter. The Federal Provincial Territorial Working Group on Prostitution (1995a, 1995b) reported that in some of Canada's smaller cities, nearly all sex work activity occurs in off-street venues such as escort agencies, and that along Canada's coasts, there are reports of boats being used as sites for sex work. One of the results of such 'hidden' sex work is that some law enforcement agencies report no knowledge of sex work in their jurisdictions. Even in the larger Canadian cities where hidden sex work is somewhat more visible, HIV and AIDS outreach has reported difficulties accessing sex workers in these venues. Jackson, Highcrest and Coates (1992) found that, for example,

> Outreach workers have indicated that some brothel agencies in Toronto maintain a strict control over interactions between prostitutes from their community and other prostitutes. It is believed that some agencies and brothels tend to be more interested in profit making than the health of the prostitutes, and that some brothel owners demand that prostitutes follow clients' wishes for sexual intercourse without the use of condoms. (Jackson, Highcrest and Coates, 1992, p. 283)

In a 1995 needs assessment involving Asian sex workers, two male respondents discussed their experiences working in a massage parlour:

> The issue of condoms on the premise could be improved. Owners have asked their workers not to have condoms with them for fear of legal incrimination . . . that some workers do practice unsafe sex in exchange for higher monetary return. Some workers do go against their employer's request of not having condoms by hiding the condoms on them during their shift. At times clients do bring their own condoms with them. (Wong, 1995, pp. 17–18)

From a legal perspective, there is a tendency to 'to lump prostitutes in with strippers, porn film performers, phone sex mates and performance artists', even though 'a porn performer cannot be charged with soliciting, a phone sex mate cannot be charged with keeping a brothel, a stripper cannot be charged with pimping. The work is not the same, the repercussions of the work are not the same, we are not all the same' (Highcrest and Maki, 1992, p. 4). Yet from a public health perspective, we have little understanding as to whether the risks associated with hidden sex work are similar to those with visible sex work. This is because little is known about the range of sexual behaviours and condom use, or the level of AIDS knowledge and beliefs, of either hidden male sex workers or their clients.

Sexual Identities

Thirty-seven per cent of respondents cited by the Badgley Committee (1984) were male. Of these, 23 per cent reported that they were heterosexual, 31 per cent homosexual and 31 per cent bisexual. An additional seven male sex workers indicated that they were undecided about their sexuality. Earls and David (1990) found that 64 per cent of male sex workers indicated that their first sexual partner had been another man, and 70 per cent indicated that their sexual orientation was either homosexual (52 per cent) or bisexual (18 per cent). Comparing a Montreal sample of male sex workers to other samples of men who have sex with men, Shaver and Newmeyer (1996) found that the sex workers were more 'diverse with respect to sexual identity: only 50 per cent (in contrast to 89 per cent and 81 per cent of the respondents in the gay men's studies) identified as homosexual, or gay. Significantly higher proportions of the hustlers identified as bisexual or heterosexual (*ibid.*, p. 9).

Many Canadian studies have found that younger men who self-identify as homosexual may be more prone to enter sex work than those who self-identify as heterosexual or bisexual. One well documented reason is that younger gay men may be drawn to the street as a means of discovering or exploring aspects of their sexuality (Badgley Committee, 1984; Mathews, 1986; Visano, 1987; Scott, 1988; Earls and David, 1990; Lowman, 1991; Tremble, 1993; Highcrest, 1997)

There is continued debate as to the influence of sexual coercion, threat or force on subsequent involvement in male sex work and/or engagement in behaviours with an increased risk for HIV. Current research, notably the Vanguard Study in Vancouver, may attempt to elaborate a possible three-way association. At the time of this writing, however, no reasonable data exist to illustrate associations between reported sexual coercion, involvement in sex work and an increased risk for HIV infection. The Badgley Committee (1984) stated that the proportion of younger male sex workers who reported sexual abuse was similar to the proportion reported by males in the general Canadian population.

HIV/AIDS Outreach

While many Canadian researchers have been slow to incorporate issues of HIV and AIDS into their investigations of male sex work, sex worker outreach groups have been proactive and vocal.

> There are many jobs that involve risks and require safety measures. Sex workers are well aware of the potential risks of their trade, including the potential for violence or infection. Because of this they ensure precautions for both themselves and their clients. Just as construction workers always wear helmets on a job site, sex workers use condoms. (STELLA, 1996)

One of the messages promoted by Maggie's Prostitutes' Safe Sex Project, is that:

> The risk of catching HIV is not from having sex for money, but from having risky sex with partners who we trust, love and play with – from people and activities that are outside the parameters of sex work. (Sex Workers Alliance of Vancouver, 1997).

Commenting on Toronto's Safe Sex Project for prostitutes (initiated by the Canadian Organization for the Rights of Prostitutes [CORP]), Danny Cockerline had this to say:

> When we first started doing this project, our approach was to find out what people knew about safe sex and offer them condoms. What we found was that a lot of people were really insulted because they knew about condoms and safe sex already. Even offering them a condom was an insult because they would say, 'Well, I've got my own condoms'. So we started a new approach where we would give them material like pamphlets to give to their customers. The whole approach was that this is material to educate your customer and it is not therefore an insult to you. That has been very successful . . . It encourages them to feel good about the fact that they are practising safe sex and promoting it with their customers. (cited in Brock, 1985, p. 16)

Also in Toronto, Street Outreach Services (SOS) have been working to serve the needs of street youth involved in, or at risk of becoming involved in, sex work since 1985. Among the services offered are HIV/AIDS education initiatives. In 1994–95, a peer education workshop, safer sex toy workshops, helped client groups to develop educational materials, pre- and post-test HIV counselling, and condom distribution. Between October 1994 and March 1995, 477 different young people accessed the SOS drop-in on a total of 3578 occasions. Seventy-five per cent of these visits were by males.

In Winnipeg, the Village Clinic's Street Outreach Project is mandated by a strategy that allows male sex workers 'to define their own needs and identify strategies to meet those needs, instead of service being delivered based on assumptions of employees and volunteers of the community clinic' (Linnebach and Schellenberg, 1996, p. 11). This project incorporates harm reduction, and provides basic health services including condoms, health information and service referrals to male sex workers in a non-judgemental manner.

Through the Commercial Sex Information Service (CSIS) of the Sex Workers Alliance of Vancouver, Canadian sex workers and their clients can access information using the Internet on a variety of issues affecting sex workers, including health concerns surrounding HIV and AIDS. Walnet, which houses the CSIS and SWAV Web sites, was first set up in December 1995. During the 15 months between then and March 1997, Walnet served up 246094 pages. In February 1996, Walnet served up 13382 pages. A year later, in February 1997, Walnet served 30906 pages, which represents a growth of 231 per cent.

Hypocrisy and Canadian Male Sex Work

The first major sweep to try to combat male sex work in Toronto's homosexual track[3] occurred in June 1987 by a 14-member undercover squad. Twenty-three men were arrested.

Despite concern about the deadly AIDS virus police taking part in the sweep took no special precautions and those arrested will not be automatically tested for the disease, police said. However, one investigator noted that, unlike female prostitutes, none of the men who were arrested carried condoms as protection against infection. (*Toronto Star*, 1987)

Throughout the 1990s, Canada's media have continued to feed stereotypes of the male sex worker as an AIDS vector. A blatant example is an opinion piece in the *Vancouver Province* concerning the ability to curb the irresponsible behaviour of sex workers and their clients. Though reporting on an HIV positive female sex worker and the repercussions that behaviours attributed to her might have on her clients and on society, the article, titled 'A Deadly Dilemma', is illustrated by a quarter-page photograph of two male sex workers and the caption 'Male prostitutes wait for customers . . . difficult issues for health officials' (*Vancouver Province*, 1990, p. 52).

After years of targeting sex workers, law enforcement agents in Toronto, Calgary and Ottawa have recently begun to target customers and clients through a programme called John School. Modelled on a San Francisco based initiative, John School provides an opportunity for the clients of sex workers to avoid prosecution for 'communicating for the purpose of prostitution in a public place'. Instead, they are fined $500, and made to attend a full day of lectures (Sex Workers Alliance of Vancouver, 1997).

Alternatives to Canada's current criminalization of prostitution-related offences include decriminalization or regulation (legalization). However, no country, city or jurisdiction in the world has ever adopted a decriminalization approach to sex work (International Conference on Prostitution and other Sex Work, 1996). The most frequently recommended approach in Canada is regulation or legalization, whereby sex work would be allowed in certain forms through either zoning or licensing. This was the recommendation of the federally appointed Fraser Committee (1985), although the recommendation was in fact never adopted. Debates about criminalization/decriminalization/regulation are volatile and current. Bastow (1996) has argued that the criminalization of sex work allows little leverage for sex workers to insist on condom use with their customers, and may in fact increase the chances of HIV transmission. For Highcrest and Maki (1992, p. 3) one of 'the biggest barriers to prostitutes accessing AIDS prevention information is the criminalization of our work'.

Associated with debates about legalization, decriminalization and licensing, is the forced or mandatory medical examination of male sex workers, including HIV antibody testing. In 1984, 69 per cent of Canadians agreed with the statement 'prostitution is a major cause of the spread of venereal disease', and 82 per cent agreed that one of the roles of government in adult prostitution was to 'require prostitutes to have medical examinations' (Peat, Marwick and Partners, 1984). However, the National Advisory Committee on AIDS in

1989 'concluded that mandatory or compulsory HIV testing is unwarranted for persons working in the sex industry because harms from such testing would outweigh any benefits for them' (cited in Jürgens and Palles, 1997, p. 174).

In their report on HIV antibody testing and confidentiality, Jürgens and Palles make reference to a document of the Ontario Law Reform Commission who state that it is not clear whether the mandatory testing of sex workers would deter high risk sexual behaviour. The commission concluded:

> Unless Canadians are willing to consider isolating indefinitely or otherwise restricting all infected workers – measures that would encourage prostitutes and others at risk to avoid HIV-related testing and other help-seeking alternatives – little could be done with the information. In short, for both the client and the sex worker the Commission believes the risk of transmission is best addressed by targeted education efforts and programs designed to encourage risk-reducing behaviour, including information about the use of condoms and clean needles. No exception to a general rule requiring voluntary, specific, and informed consent for all HIV-related testing is justified with respect to male or female sex workers. (cited in Jürgens and Palles, 1997, p. 179)

Calgary Alderperson Beverly Longstaff has suggested that the mandatory testing of sex workers

> may result in unintended consequences. The clients may pressure sellers to engage in unprotected sex on the supposition that the prostitutes are somehow medically certified. This would be dangerous for everyone involved. (Longstaff, 1993, pp. 5–6)

By conceiving of male sex work as an occupation, in which the risk of HIV and AIDS is little more than one of a number of occupational hazards, it may be possible for law enforcement and policy-makers to turn from current tactics towards occupational safety and the promotion of healthy sexuality. However, despite evidence which does not support the 'exaggerated link between male sex work and HIV/AIDS, policies directed at the sanitary policing of prostitutes are still evident today' (Shaver, 1996, p. 42).

Conclusions

In 1985 the Fraser Committee issued the statement, 'Prostitutes are very aware of the dangers of sexually transmitted diseases (STDs) and the reputation prostitutes have for the spread of such diseases'. It then went on to qualify this statement by noting that 'this reputation is unsubstantiated by epidemiological researchers' (Fraser Committee, 1985, p. 384).

Reviewing the behavioural and epidemiological data set out earlier in this chapter, it is clear that any consensus on male sex work and the risk of HIV infection and transmission in Canada is going to be hard to achieve. Studies have inquired into the experiences of male sex workers with STDs, health care utilization, injecting drug use, HIV testing, HIV/AIDS knowledge, attitudes and beliefs, sexual behaviour with clients and with partners, and, occasionally, HIV status. Overall there is little consistency in terms of measurement or sampling. However, the majority of studies have included questions on the use of condoms, and it is this measure that is most likely to allow any estimate of the risk of HIV infection in male sex work in Canada today.

The Badgley Committee (1984) reported that 18 per cent of male sex workers used condoms for oral sex, and 19 per cent for anal sex. Read *et al.* (1993) reported that 54 per cent of their sample always used condoms with male clients, and 68 per cent with female clients. MacDonald *et al.* (1994) found that 55 per cent of male sex workers always used condoms. Baskerville, Leonard and Hotz (1994) report that 72 per cent of their sample had always used a condom for anal sex with a client in the previous three months. Millson *et al.* (1994) report that condoms were always used for anal sex with male clients by 40 per cent of their sample, and by 34 per cent with female clients. They also report that condoms were always used for anal sex with male clients by 40 per cent, by 67 per cent and by 77 per cent in 1991–92, 1992–93 and 1993–94. For vaginal sex with female clients, condoms were reportedly used all the time by approximately 50 per cent of respondents in each of the three time periods. Finally, Shaver and Newmeyer (1996) report that 71 per cent of male sex workers used condoms most or all of the time for oral sex with clients, 45 per cent for oral sex with partners, 92 per cent for anal sex with clients, and 71 per cent with partners. The authors found that these figures were comparable to those for temporally and geographically similar samples of men who have sex with men. In a 1985 research review on sex work in Canada, Sansfaçon stated that only 30 to 40 per cent of male sex workers used condoms. Our findings suggest that this figure no longer applies. Taken together, our review of findings on reported condom use do suggest a trend towards greater use over time: that Canadian male sex workers are increasingly protecting themselves and their clients from infection and transmission of HIV and other STDs.

Although prostitutes do contract STDs, the public's strongly held belief (held by 69 per cent of the survey respondents) that prostitutes are a major cause of the spread of such diseases, is not substantiated. Epidemiological studies indicate that prostitutes are not a prime factor in the spreading of STDs. This occurs as a consequence of sexual mores changing throughout society and cannot be seen as the result of the behaviour of one relatively small group of people. As indicated, prostitutes, of all people in society, have a real interest in seeing that they are not infected. (Fraser Committee, 1985, p. 395)

Arriving at a more accurate understanding of the relationship between male sex work and HIV/AIDS in Canada will clearly require further work as well as the realization that, for all we know, there is at least as much that we have missed. Much of what we know in terms of male sex work and HIV and AIDS predates current social, behavioural and epidemiological measures of sexuality and its expression. With few exceptions, most samples of male sex workers have been subsamples of other larger populations, or have been small in size. Rarely have the same methods and measurements for the study of male sex work been utilized in cities of different sizes across the country. There are little longitudinal data on male sex work, and even less multi-site data. We know virtually nothing of male sex work other than visible street prostitution. The exchange of sex for goods other than money has, to our knowledge, never been studied in Canada, and at present we have little insight into the behaviours, attitudes and beliefs of either clients or partners of male sex workers and how these relate to HIV and AIDS. We lack a solid understanding of how male sex workers who are also injecting drug users differ from male sex workers who are not injecting drug users. Possible associations between reported sexual coercion, involvement in sex work and an increased risk for HIV infection should be further explored, and we need to better understand the relationship between sexual identity, social environment, internal and external homophobia and the experiences of younger male sex workers.

Often, when male sex work has been investigated in Canada, it has been conceptualized as a social problem rather than a social fact. It is vital to recognize that in Canada male sex work *is* a social fact. Regardless of morality, politics or the law, male sex work exists today and will continue into the future. This being the case, are we not obliged to help make certain that for the individuals that male sex work involves, their future is a safe and healthy one? Sex in exchange for money or kind need not be unsafe nor dangerous, as Danny Cockerline has observed: 'Most people who become infected with HIV are getting it for free' (cited in Brock, 1985, p. 14).

Only a small portion of the rich literature on sex work in Canada is included in this chapter. Yet the historical literature tells us that sex work, like the railroad, followed Canada's history of colonization and settlement. In essence, sex work is a founding occupation, an occupation that crosses our past, present and future histories, and an occupation whose public façade continues to be built upon hypocrisy.

The thing is we will always be here, and we will always be here because you will always need us. You need us because you need sex, at times, when it is not possible or convenient to get it from anybody else. So you can choose. You can choose to damage us with laws. You can choose to damage yourselves in the process because hypocrisy always brutalizes. You can choose to damage your institutions, you can choose to damage the communities in which we live, or you can choose to accept . . . the choice is really up to you. (Hannon, 1996)

Acknowledgements

We would like to thank the following who assisted in locating many of the materials referred to in this chapter: John Lowman, Fran Shaver, Augustine Brannigan, Jacqueline Nelson, John Schellenberg, Ki Namaste, Raj Maharaj, Carol Strike, Sandra Houston, Kyle Rae, The Canadian Lesbian and Gay Archives, City of Toronto Department of Public Health, City of Vancouver Archives, The National AIDS Clearinghouse, Laboratory Centre for Disease Control-Health Canada, and especially Andrew Sorfleet and the invaluable resources made available through CSIS and SWAV.

Notes

1 Twenty-five per cent of the sample were transgendered sex workers who self-identified a gay.
2 The question did not differentiate between the role of the respondent as either a sex worker or a client.
3 The track or a track is a geographic location, usually a street that is known for sex work.

References

ACHILLES, R. (1995) *The Regulation of Prostitution*, background paper presented to the City of Toronto Board of Health, Toronto: City of Toronto Public Health Department, 24 April.
BADGLEY COMMITTEE (COMMITTEE ON SEXUAL OFFENSES AGAINST CHILDREN AND YOUTH) (1984) *Sexual Offenses against Children*, Ottawa: Department of Supply and Services.
BASKERVILLE, B., LEONARD, L. and HOTZ, S. (1994) *Evaluation of the SITE: A Pilot HIV Prevention Programme for Injection Drug Users*, Ottawa: Ottawa–Carleton Health Department.
BASTOW, K. (1996) 'Prostitution and HIV/AIDS', *Canadian HIV/AIDS Policy & Law Newsletter* **2**, 2, pp. 12–14.
BROCK, D. (1985) 'Prostitutes are scapegoats in the AIDS panic', *Resources for Feminist Research*, **18**, 2, pp. 13–17.
BUREAU OF MUNICIPAL RESEARCH (1993) *Cities*, Toronto: Toronto Bureau of Municipal Research.
DUFOUR, A., ALARY, M., POULIN, C., ALLARD, F., NOEL, L., TROTTIER, G.,

HANKINS, C. and LEPINE, D. (1995) 'HIV prevalence and risk behaviours among inmates of a provincial prison in Quebec City', presentation at the 5th Annual Canadian Conference on HIV/AIDS Research, Winnipeg.

EARLS, C.M. and DAVID, H. (1989) 'A psychosocial study of male prostitution', *Archives of Sexual Behavior*, **18**, 5, pp. 401–19.

EARLS, C.M. and DAVID, H. (1990) 'Early family and sexual experiences of male and female prostitutes', *Canada's Mental Health*, **38**, 4, pp. 7–11.

FEDERAL PROVINCIAL TERRITORIAL WORKING GROUP ON PROSTITUTION (1995a) *Dealing With Prostitution in Canada: A Consultation Paper*, Ottawa: Department of Justice.

FEDERAL PROVINCIAL TERRITORIAL WORKING GROUP ON PROSTITUTION (1995b) *Results of the National Consultation on Prostitution in Selected Jurisdictions, Interim Report*, Ottawa: Department of Justice.

FLEISCHMAN, J. (1989) *The Evaluation of the Street Prostitution Legislation: A Summary of Research Findings*, Ottawa: Department of Justice.

FORBES, G.A. (1977) *Street Prostitution in Vancouver's West End: Prepared for Vancouver Police Board and Vancouver City Council*, Vancouver: Vancouver Police Department.

FRASER COMMITTEE (SPECIAL COMMITTEE ON PORNOGRAPHY AND PROSTITUTION) (1985) *Pornography and Prostitution in Canada*, Ottawa: Department of Supplies and Services.

GEMME, R. and PAYMENT, N. (1992) 'Criminalization of adult street prostitution in Montreal: evaluation of the law in 1987 and 1991', *Canadian Journal of Human Sexuality*, **1**, 4, pp. 217–20.

GILBERT, S. (1986) 'Hustling: a theatrical investigation into male prostitution', unpublished manuscript, Toronto: Buddies in Bad Times Theatre.

GODIN, G., CARSLEY, J., MORRISON, K. and BRADET, R. (1993) *Entre hommes – 91/92: Les Comportements Sexuelles et L'environment Social des Hommes Ayant des Relations Sexuelles Avec D'autres Hommes*, Quebec: COCQ-sida.

HANNON, G. (1996) 'St. Lawrence Centre Forum. Prostitution A Profession Like Any Other?' a discussion sponsored by the Canadian Organization for the Rights of Prostitutes, Toronto, 29 October.

HAUG, M. and CINI, M. (1984) *The Ladies (and Gentlemen) of the Night and the Spread of Sexually Transmitted Diseases*, Working Papers on Pornography and Prostitution, Report No. 7, Ottawa: Department of Justice.

HEALTH CANADA (1998) *HIV and AIDS in Canada, Surveillance Report to December 31, 1997*, Division of HIV/AIDS Surveillance, Bureau of HIV/AIDS and STD, Laboratory Centre for Disease Control, LCDC Health Canada, Ottawa: Health Canada.

HIGHCREST, A. (1997) *At Home on the Stroll. My Twenty Years as a Prostitute in Canada*, Canada: Alfred A. Knopf.

HIGHCREST, A. and MAKI, K. (1992) 'When love is illegal, AIDS prevention in the context of the private sex lives of prostitutes', presentation at the VIII International Conference on AIDS, Amsterdam, July.

INTERNATIONAL CONFERENCE ON PROSTITUTION AND OTHER SEX WORK (1996) Participation Kit, Montreal: Quebec Public Interest Research Group at McGill University.

JACKSON, L., HIGHCREST, A. and COATES, R. (1992) 'Varied potential risks of HIV infection among prostitutes', *Social Science and Medicine*, **35**, 3, pp. 281–6.

JÜRGENS, R. and PALLES, M. (1997) *HIV Testing and Confidentiality: A Discussion Paper*, Montreal: Canadian AIDS Society and Canadian HIV/AIDS Legal Network.

KINSMAN, G. (1994) 'Constructing sexual problems: "These things may lead to the tragedy of our species"', in L. SAMUELSON, (Ed.) *Power and Resistance, Critical Thinking About Canadian Social Issues*, Halifax: Fernwood Publishing.

LABORATORY CENTRE FOR DISEASE CONTROL (1994) *The Proceedings of the Meeting on HIV Infection among Injection Drug Users in Canada*, Montreal, Quebec, 12–13 December, Ottawa: Health Canada.

LAMOTHE, F., BRUNEAU, J., FRANCO, E., LACHANCE, N., DESY, M., SOTO, J. and VINCELETTE, J. (1996) 'Risk factors for HIV seroconversion among injection drug users in the Saint-Luc cohort. Montreal 1988–1995', presentation at the XI International Conference on AIDS, Vancouver, BC, Canada, July.

LINNEBACH, K. and SCHELLENBERG, J. (1996) 'Street outreach with MSM sex trade workers allows clients to define their needs', *Canadian AIDS News*, **9**, 2, p. 11.

LONGSTAFF, B. (1993) *Report of Subcommittees on Prostitution to the Federation of Canadian Municipalities Big Cities Mayor's Caucus*, Calgary: Federation of Canadian Municipalities.

LOWMAN, J. (1986) 'Prostitution in Vancouver: some notes on the genesis of a social problem', *Canadian Journal of Criminology*, **28**, 1, pp. 1–16.

LOWMAN, J. (1987) 'Taking young prostitutes seriously', *Canadian Review of Sociology and Anthropology*, **24**, 1, pp. 99–116.

LOWMAN, J. (1990) 'Street prostitutes in Canada: an evaluation of the Brannigan–Fleischman opportunity model', *Canadian Journal of Law and Society*, 6, pp. 137–64.

LOWMAN, J. (1991) 'Prostitution in Canada', in M.A. JACKSON, C.T. GRIFFITHS and A. HATCH (Eds) *Canadian Criminology: Perspectives on Crime and Criminality*, Toronto: Harcourt Brace Jovanovich.

LOWMAN, J. (1992) 'Street prostitution', in V.F. SACCO (Ed.) *Deviance: Conformity and Control in Canada*, 2nd edn, Scarborough, Ontario: Prentice-Hall Canada.

MACDONALD, N.E., FISHER, W.A., WELLS, G.A., DOHERTY, J.A. and BOWIE, W.R. (1994) 'Canadian street youth: correlates of sexual risk-taking activity', *Pediatric Infectious Disease Journal*, **13**, 8, pp. 690–97.

MATHEWS, R.F. (1986) 'Mirror to the night: a psycho-social study of adolescent prostitution', unpublished PhD thesis, Department of Education, University of Toronto.

MILLSON, M., COATES, R., RANKIN, J., MYERS, T., MCLAUGHLIN, B., MAJOR, C. and MINDELL, W. (1991) 'The evaluation of a programme to prevent human immunodeviciency virus in injection drug users in Toronto', Final Report presented to the City of Toronto Board of Health, Toronto: University of Toronto, September.

MILLSON, P., MYERS, T., RANKIN, J., FEARON, M., MAJOR, C., and RIGBY, J. (1994) 'Drug injection and risk of HIV study update – Toronto', in LABORATORY CENTRE FOR DISEASE CONTROL (Ed.) *The Proceedings of the Meeting on HIV Infection Among Injection Drug Users in Canada*, Montreal, Quebec, 12–13, December, Ottawa: Health Canada.

MOYER, S. and CARRINGTON, P.J. (1989) *Street Prostitution: Assessing the Impact of the Law, Toronto*, Ottawa: Minister of Justice.

MYERS, T., GODIN, G., CALZAVARA, L., LAMBERT, J. and LOCKER, D. (1993) *Canadian Survey of Gay and Bisexual Men and HIV Infection: Men's Survey*, Ottawa: Canadian AIDS Society.

MYERS, T., ALLMAN, D., STRIKE, C., CALZAVARA, L., MILLSON, P., MAJOR, C., GRAYDON, M. and LEBLANC, M. (1997) 'Bisexual men and HIV in Ontario: sexual risk behaviour with men and with women', Sixth Annual Canadian Conference on HIV/AIDS Research Ottawa, May.

NAMASTE, K. (1995) *HIV/AIDS and Transgerder Communities in Canada: A Report on the Knowledge, Attitudes and Behaviour of Transgerdered People in Canada with Respect to HIV and AIDS*, Toronto: Lenderpress.

PARENT, R., NOEL, L., ALARY, M., CLAESSENS, C., MARQUIS, G., GAGNON, M., DESLAURIERS, D. and MARCOUX, N. (1994) 'Evaluation de la prevalence des infections au VIH et de certains comportements d'injection et sexuels chez les utilisateurs de drogues par injection frequentant le programme point de reperes', in LABORATORY CENTRE FOR DISEASE CONTROL (Ed.) *Proceedings of the Meeting on HIV Infection Among Injection Drug Users in Canada*, Montreal, Quebec, 12–13 December, Ottawa: Health Canada.

PEAT, MARWICK AND PARTNERS (1984) *A National Population Study of Prostitution and Pornography*, Ottawa: Department of Justice.

PROSTITUTES' SAFE SEX PROJECT (1991) *Prostitutes' Safe Sex Project, What Is It and How Does It Work*, Toronto: Prostitutes' Safe Sex Project.

READ. S., DEMATTEO, D., BOCK, B., COATES, R., GOLDBERG, E., KING, S., MAJOR, C., MCLAUGHLIN, B., MILLSON, M. and O'SHAUGHNESSY, M. (1993) *HIV Prevalence in Toronto Street Youth*, Toronto: The Hospital for Sick Children.

REKART, M. (1993) 'Trends in HIV seroprevalance among street-involved persons in Vancouver, Canada, 1988–1992', presentation at the IX International Conference on AIDS, Berlin, Germany, June.

REKART, M.L. and MANZON, L. (1989) *Knowledge, Attitudes and Behaviours of Street-Involved Persons in Vancouver*, Ottawa: National AIDS Clearinghouse, Canadian Public Health Association.

ROY, E., HALEY, N., BOIVIN, J.F., FRAPPIER, J.Y., CLAESSENS, C., LEMIRE, N., GAGNON, C., GAOUTTE, M., PAGE, V. and SAMUELSON, J. (1996) *HIV Infection Among Montreal Street Youth*, Montreal: Groupe de Recherche Sur les Juenes de la Rue et L infection au VIH.

SASFAÇON, D. (1985) *Prostitution in Canada, A Research Review Report*, Ottawa: Department of Justice.

SCOTT, V. (1988) 'The role of sex worker representative organisations', presentation at the First National Sex Industry Conference, 25–27 October, Melbourne, Australia.

SEX WORKER'S ALLIANCE OF VANCOUVER (1997) Interret site <http://www.walnet.org/csis/groups/swav/>.

SHAVER, F. (1993) 'Prostitution: a female crime?', in E. ADELBERG and C. CURRIE (Eds) *In Conflict With the Law: Women and the Canadian Justice System*, Vancouver: Press Gang Publishers.

SHAVER, F. (1994) 'The regulation of prostitution: avoiding the morality traps', *Canadian Journal of Law and Society*, **9**, 1, pp. 123–45.

SHAVER, F. (1996) 'Prostitution: on the dark side of the service industry', in T. O'REILLY-FLEMING (Ed.) *Post-Critical Criminology*, Scarborough: Prentice Hall Canada.

SHAVER, F.M. and NEWMEYER, T. (1996) 'Men who have sex with men: a comparison of the sexual practices and risk-taking behaviour of gay and bisexual men and male prostitutes', presentation at Sida, Jeunesse et Prevention. Au-dela du Discours, des Actions! Dans le Cadre du 64e congres de l'ACFAS. Université McGill à Montreal, 14–16 May.

STATISTICS CANADA (1997) *Street Prostitution in Canada*, Catalogue No. 85–002–XPE, 17, 2, Ottawa: Canadian Centre for Justice Statistics.

STELLA (1996) *Some Myths About Sex Work*, pamphlet, Montreal.

STREET OUTREACH SERVICES (1995) *Submission by Street Outreach Services (SOS) to the Board of Health*, Toronto: Street Outreach Services, 14 June.

TASK FORCE ON CHILDREN INVOLVED IN PROSTITUTION (1997) *Children Involved in Prostitution*, Alberta: Minister of Family and Social Services.

THE TORONTO PROSTITUTES COMMUNITY SERVICE PROJECT (1994) Maggie's, unpublished manuscript.

TORONTO STAR (1987) '23 arrested in sweep of homosexual prostitutes', 5 June.

TREMBLE, B. (1993) 'Prostitution and survival: interviews with gay street youth', *Canadian Journal of Human Sexuality*, **2**, 1, pp. 33–45.

VANCOUVER PROVINCE (1990) 'A Deadly Dilemma', October 5.

VANCOUVER SUN (1980) 'Chrétien Promises New Prostitution Law', 23 July.

VISANO, L. (1987) *This Idle Trade*, Concord: Visano Books.

VISANO, L. (1991) 'The impact of age on paid sexual encounters', *Journal of Homosexuality*, **20**, 3–4, pp. 207–26.

WONG, S.K.H. (1995) 'Needs assessment of Asian sex trade workers in Toronto, final report', Toronto: Asian Community AIDS Services.

Chapter 5

Social Environment and Male Sex Work in the United States

Edward V. Morse, Patricia M. Simon and Kendra E. Burchfiel

In little over a decade, medical science has advanced significantly in its ability to detect, treat, and in many cases sustain the lives of persons infected with human immunodeficiency virus (HIV). Similarly, public health educational efforts in Europe and North America have significantly increased public awareness and knowledge regarding infection and transmission. With the introduction of protease inhibitors, medical science cautiously embraces combination drug therapy, which is likely to result in positive treatment gains and increased survival for HIV infected individuals, some of whom will now have the opportunity to return to their previous lifestyles. Simultaneously, however, these same medical advances may have a latent negative consequence of restoring health to various HIV infected marginalized populations, who have not historically participated in HIV prevention and intervention efforts. Many of these individuals, left within their current uncompromising social environments, may continue to engage in health threatening HIV-related high risk sexual and drug use behaviour patterns in order to survive. In the United States, male street sex workers[1] are one such population. Studies of HIV seroprevalence among male sex workers in the United States report rates ranging from 17.5 per cent (Morse *et al.*, 1991) to 29.4 per cent (Elifson, Boles and Sweat, 1993), thus confirming their identity as a highly vulnerable group. With improved medical outcomes, it is now more important than ever to understand the HIV-related social risk behaviour and medical profiles of male sex workers and their customers, as well as the social contexts within which these behaviours occur. Utilizing this knowledge is critical to the design of effective prevention and intervention efforts aimed at arresting future HIV transmission.

Drawing on current and past research of male street sex worker culture in the United States, this chapter explores a wide range of psychological, behavioural, social and economic dimensions of male sex work in an effort to understand its public health implications. In order to appreciate the multifaceted issues, it is useful to first understand who is involved. In aggregate, any particular urban population of male sex workers might differ significantly by race, ethnicity and language spoken. However, few if any critical geographically based determinants specific to the sex worker's world have been found to be particularly predictive of or significant with respect to HIV transmission.

Thus, while the majority of material presented in this chapter draws extensively from data the authors gathered in the southern United States over the last decade, and that of other North American based research studies, it is expected that implications for HIV prevention, drawn from the behaviour patterns discussed, are generalizable.

In this chapter, attention focuses first on the sexual dimensions of the male sex worker or male street sex worker including sexual orientation, sexual acts performed, and safe sex practices. Second, male sex workers' patterns of substance use, including types and frequency of substances used, the trend towards polysubstance use, and the relationships among substance use, safe sex and mental health status are examined. Third, the economic dimensions of street sex work are described, including questions of easy money, unskilled work in an always open sex market, and the demand for services in terms of the number, frequency and types of tricks performed for money, drugs, or other items of economic value. Fourth, health issues specific to the workers themselves are examined including the prevalence of HIV and other STDs; knowledge of HIV transmission and prevention in general; and the intricate relationships between knowledge of disease risk, risk taking, perceptions of risk specific to the hustling situation, and polysubstance use. Finally, attention is focused on possible policy implications.

We will begin, however, by first defining what is meant by the term male street sex worker, or in more common parlance a male prostitute, or male hustler. Excluding minor variation and elaboration, a male street sex worker is defined as an individual who walks the streets and open landscapes of urban areas for the purposes of establishing contact with other men who wish to engage in a diversity of sexually defined acts in exchange for money, drugs, and/or other items of monetary value. A number of researchers have attempted to construct behavioural matrixes in order to present a typology of male sex workers that might facilitate understanding of the differential complexities of their occupation (Caulkins and Coombs, 1976; Fisher, Weisberg and Marotta, 1982; Gandy, 1971; Pieper, 1979; Raven, 1960; Ross, 1959). However, over the past decade we have found little to be gained by trying to fit aberrant behaviour patterns into inflexible boxes. Collective observations of street life, as well as hundreds of hours of personal interviews with male sex workers across the country, indicate that although some male sex workers hustle on the street (street hustler), some in a bar (bar hustler or dancer), some are kept by a single individual for a period of time (kept boy), and some work for an escort service (call boy), male sex workers move across all of these categories, occupying one or several during any given period of time (Morse *et al.*, 1991).

In the United States, and in the settings we have investigated in Louisiana, the only factors determining the particular role set the sex worker takes on at any one moment appear to be the amount of money in his pockets and where he happens to be standing. All other nuances of the sex worker's role set are more or less coincidental. The major reasons for a sex worker to be in one physical location rather than another are usually based on weather conditions, the distribution of potential customers cruising at the particular moment, the ability to remain anonymous and out of the way of proprietors and property owners, or the need to escape the grasp of law enforcement officers who would rather shake the sex workers down than arrest them. Many call boys, kept boys, and massage parlour workers are likely, at one time or another in the past, to have worked as street hustlers (Luckenbill, 1986; Morse *et al.*, 1991).

The clandestine nature of the environment in which the male sex worker lives and works has made it difficult to gain access, to systematically study, and to gather the data necessary to design effective health intervention programmes. Although ethnographic descriptions of the male sex workers' world dominate the literature (Raven, 1960; Reiss, 1964; Weisberg, 1985), few North American studies have used rigorous methods to examine the relationship between male sex work and the prevalence of STDs, in this case HIV/AIDS. The authors have melded a variety of ethnographic and interviewing strategies into a set of successful field techniques to contact, interview and take blood samples from hundreds of male sex workers and their customers (Morse *et al.*, 1991; Morse and Simon, 1994). Most of the data cited in this chapter were derived from the authors' study of 211 male street sex workers and their customers surveyed in New Orleans, Louisiana between 1988 and 1993. These data, in combination with observations drawn from major urban areas across North America, provide the detail necessary not only to gain a better understanding of who may be involved in sex work, but also to more clearly describe the prevalence of HIV in the population as well as the social context within which HIV-related prevention and intervention efforts need to take place. The first question to ask is, Who enters the occupation of male street sex worker?

Socio-demographics

The male street sex workers the authors have observed in urban areas including the East Coast, the Deep South, and the West Coast, as well as those reported on in the literature, all possess a very similar socio-demographic profile (Butts, 1947; Churchill, 1967; Cory and LeRoy, 1963; Elifson, Boles and Sweat, 1993; Ginsburg, 1967; McNamara, 1965; Morse *et al.*, 1991; Raven, 1960; Reiss, 1964; Russell, 1971). The vast majority of persons in this occupation are relatively young. A comparison of field observation notes, data from face-to-face interviews, and the general literature suggests that most male sex workers are between the ages of 18 and 40, and have been selling sex for an average of eight years. However, the existence of two other age cohorts with relatively significant presence in the street are both surprising and problematic in terms of the challenges they pose for public health intervention. It seems that there is still room in the street for the few older sex workers whose ages extend well into the late fifties and early sixties. These 'long-term survivors', many of whom may have been sex workers for over 20 years, are consistently the least open to health messages, and by far the most reticent to become involved with any outreach efforts that appear to be health-related. Of even greater concern, however, are the very young male sex workers, variously called *chickens* if they are teenagers or *pin feathers* if they are even younger. This cohort ranges in age from six to about 16. At the upper end of the age range, they may present themselves as street-wise and tough. Interestingly, they are also some of the most eager to learn about the availability of free health services. At the other end of the age range are the very young children, all of whom report that they sell sex in the streets not only with their parent's knowledge and consent, but that they provide expected sources of family income.

While on the one hand the youngest are far less recalcitrant than their more elderly counterparts, their family's economic dependency on their monetary earnings derived from sex work, make them equally difficult to reach with preventive health care messages. This is especially the case with HIV, where the messages being transmitted directly encourage altering or refraining from participation in sexual behaviours their customers may seek. The specific social environment and needs of *pin feathers* are critical to address for both ethical and programmatic reasons. Removing young male sex workers from the streets can only come about by working with children and families to help them explore alternate means of coping with economic deprivation. In addition, municipalities must be encouraged to enforce existing child abuse statutes and other local ordinances. These two efforts are important ways of preventing young male sex workers from acquiring HIV.

The racial/ethnic composition of the urban male sex worker population tends to mirror that of the particular urban area in which they are working. However, the racial/ethnic composition of the male sex workers' customers tends to be predominately white and of all social classes (Morse *et al.*, 1991). Although white customers tend to use the services of white male sex workers, black customers, who also come from all levels of society, tend to hire both black and white sex workers in almost equal proportions.

Contrary to what one might imagine, many male sex workers are relatively well educated. Over one-third of the male sex workers we have interviewed have earned either a High School Diploma or a General Equivalency Diploma. In fact, many complete their education while imprisoned for violating the local ordinance against prostitution. A number of them have enrolled in trade school programmes or taken college courses, though most male sex workers typically report leaving trade school before completing even the shortest of programmes. Almost all the male sex workers we have encountered are able to read, and in fact are well informed about their socio-political environment. Many report reading a newspaper, magazines and books on a regular basis. Reading and going to the movies are two ways street sex workers deal with boredom and loneliness. Sex workers' facility at reading and attention to their social environment are likely to account in part for their accurate AIDS knowledge. On the other hand, for reasons to be explained shortly, little if any of this HIV-related high risk behaviour modification information is ever integrated into their sexual behaviour practices. In addition to the age, race and educational distribution of the sex workers, their social class background is important to keep in mind when developing public health policy.

Anticipating and understanding interaction patterns are greatly facilitated by knowing a person's social class background. The father's occupation was used as a crude indicator of the social class of the 211 male sex workers interviewed by the authors. Among these male sex workers, just over one-third (34.6 per cent) had fathers who worked as unskilled labourers and more than 50 per cent identified their fathers as working in relatively higher status positions: 25.1 per cent skilled workers, 10 per cent professionals, 11.8 per cent business or managerial positions and 6.2 per cent in the armed services. For 12 per cent of the sex workers, it could be reasonably surmised that the social class of their families was extremely low or that they had been estranged long enough from their families so as not to know their father's occupation: 2.4 per cent had fathers who worked in illegal occupations (for example drug pushers, car thieves, gamblers), 2.4 per cent reported their fathers had never worked, and 7.6 per cent stated they had never known their fathers.

Problems were to be noted in the family backgrounds of many male sex workers. Over 40 per cent of the male sex workers interviewed stated that they had left home by age 16. Of those leaving home before age 16, 60 per cent indicated that domestic violence or trouble with the law had been their primary reason for leaving. A history of physical and sexual abuse is commonly cited in studies of male sex workers (Caulkins and Coombs, 1976; Craft, 1966, 1968; Elifson *et al.*, 1993; Morse *et al.*, 1991). The public policy implications of this trend in the data are quite harsh. The data suggest that in most instances, the sex workers' families cannot be engaged as a source of social or economic support while attempting by programmatic means, such as job training, to rehabilitate sex workers.

In terms of HIV health policy, the key question has less to do with sex workers' family than with the living arrangements they later construct for themselves, some of which tend to reflect earlier arrangements. We have found that a substantial number of sex workers, finding it difficult to sustain long-term relationships, end up living alone (51 per cent) (Simon *et al.*, 1992). On the other hand, 7.1 per cent lived with parent(s) and more than 40 per cent lived with a friend, wife or girlfriend. Most reported having never married (70 per cent), while 24 per cent indicated that they were divorced or separated. Forty-two per cent reported knowingly having fathered at least one child. Of those in relationships with women, the vast majority of the latter were themselves sex workers, some of whom often shared their customers with their personal partners. Relationships were often transitory and psychologically if not physically abusive on the part of both partners, and frequently were established for economic convenience, protection, or as a way to consolidate access to a regular supply of illicit drugs. Overall, it was clear that the disorganized family background into which many sex workers were originally socialized was mirrored in later ways of accommodating life's immediate demands.

Most male sex workers report having a social network of six to seven friends, 90 per cent of whom sell sex themselves. Overall, and on the basis of our work, male street workers in the United States tend to live in marginalized social environments which only exacerbate their previously socially reinforced tendencies to seek out a pleasure-oriented existence surrounded by peers who support and encourage engagement in risk-taking behaviour. In terms of socio-demographics in general, the male street sex worker is likely to be young, socialized in a violent home environment, well enough educated to function in our society, but for a variety of reasons he exhibits a strong propensity to seek out short-term, easy solutions to problems through the sale of sex and through substance use. We turn next to various dimensions of sex worker lifestyle as they might be relevant to shaping more effective HIV-related health policy. The most practical place to begin is with the male sex worker's sexual orientation.

Sexual Orientation

Conceptually, sexual orientation can become rather problematic when applied to a sample of practising male street sex workers. Obviously all of them by their role definition when working, have sex with men and thus would be labelled homosexual based on their sexual behaviour practices. Using behaviour as a basis for defining sexual orientation, even if defensible, leads to much confusion when attempting to interpret the concordance or discrepancy between self-image and the tendency to have sex with other men. A more useful distinction regarding sexual orientation can be made by simply defining orientation according to the sex worker's own self-identification. Thinking of sexual orientation in this fashion, we have found that approximately 40 per cent of male sex workers identify themselves as heterosexual, 40 per cent identify themselves as bisexual, while only 20 per cent consider themselves to be exclusively homosexual. Noteworthy is the fact that nearly 80 per cent of male sex workers report engaging in sexual activity with men and/or women. However, for the male street sex worker, sexual contacts with women are almost wholly limited to contexts outside of work. This fact does not diminish the need to design public health policies that address the differing health needs of both male and female partners.

Male sex workers' sexual orientation has also been found to be significantly associated with levels of HIV infection (Elifson, Boles and Sweat, 1993; Morse *et al.*, 1991; Simon *et al.*, 1994). In US studies, those who identify themselves as homosexual are more likely to be HIV seropositive than those who identify themselves as bisexual or heterosexual. Of the 211 male sex workers we interviewed, 33.3 per cent of those who identified themselves as homosexual were HIV positive. In comparison, 20.7 per cent of those who identified themselves as bisexual were HIV positive, while only 6.1 per cent of those who identified themselves as heterosexual were HIV positive.

The data discussed in the following section suggest that heterosexual male sex workers are at lower HIV risk because they are less likely to engage in those sexual behaviours believed to place them at greatest risk for HIV infection. On the other hand, while the heterosexual male sex worker is at lower risk for contracting HIV, once infected, he is more likely to transmit to other heterosexuals through his female partners (Morse *et al.*, 1991). To be effective, HIV prevention and intervention programmes for male sex workers must be designed so as to take into consideration the sexual orientation of the sex workers and their differential proclivities to willingly participate in risky sexual acts. What, then, are the sexual acts that the male sex workers participate in with their customers?

Sexual Activities

As a group, male sex workers, because of the very nature of the work their occupation entails, tend to be exposed to a wide variety of HIV-related sexual risk behaviours. The range of sexual activities offered for sale and the role played in these activities are in large part shaped by sexual orientation. For instance, sex workers who identify themselves as homosexual are more likely to be the receptive partner during anal sex than those who identify themselves as heterosexual or bisexual, and are thus at greater risk for contracting HIV. More specifically, in our study, the data revealed that 78.7 per cent of male street workers identifying themselves as homosexual reported being the receptive partner during anal sex. In comparison, only 11 per cent of self-identified heterosexual and 36.8 per cent of self-identified bisexual male street sex workers reported this to be the case.

The data also reflected similar tendencies towards participating in other high risk sexual acts on the part of those who self-identify as homosexual. In a general sense, self-identified homosexual sex workers were more likely to report engaging in internal water sports, fisting, faeces play (scat), and rimming. Contact with body fluids may result in HIV transmission. Male sex workers who self-identified as homosexual were also more likely to report gaining sexual pleasure and general enjoyment from engaging in sex with customers. Similarly, those who reported enjoying sex while hustling were also more likely to engage in high risk sexual acts. When considered within the context of developing health care policy, the sexual acts a sex worker offers to his customers and the pleasure he derives from engaging in these acts are likely to be neither mutable nor easy to control within the confines of the law. On the other hand, health policies written in this area can be far more effective if they focus on understanding why some male sex workers do not employ safer sex techniques while practising their trade.

Edward V. Morse, Patricia M. Simon and Kendra E. Burchfiel

Safe Sex

When we asked male sex workers and their customers to indicate on a three-point scale (never, sometimes, always) the frequency with which they used condoms while hustling or engaging a male sex worker, only 19.9 per cent of sex workers and 10.4 per cent of customers reported always using condoms. Of those sex workers who engaged in high risk sexual activities such as receptive anal sex, the majority (75.8 per cent) reported using condoms infrequently or never. According to the sex workers, the majority of customers (54.7 per cent) seldom or never used condoms when engaging in anal sex. Of serious concern is the fact that sex workers suggested that few customers ever requested that the sex worker wear a condom. In fact, only 3.8 per cent of the male sex workers reported that customers always asked them to wear a condom. Equally telling are data gathered from customers confirming that safer sex is neither requested nor practised. Two-thirds of the customers sampled stated emphatically that they would cancel a sexual transaction and seek out another male sex worker if the latter demanded that a condom be worn (Morse *et al.*, 1992a).

Curiously, although sex workers and customers report rarely using condoms, our data indicated that condoms were readily available in the hustling situation (Simon *et al.*, 1993). In fact, the number of male sex workers who carry condoms while they are hustling was relatively normally distributed. When interviewed, 46.4 per cent of the male sex workers reported that they never or seldom carry condoms while hustling, 9.5 per cent carry them about half the time, and 44 per cent carry them very frequently or always. Approximately half of the male sex workers were likely to carry condoms a majority of the time they were working. Although the data indicated that condoms were present during about half of the hustling transactions, they also show that condoms are not being used.

Frequency of condom use in other groups has been shown to be a protective factor for HIV transmission, yet no similar trend was found within the male sex workers population (Simon *et al.*, 1993). No significant differences were found in HIV seroprevalence rates between those sex workers reporting consistent condom use during anal sex and those reporting that they never used condoms. That male sex worker condom use was not significantly related to HIV serostatus appears to arise from a variety of interrelated factors, each with important policy implications. First, the majority of the sex workers sampled reported that neither themselves nor their customers wore condoms even if they had them. Second, belief in the efficacy of condoms to protect them from disease was positively related to their engagement in HIV-related risk behaviour. The male sex workers who indicated that use of condoms would protect them from contracting HIV were also the same men who were more likely to engage in anal sex (Simon *et al.*, 1993).

The male sex workers' reasons for not carrying condoms shed light on potential barriers to engagement in safer sex practices. In addition to the usual complaints about fit, comfort and reliability of condoms, most of the male sex workers interviewed stated two main reasons for not carrying condoms while out hustling. First, many sex workers told of altercations with the police when they were found to have pockets full of condoms. According to the sex workers, the police used the presence of condoms as evidence of the sex workers' occupation. Many male sex workers felt that carrying condoms contributed to the likelihood of their arrest. Second, they perceived that carrying condoms could have a negative effect on their trade. Male sex workers reported being concerned that carrying condoms would be an indication to customers that the sex worker was either HIV infected or infected with some other STD. The sex workers' belief that carrying condoms restrains trade and contributes to arrest indicates that no simple educational programme targeting sex workers is likely to have significant impact in terms of enhancing safer sex practices. Yet, the data strongly suggest that interventions might well be effective if aimed at encouraging safer sex practices on the part of customers.

Finally, of no less importance in regard to condom use and the transmission of HIV is the inconsistent use of condoms or other barrier methods of disease protection with female partners outside the work environment. Of the male street prostitutes identifying themselves as heterosexual or bisexual, 42.3 per cent reported having a steady female partner (a wife, married or common-law, and/or a girlfriend). Seventy-four per cent of these men reported consciously choosing never to wear a condom during sexual intercourse with their female partners. In addition, none of the male sex workers ever wore a glove or used a dam during sexual activities with their female partners. This information, coupled with the fact that 40 per cent of these wives and girlfriends were themselves sex workers, suggests that there is a risk of HIV transmission from male to female sex workers, and hence to the clients of the latter.

In terms of employment of safer sex practices, and specifically condom use, most male sex workers interviewed by the authors felt that they had no real power or control over the hustling situation. Without this control, they felt they had no influence over the practice of safe sex while they were working. The male sex workers who reported that they were in control of the hustling situation were more likely to engage in HIV risk reduction behaviour, such as safe sex, than those who reported that they were not in control. Sex workers' perceptions of lack of control while hustling sex is an important barrier to HIV risk reduction, which should be kept in mind when developing health care policy. Perceptions of lack of control over the hustling situation are also influenced by the sex workers' heavy reliance on alcohol and drugs, as well as their economic dependence on hustling sex, which in turn contributes to their participation in risk related sexual activity.

The Male Sex Worker as a Polysubstance User

Substance use by male sex workers interviewed was almost universal. Over 95 per cent of those interviewed reported at least weekly use of alcohol and/or other drugs. The data also indicated that polysubstance use by male sex workers was normative. Seventy-nine per cent of male sex workers reported using two different substances at least twice a week. Additionally, 48.8 per cent used three or more different substances twice a week or more. Many male sex workers engaged in daily polysubstance use: 43 per cent used two different substances daily and 16 per cent used three or more substances daily (Morse *et al.*, 1992b).

Substance use while directly engaging in sex work was also found to be common. Over 68 per cent reported that they were usually high on drugs or alcohol while hustling. Only 15 per cent stated that they were never high on drugs or alcohol while they engaged in sex work (Simon *et al.*, 1993). It may be surmised, then, that impaired decision making characterized by substance use during sex work is likely to be a major deterrent to safer sex and thus places the male sex worker and his customer at increased risk.

Alcohol, marijuana and crack/cocaine by themselves or in combination are the substances that nearly all (98.1 per cent) male sex workers chose to use (Morse *et al.*, 1992b). Less than 15 per cent reported frequently using other substances such as stimulants, inhalants, sedatives, heroin and hallucinogens. The researchers had no trouble locating and interviewing over 100 male sex workers who were also injecting drug users. Both the quantity and frequency of substance use, as well as whether the male sex worker was high while working, were significantly associated with injecting drug use. Those who were frequent polysubstance users and often high while hustling sex were more likely to be injecting drug users (Morse *et al.*, 1992b). Among the injecting drug using sex workers, a little more than half (56 per cent) shared needles and 28 per cent injected and shared needles with their customers. Besides type of substance used and route of administration, a critically significant dimension of sex workers' substance use is its relationship to engagement in HIV-related sexual risk behaviour.

Although the frequency with which a sex worker engaged in substance use while actually working was associated with increased engagement in high risk behaviour, a significant inverse relationship was found between the frequency and quantity of substance use in general, and engagement in HIV-related sexual risk behaviour. Contrary to predictions that substance use would cause disinhibition and thus increase risk behaviour, the authors found that frequent use of several substances actually served as a protective factor for engagement in high risk sexual behaviour. Instead of enhancing desire, it is possible that frequent substance use interferes with a sex worker's ability to work by causing disinterest in sexual activities and sex work. This finding has positive implications for programmatic intervention, in that those male sex workers who are most likely to engage in high risk sexual behaviour are also those who are less likely to be frequent polysubstance users and, therefore, to be more open or reachable for prevention efforts. The relationship between substance use and psychological state among male sex workers also has implications for the design of intervention programmes.

Polysubstance use was found to be associated with the male sex worker's psychological distress, his feelings about homosexuality, and his self-identified sexual orientation. Increased hostility, one element of psychological distress, was significantly associated with increased substance use. In addition, Simon *et al.* (1992) found a cluster of psychological dimensions of distress, as measured by various sub-scales of the SCL90-R, that were significantly associated with the use of substances while hustling sex. These dimensions were obsessive-compulsivity, interpersonal sensitivity (feelings of personal inadequacy and inferiority), depression and anxiety.

The relationship between having negative feelings about homosexuality and being high while hustling sex approached statistical significance. Further, the self-identified sexual orientation of sex workers was found to be relevant to both overall substance use and substance use while hustling sex, though not statistically significant. Heterosexual male sex workers were more likely to use alcohol and other drugs more frequently, and in greater quantities in general and while hustling sex, than bisexual or homosexual male sex workers. The authors contend that substance use may be a type of self-medication which enables male sex workers to cope with the psychological difficulties and dangers associated with sex work (Morse *et al.*, 1992b). Seemingly, to practise the trade, some sex workers have to have drugs, and to have drugs they must sell sex.

Substances are often obtained using the income from sex work or are given as payment from customers to workers for sexual activities. Although the direction of a causal relationship between substance use and sex work is not likely to be determined, it is clear that substance use and sex work are strongly associated. Substance use may encourage men to sell sex or the sexual activities involved in sex work may drive male sex workers to substance use; either way, both issues must be addressed simultaneously in any intervention programme targeting male sex workers. Drug use also frames the next important policy determinant to explore, the economics of sex work.

Sex for Sale

In our data, a sex worker's economic dependence on sex work is all too often intertwined with substance use or polysubstance use. Approximately 64 per cent of the male sex workers surveyed, depended on sex work for all or most of their expenses, and an additional 26 per cent depended on it for at least half of their expenses. Only 10 per cent reported that they depend on sex work for very little of their expenses. Being economically dependent on sex work was also significantly correlated with spending discretionary income (that which is not spent on food and rent) on alcohol and other substances, in some cases to the exclusion of all other items. In addition, 45 per cent stated that they had accepted drugs or alcohol as direct payment for sexual services.

In the United States, the aspects of male sex work we have looked at cultivate a work environment which not only tolerates, but also encourages and facilitates substance use professionally and socially. As long as illicit drugs remain continuously accessible in most urban American communities, sex work will flourish, and so too will the spread of HIV. As one male street sex worker quipped, 'Even while high on drugs, a man can make easy money as a prostitute.'

Sex Work Delivers Easy Money

The occupation of sex work, unlike many others, is open to men possessing few formally certified skills, many addictions and extensive criminal records. In short, sex workers face few job-related constraints. As long as an activity or characteristic of the sex worker does not interfere with his sexual functioning, it will not interfere with his work or the ability to make money. In fact, the male street workers interviewed overwhelmingly stated that *easy money* is the reason they have chosen the profession.

Even though over one-third (39.3 per cent) of the male sex workers we contacted had earned a High School Diploma or a General Equivalency Diploma, most lacked marketable job skills. Almost all have extensive criminal records and a history of substance use. Given these constraints, the job opportunities for male sex workers outside of sex work are typically low-paying menial jobs and of short duration. In comparison, sex work is a much more lucrative option. The majority (85 per cent) of the sex workers we interviewed, report receiving between $20 and $50 per trick, averaging about $35 for 15 minutes of work. Considering other job options, it is no wonder almost one-half (47.4 per cent) of the sex workers reported themselves to be full-time sex workers. The remaining sex workers supplemented their sex work income by working as unskilled labourers or by engaging in other illegal ventures such as selling drugs and stealing. For men with heavy substance needs and few work skills, sex work is hard to pass up, if for no other reason than economics.

Unfortunately, the economic value of sex work in the United States serves as a strong barrier both to leaving the profession and to HIV risk reduction. This relationship is demonstrated by the direct connection between increased risk taking behaviour by the male sex workers and their increased economic dependence on hustling sex. The more dependent male sex workers were on sex work for their basic sustenance, the more likely they were to engage in high risk sex. Without job retraining and job opportunities tailored specifically to this very marginalized population, little progress can be made to reduce engagement in sex work and, thus, the prevalence of HIV and other STDs.

The Prevalence of HIV

There are few published studies employing antibody testing that report the prevalence of HIV among male sex workers in the United States, yet those that do exist clearly demonstrate the magnitude of the health problems. One study conducted in Atlanta, Georgia found a seroprevalence rate of 29.4 per cent among a sample of 235 male street sex workers (Elifson, Boles and Sweat, 1993). The HIV seroprevalence rate found in the authors' Louisiana sample of 211 male sex workers was 17.5 per cent or 175 per 1000 (Morse *et al.*, 1991). When compared with the rate among female sex workers reported by the Centers for Disease Control (12 per cent or 120 per 1000), the rate for males is notably higher (CDC, 1987).

In the authors' Louisiana study, no statistically significant differences between race (black versus white), injecting drug use patterns (injectors versus non-injectors), or age (younger than 25 versus older than 25) were found among the HIV seroprevalence rates of the male sex workers. However, when age, race and injecting status are considered in combination a very different picture of prevalence appears. Seroprevalence rates range from a high of 25 per cent for young black injecting drug users and older white injecting drug users, to a low of 8 per cent for older black non-injecting drug users. In addition, the presence of other STDs in the sample was very high. Of the male sex workers interviewed, 41.7 per cent reported a history of gonorrhoea, 18.5 per cent of syphilis, and 14.2 per cent of hepatitis. Laboratory confirmation of syphilis in this sample found 22.5 per cent of the male sex workers positive for syphilis, while 7.7 per cent of the total sample was both syphilis and HIV positive.

Several simple calculations based on the male sex workers' reported frequency of commercial sex illustrate the potential impact of their potential to spread HIV. The 211 male street sex workers interviewed sold more than 164 000 sexual acts per year. More importantly, the 37 HIV infected sex workers in the sample reported an estimated 30 992 infected sexual contacts per year, amounting to approximately 2.3 tricks per day per male sex worker. Because few encounters employed safer sex practices, most of these contacts could potentially result in HIV transmission. When one realizes these figures represent the number of infectious acts performed in only one American city, the need for radical health policy intervention is clear. While the need is clear, the nature of what programmatic course to follow is murkier.

Male Sex Workers' Knowledge of HIV and Perception of Risk

By far the most familiar forms of health intervention are those that call for mass distribution of health information and education to target populations. Traditional thought dictates that increased knowledge of a particular health condition positively affects attitudes and practices that will reduce risk and move targeted groups towards health. This so-called knowledge, attitudes, and practices model (KAP) forms the basis of many risk reduction efforts. By the 1990s, however, it is clear that programmatic interventions based on this model produce few behavioural changes. The relationship between male sex workers' fund of HIV-related knowledge and their high risk sexual practices is illustrative of the failure of the KAP model. Male sex workers' general fund of knowledge regarding prevention and transmission of HIV is very high. Of the 211 male sex workers interviewed, 96 per cent received a perfect score on an HIV knowledge inventory. Similarly, the male sex workers overwhelmingly perceived HIV/AIDS as a very serious disease (94 per cent think HIV is serious), and 94 per cent perceived themselves as having a greater than 50 per cent chance of contracting HIV. Most important, however, is the fact that perceptions of increased severity, personal susceptibility and knowledge of prevention and transmission of HIV do not deter the male sex worker from engaging in high risk sexual behaviour associated with contracting HIV. In addition, neither age, education, race, nor number of years as a sex worker were significantly associated with engagement in HIV-related risk behaviours (as defined by engagement in unprotected anal sex). It is, therefore, possible that the male sex worker feels that he is already infected and needs no protection, or although he sees himself as potentially susceptible to HIV, he may feel that he will be lucky and escape infection (that is, optimistic bias or denial). Feelings of invulnerability or pessimism about contracting HIV, coupled with the strong economic pull of sex work, make these kinds of preventive interventions very difficult. The key questions then are, what are the significant barriers to HIV prevention in this population, and how can public health policy be utilized to overcome these barriers.

The authors have identified four major barriers to male sex workers' risk reduction. Male sex workers who engaged in HIV-related high risk sexual behaviours were more economically dependent on sex work for basic survival, perceived themselves to have less control over the hustling situation, felt increased pleasure from sexual activity with customers, and reported frequent substance use while directly engaged in sex work (Simon *et al.*, 1993).

Implications of the Sex Workers' Knowledge and Perceptions on Health Policy

What are the implications of these data trends for HIV prevention and intervention health policy? It should be clear from the preceding discussion that education programmes aimed at increasing male sex workers' knowledge of HIV prevention and transmission are not sufficient, in and of themselves, to result in any serious reduction of HIV-related risk behaviour. Equally poignant to note, is that education designed to instill fear of HIV/AIDS by stressing the seriousness of these conditions is not necessary, as virtually all male sex workers already view HIV/AIDS as a very serious health condition.

Simply sensitizing male sex workers to their vulnerability to HIV may only serve to increase HIV-related risk taking. The data suggest that although male sex workers may be able accurately to assess their increased vulnerability to HIV infection, feeling there is nothing to lose, they do not protect themselves by employing risk reduction practices. Whether male sex workers are overly optimistic, in denial, face social and economic barriers they feel powerless to overcome, or are simply so pessimistic that they assume risk reduction is not necessary because they are already infected, is a research question of extreme importance that should be addressed. It is critical to examine the social and psychological factors affecting male sex workers' perceived susceptibility to HIV and their risk taking behaviour in order to design more effective prevention programmes.

As previously discussed, those male sex workers who perceive condoms as being beneficial in protecting them against HIV infection are more likely to engage in HIV-related risk behaviour. This finding further demonstrates that educational programmes about the effectiveness of condoms, intending to create a safer environment for sexual activity while imparting knowledge, cannot insure that male sex workers will wear condoms during risky sexual activities. The reluctance of sex workers who recognized the potential benefits of condoms to actually use them is probably due to competing constraints, as many customers indicated that they would cancel the transaction if the sex worker insisted that a condom be worn. Therefore, intervention aimed at increasing condom use must target both sex worker and customer. Sex workers can be taught techniques that will help them eroticize the use of condoms and thus possibly make them more appealing to customers. On the other hand, because customers have the economic power to determine the conditions under which sex will occur, it is the customer who needs to be the prime target of prevention and safe sex intervention efforts.

The fact that many male sex workers derive enjoyment and sexual pleasure from sex work is a very difficult perception to mediate or significantly alter. Under closer examination, gaining sexual pleasure and enjoying sex work have at least two serious negative consequences. First, the degree to which the male sex worker enjoys his work is directly proportional to the frequency with which he engages in sex work. Second, increased enjoyment is directly related to engaging in high risk sexual acts such as receptive anal intercourse. Programmatic attempts to encourage the employment of safer sex techniques must find ways of reframing the use of condoms from negative perceptions to more erotic and pleasurable ones. A 'harm reduction' methodology that focuses on gradual use of safer sex techniques rather than an 'all or nothing' approach can slowly introduce sex workers to the enjoyment of safer sex.

Substance Use Treatment and Needle Exchange

Any programme of HIV prevention or intervention involving male sex workers such as those we interviewed must take into consideration the strong relationship between substance use and sex work. Substance use programmatic intervention efforts coupled with programmes encouraging the employment of safer sex techniques will best serve not only the needs of male sex workers and their customers, but also potentially reduce the spread of HIV to the larger society. Three types of substance use treatment programmes need to be made available to male sex workers: needle exchange and other 'harm reduction' programmes, abstinence-based programmes, and dual diagnosis programmes that can respond to both mental health issues and substance use.

For male sex workers who use injecting drugs and cannot or do not access abstinence-based substance use treatment, the employment of harm reduction methods such as needle exchanges and distribution of bleach kits will assist HIV prevention efforts. Better yet, is the hope that additional states in the United States will pass legislation allowing needles to be purchased at pharmacies without prescriptions. The fact that only about one-half of male sex workers residing in Louisiana (where there is no restriction on syringe purchases) reported needle sharing, suggests that availability of syringes through open access may reduce the likelihood that needle sharing will occur.

All too often abstinence-based substance use and chemical dependency treatment programmes are not designed for, or sensitive to, the lifestyles of male sex workers. Yet, substance use treatment programmes that address the needs of this population without invoking additional stigma on them must be made a priority if any real inroads are to be made in HIV risk reduction.

Finally, the positive correlation between male sex workers' substance use and the presence of identifiable psychological symptoms strongly suggests that any efforts to reduce risk behaviour and substance use must also address mental health problems. If, as the authors surmise, male sex workers use substances as a way of self-medicating in response to psychological distress, before this band-aid is removed, psychological concerns will need to be explored and addressed. Failure to provide dual diagnosis treatment programmes combining substance use treatment with mental health treatment will seriously retard HIV risk reduction efforts and may even render intervention programmes ineffective. As one might suspect, substance use treatment programming for male sex workers might be significantly more successful if it incorporated or was linked to a job training environment.

The evidence presented in this chapter clearly demonstrates that there is a strong economic motivation for sex work. Lack of job skills, a criminal record and poor education typically result in job opportunities that are low paying and of short duration. The minimum wage cannot compete with the *easy money* of sex work. Providing the male sex worker with job training and placement programmes is the only realistic way to compete with the economic motivation for engaging in HIV-related risk behaviour.

Interventions with Customers

Finally, it is important to remember that the customers of male sex workers, because of their economic power over the worker, are a major factor affecting risk reduction. Because the customer of the male sex worker has the balance of control over the hustling situation, it is logical to suggest that customers could, if they wanted, demand and receive safer sexual encounters. While accessing groups of customers who employ sex workers may be thought to be difficult, in fact in our own research, contact with customers was found to be relatively easy if done in a confidential and relatively clandestine way (Morse *et al.*, 1992a). Where contact can be made, programmatic interventions can be built. Ideally, then, intervention programmes aimed at strengthening the customers' bargaining power during the purchase of sex should serve to reduce HIV-related risk for both sex worker and customer.

Programmatic efforts aimed at the reduction of HIV-related risk behaviours among male sex workers must be multi-modal if they are to be effective. The balance between the perceived benefits to sex work and the benefits to HIV risk reduction must be tilted in favour of HIV prevention. Intervention programmes and public policy that simultaneously target the psychological, economic and substance use needs of the male sex worker are essential to the success of any risk reduction programme.

Acknowledgement

Funding for this work was provided in part by CDC Cooperative Agreement U64/CCU613329–01.

Note

1 In this chapter, the terms 'male sex worker', 'male prostitute' and 'hustler' are used interchangeably.

References

BUTTS, W.M. (1947) 'Boy prostitutes of the metropolis', *Journal of Clinical Psychopathology*, **8**, pp. 673–81.

CAULKINS, S.E. and COOMBS, N.R. (1976) 'The psychodynamics of male prostitution', *American Journal of Psychotherapy*, **30**, pp. 441–51.

CENTERS FOR DISEASE CONTROL AND PREVENTION (CDC) (1987) 'Antibody to human immunodeficiency virus in female prostitutes, *Morbidity and Mortality Weekly Report*, **36**, pp. 157–61.

CHURCHILL, W. (1967) *Homosexual Behavior Among Males: A Cross-Cultural and Cross-Species Investigation*, New York: Hawthorn Books.

CORY, D.W., LEROY, J.P. (1963) *The Homosexual and His Society: A View From Within*, New York: Citadel Books.

CRAFT, M. (1966) 'Boy prostitutes and their fate', *British Journal of Psychiatry*, **112**, pp. 1111–14.

CRAFT, M. (1968) 'Law, practice, and results among a group of boy prostitutes', presentation at the annual meeting of the American Psychological Association.

ELIFSON, K.W., BOLES, J. and SWEAT, M. (1993) 'Risk factors associated with HIV infection among male prostitutes', *American Journal of Public Health*, **83**, pp. 79–83.

FISHER, B., WEISBERG, D.K. and MAROTTA, T. (1982) *Adolescent Male Prostitution*, San Francisco: Urban and Rural Systems Associates.

GANDY, P. (1971) 'The prostitute: developing a deviant identity', in J.M. HENSLIN (Ed.) *Studies in the Sociology of Sex*, New York: Appleton-Century-Crofts.

GINSBERG, K.N. (1967) 'The "meat-rack": a study of the male prostitute', *American Journal of Psychotherapy*, **21**, pp. 170–85.

LUCKENBILL, D.F. (1986) 'Deviant career mobility: the case of male prostitutes', *Social Problems*, **33**, pp. 283–96.

McNAMARA, D.E.J. (1965) 'Male prostitution in American cities: a socio-economic or pathological phenomenon?', *American Journal of Orthopsychiatry*, **35**, p. 204.

MORSE, E.V. and SIMON, P.M. (1994) 'Resolving the hustle: the first step to an ethnographic study of clandestine street sex behavior patterns', *NIDA Monograph*, pp. 411–16.

MORSE, E.V., SIMON, P.M., OSOFSKY, H.J., BALSON, P.M. and GAUMER, H.R. (1991) 'The male street prostitute: a vector for transmission of HIV infection into the heterosexual world', *Social Science and Medicine*, **32**, pp. 535–9.

MORSE, E.V., SIMON, P.M., BALSON, P.M. and OSOFSKY, H.J. (1992a) 'Sexual behavior patterns of customers of male street prostitutes', *Archives of Sexual Behavior*, **21**, pp. 347–57.

MORSE, E.V., SIMON, P.M., BAUS, S.A., BALSON, P.M. and OSOFSKY, H.J. (1992b) 'Cofactors of substance use among male street prostitutes', *Journal of Drug Issues*, **22**, pp. 977–94.

PIEPER, R. (1979) 'Identity management in adolescent male prostitution in West Germany', *International Review of Modern Sociology*, **9**, pp. 239–59.

RAVEN, S. (1960) 'Boys will be boys', *Encounter*, **86**, p. 19.

REISS, A.J. (1964) 'The social integration of queers and peers', in H.S. BECKER (Ed.) *The Other Side: Perspectives on Deviance*, New York: Free Press.

ROSS, H.L. (1959) 'The "Hustler" in Chicago', *Journal of Student Research*, **1**, pp. 13–19.

RUSSELL, D.H. (1971) 'On the psychopathology of boy prostitutes', *International Journal of Offender Therapy*, **15**, p. 49.

SIMON, P.M., MORSE, E.V., OSOFSKY, H.J., BALSON, P.M. and GAUMER, H.R. (1992) 'Psychological characteristics of a sample of male street prostitutes', *Archives of Sexual Behavior*, **21**, pp. 33–44.

SIMON, P.M., MORSE, E.V., BALSON, P.M., OSOFSKY, H.J. and GAUMER, H.R. (1993) 'Barriers to human immunodeficiency virus related risk reduction among male street prostitutes', *Health Education Quarterly*, **20**, pp. 261–73.

SIMON, P.M., MORSE, E.V., OSOFSKY, H.J. and BALSON, P.M. (1994) 'HIV and young male street prostitutes: a brief report', *Journal of Adolescence*, **17**, pp. 193–7.

WEISBERG, D.K. (1985) *Children of the Night: A Study of Adolescent Prostitution*, Toronto: Lexington.

Chapter 6

Aspects of Male Sex Work in Mexico City

Ana Luisa Liguori and Peter Aggleton

Finally, Hercules killed the Hydra of Lerna, a monstrous serpent with seven heads which grew back every time they were cut off, if they were not all cut off by a single blow. (Greek myth)

The forces of conservatism that promote repression, censure and intolerance, and the homophobia that denies individuals the freedom to fully express and develop their sexuality are like the Hydra of Lerna. They rear their ugly heads in all spheres of life. Without doubt, however, one of their most belligerent faces is reserved for male sex work.

One of the most visible instances of social intolerance in Mexico in recent years is shown by the murder of *travestis* involved in sex work. These murders differ dramatically from the homicides of female sex workers. Whereas the latter tend to be committed by one man, the former are most usually perpetrated by a group of individuals, and they are indescribably brutal. The most publicized recent cases were the murders committed in Tuxtla Gutiérrez, Chiapas between June 1991 and February 1993 when at least 13 people were killed (Ronquillo, 1994). Similar cases have been reported in Culiacán, where 13 deaths were documented between February and December 1992 (Navarro, 1993), as well as in Oaxaca. In Mexico City itself, Liborio Cruz, a 19-year-old *travesti* was beaten to death on a public street by 15 individuals in June 1995 (*La Jornada*, 1995). These crimes have largely gone unpunished, and only in the case of Chiapas where a strong and organized response occurred, has anyone been arrested and charged with the murders, although according to Ronquillo (1994) they are most likely scapegoats identified by local government. These recorded incidents are only the tip of the iceberg. In the context of AIDS, it is also a crime not to provide people with access to the resources to protect themselves, and their partners, against infection.

When we began the study described in this chapter, we were surprised by how little attention both government and AIDS activist groups had given to men involved in sex work in Mexico. Although the AIDS epidemic began in Mexico in 1983, and by 1997 it was calculated that there had been more than 42000 cumulative cases, there have been few studies and interventions involving this important population. This is a little surprising when it has recently been estimated that the prevalence of HIV among male sex workers in Mexico City alone, rose from 7 per cent in 1986, to 14 per cent in 1989, to 24 per cent in 1990, to between 20 and 30 per cent today (Valdespino *et al.*, 1995).

The Study

A chapter such as this cannot hope to capture the full diversity of male sex work. Instead, we have aimed to examine two contrasting types of male sex work in Mexico City: *travestis* and *masajistas* (men who work as masseurs in public baths and saunas). Even though in both cases the men involved are of low socio-economic status, their experiences and work practices are very different. We will focus here on social and work contexts as well as attitudes, behaviours and prevention practices with respect to HIV and AIDS.

We decided to examine the work of *travestis* because of their numerical importance in sex work and because they constitute a very visible form of male sex work. *Masajistas*, on the other hand, are not so significant numerically, but offer a radical contrast in terms of identity and work practices. Our interest lay in demonstrating the variability of male sex work in Mexico today, along with the diversity of sexual identities constructed in specific cultural contexts. The fieldwork reported here was largely qualitative in nature and involved in-depth interviews with sex workers and key informants, including AIDS activists, government authorities and health workers in HIV information and testing centres.

Travestis

The information in this chapter contains a number of biases determined by the first author's professional and personal relationships with two pioneer activists in the struggle for gay rights in Mexico, who have been much involved in HIV/AIDS-related activities since the beginning of the epidemic: Gerardo Ortega and Juan Jacobo Hernández. The majority of interviews were conducted in Ciudad Nezahualcóyotl in groups facilitated by Gerardo Ortego and the first author. Approximately 15 *travestis* participated in these group discussions, which were complemented by three individual in-depth interviews conducted at a later date.

Masajistas

Access to the *masajistas* was facilitated by Juan Jacobo Hernández, who has been undertaking AIDS education with young men working in Mexico City saunas for some years. A colleague also helped arrange the interviews which were conducted in one particular bath house on three separate occasions. On the first occasion, four *masajistas* were interviewed; on the second, more detailed interviews were conducted with two of the original informants and a first interview was completed with a further respondent. On the third occasion, informal discussions were held with the manager of the sauna. Observation also took place.

Clients

Not a great deal is known about the clients of male sex workers in Mexico, since they are not easily accessed. Paying for sex is a stigmatized behaviour, especially so in the case of male sex work. Moreover, many clients use male sex workers in order to protect their privacy and anonymity in a way not possible were they to make sexual contact on the gay scene. As a result, the information available derives indirectly from the observations and reflections of male sex workers themselves.

Existing Literature

Before this study of male sex workers' sexual behaviours and practices, very little research had been conducted in this field. A review of existing studies on male sexuality, homo/bisexuality, AIDS and STDs revealed few references to male sex work. Gómezjara and Barrera (1978), however, in *The Sociology of Prostitution* offer an explanation of male sex work in terms of the injustices of the capitalist system. While sex work offers better economic opportunities to young men than those that can be found in the labour market, it requires participants to confront social intolerance as they leave the protection offered by the norms of heterosexuality. However, very little hard data is offered to support this particular analysis.

There exist, however, a few studies conducted among *travestis* in which sex work is mentioned tangentially. The work of Annick Prieur (1994a, 1994b) is probably the most important here, but only two articles detail in English the work she carried out in Mexico, and neither of these focuses specifically on sex work. Nevertheless, her doctoral thesis (currently being translated from Norwegian) offers a lot of useful information on these issues, since the majority of informants in her study were involved in sex work.

Occasional references to male sex work can be found in studies of machismo in Mexico and in some literature on homosexuality, but in both cases sex work is not central to the questions being addressed. Gutmann (1996) in *The Meanings of Macho* examines such concerns briefly in his chapter on male sexuality. He cites earlier work conducted by Patricio Villalva involving more than 300 interviews with '*prostitutos*' working in the Alameda park. Almost all their clients came from the middle and upper classes. *Prostitutos* were said to be 'young men, most usually dark-skinned migrants from the countryside who visited the park in order to have sex with other, usually fairer skinned people'.

Many of the young men interviewed came to Mexico City to find work but reported having been accosted at the main bus station by men who offered them work, food and somewhere to say. Once initiated into sex work, they made from 50 to 150 dollars a day. A good proportion of the men were married and had children, yet continued to work as *prostitutos*, not considering themselves to be either homosexual or bisexual. They saw themselves as men first and foremost, men who had sex with homosexuals or gays. For *prostitutos*, definitions of homosexuality were determined primarily by the reasons *why* they had sex with other men, and only secondarily were they linked to the nature of the sexual relationship. Almost always, clients wished to be penetrated. According to Villalva, *prostitutos* are distinguishable from *chichifos* or homosexual men involved in sex work.

In *De los Otros*, Carrier (1995) describes findings from participant observation in Mexico over the last 25 years. Fieldwork took place primarily in Guadalajara where Carrier describes his observations and experiences of homosexually active men in bars, drinking places, cabarets and red light zones in the various towns he stopped in while travelling by land between California and Guadalajara. He differentiates between two types of men who have sex with men but who also have sex with women: *mayates* and *chichifos*. *Mayates* tend to come from the lower middle class and have sex with men largely as a substitute for women when they are unattached or not in a relationship. *Chichifos*, on the other hand, tend to be from the lower social classes, and have sex with men largely as a means of earning a living or in order to supplement the family income. According to Carrier's informants, *chichifos'* clients tend to be married heterosexual men, rich elderly *maricones* (rich old queens), and American tourists.

With the advent of AIDS, it might be supposed that there would have been an abundance of studies on male sex work in Mexico. However, only a very few have been conducted, and only the briefest reference is made to this important aspect of sexual life in abstracts and presentations at national and international meetings. Palacios-Martínez *et al.* (1992) have, however, interviewed 110 men recruited in the street, bars, public places, metro stations and *cantinas*. The majority of interviewees were aged 12 to 23 and came from low socio-economic backgrounds. They tended to be migrants with a low level of education, a history of family breakdown, a high level of risky sexual behaviour, and a low frequency of condom use both with clients and regular partners. Many interviewees reported using drugs.

While several recent international conference abstracts looking at male sex work state that the purpose of the studies was to facilitate the design of subsequent interventions, it is possible to count the number of prevention initiatives for men who sell sex on the fingers of one hand. This is alarming since male sex workers face high risks in their work, and may in turn infect clients unwilling to protect themselves. Additionally, many clients of male sex workers also have sex with women.

Contextual Concerns

So I said to myself, 'Well if there are people who'll pay for this, I'll do it.' (Luis Zapata, 1979)

In order to fully understand the nature of male sex work and its HIV-related dimensions, it is necessary to be aware of the economic and political context of Mexico today. The country is currently going through the most serious economic crisis it has seen in the past 50 years. Ordinary workers have been particularly badly affected, and finding enough money to survive gets more difficult every day. The economic crisis has been accompanied by a severe political crisis. The internal power struggles of the PRI,[1] the modernization of the Mexican state, corruption, political assassinations, insurrection in Chiapas and political scandals have challenged the traditional structures of government. In the process of democratic transition, the corporate base on which the political power of the PRI was built has been shaken. The Conservative Party has taken advantage of the situation, helped by a loose alliance of conservative forces across the country. The growing efforts of the right to promote their morality as the only valid one have been accompanied by growing social intolerance, especially towards sex workers. Although it is difficult to quantify precisely, the present crisis has brought with it an increase in the amount of sex work. In Mexico this kind of activity, in contrast to living off the earnings of a prostitute, is not specifically mentioned in the penal code. Nevertheless, minor regulations such as those governing policing and public order are used against sex work activities. These regulations, dealing largely with issues of public morality and scandal in public life, allow the police to arrest, detain, harass and imprison sex workers.

Sex work can generate large quantities of money for those involved. Some of this accrues to the owners and managers of bars, hotels and nightclubs, but much circulates between the police and government authorities, who exploit and extort sex workers and their clients. This in part explains the somewhat ambivalent attitude that is often expressed towards sex workers, usually more tolerant in the case of women than men. Recent months have, however, seen a growing intolerance of male sex work linked to its association with delinquency – a topic we will return to later – and to homophobia.

In reality there are many different types of male sex worker. The most common are *travestis* working the streets; *travestis* who meet their clients in cabarets; masculine-looking men who pick up their clients in the street, bars and gay discotheques; those who publicize their services in magazines and newspapers; sauna *masajistas*; and young people living on the street. Street-based sex workers usually work in certain neighbourhoods and zones. When repression intensifies, however, they tend to become more dispersed and less visible. Not that long ago, it was possible to observe groups of *travestis* or groups of masculine-looking men selling sex in the streets in clearly defined areas. The latter, for example, generally worked in the Reforma in front of Sanborn's and VIP's near the Ángel. The former could be found in the Calle de Campeche in the Hipódromo neighbourhood, in the Calle de Puebla near Insurgentes, on the Avenida Nuevo León, and in Hundido park (Ligouri and Ortega, 1989). At the time this study was conducted, however, it was much more difficult to find sex workers on the street and we therefore decided to use existing contacts in order to carry out the research.

Vestidas: The Most Beautiful of All

Everything about him that was vulgar when he was a male hustler he disposed of when he became a woman, when he began to dress as a woman and was more feminine than any women ... he was the most feminine of all, right? The prettiest of them all. (Luis Zapata, 1979)

The most visible form of male sex work is that undertaken by *travestis* or *vestidas*, men who have transformed themselves into women by cross-dressing. *Travestis* generally learn the tricks of the trade from other more experienced friends with whom they identify and eventually work. As Gerardo explained: 'You always enter prostitution through apprenticeship. One person initiates the next. First you learn how to dress, wear make-up and carry yourself, then how to work the streets. Networks are created, groups formed and lasting friendships are made.' According to Gerardo, *vestidas* generally see themselves as homosexual. The prior struggles they have had with their family over this often provide an inner strength which is useful later in sex work. Rafael (Francesca), for example, used to work as a barman in a gay bar in the centre city. She describes how she came to the beauty shop owned by Chetos and then they became friends. 'She was the one who told me how to dress and helped me learn. A little later she helped me work the streets.' In relation to this process of transformation, Francesca said 'When I began, I didn't know how to make myself look good. Now, however, I'm brilliant at it. People say I pass very well'. Chetos intervened in the conversation, explaining 'At night you put on this fantastic body, big hips, huge tits, a beautiful wig and a doll's face. You use make-up, false hair, and foam rubber to shape the body.' *Vestidas* are very skilful at using foam rubber to shape their bodies beneath their clothes. Of course, there are also more invasive ways of doing this such as injecting mineral oil in the buttocks and thighs,[2] or surgery and hormones.

The area where *vestidas* work is usually clearly defined, making it difficult for a client to be confused and pick up a man thinking he is a woman. *Travestis* rarely work alone, and even if one might easily pass as a woman, the majority do not. Moreover, generally speaking, the appearance of women working the streets is not so eye-catching as that of *travestis*.

When a *travesti* knows that a client really does not understand the situation, she has two options. She can make it clear she is a man or try to pass as a woman. Trying to pass as a woman is called *meter balín*. The option chosen depends on a number of factors. Primarily, she will want to continue the interaction because of the money involved, and if a customer is drunk or shy, she may feel able to control things. As Chetos explained:

Yes, it has happened to me. Sometimes they ask you if you are a woman and I say 'What do you see?' And he says 'Can I have a feel?' I say 'Go ahead, have a feel.' As they can't find anything, they go with you. But I don't like passing in this way. Nayeli, on the other hand, is very good at it. She uses super glue to make her penis into the shape of a woman's organs (she has injected so many hormones that she doesn't get an erection) and it really looks like one.

But few *travestis* like to take these kinds of risks because they can find themselves in violent situations. Some men, if they discover they have gone with a *vestida*, become aggressive and violent. As Chetos explained, 'Sometimes when a client finds out the truth, he gets really angry and you end up in a fight.' Because of this, many *travestis* try to make the situation clear at the start. Almendra, an 18-year-old *travesti*, explained: 'If clients ask me if I am a woman, I say "No, if you want a woman, I'll go and get you one." They usually give me 30 or 40 pesos and then I go and get them a woman.' As a result, problems of confused identity rarely occur, and the majority of clients know they are picking up a man.

For some clients, though, one of the most exciting things about *travestis* is that although they appear to be women, they are really men. As Gerardo said, 'The excitement and fascination about *travestis* is that they are men dressed up as women. For someone who can't accept his homosexual feelings, it is easier to pick up someone who looks like a woman than it is to get off with a man. It seems more important to fool themselves than anyone else.'

Men who pick up *travestis* in Colonia Condesa and the Zona Rosa generally come from the middle or upper classes because only they can pay the prices charged in these neighbourhoods. In more suburban areas, prices tend to be lower and there working-class men may be found. As we will see later, a key feature of the sex work conducted by non-*travestis* concerns negotiations over the price to be paid. The prices of different sexual acts are openly discussed, for example, whether the client wishes to penetrate or be penetrated. In the case of *travestis*, however, the only question the client is asked is whether he wishes fellatio (which generally takes place in his car), or whether he would like the 'full service' (which usually takes place in a hotel). The phrase 'full service' implies that the client will later fuck the *travesti*.

Nevertheless, once they get back to the hotel, things can change. All interviewees reported that they knew when a man wanted something more. As Chetos says, 'There are men who start grabbing your cock when you're having sex. And then they say, now it's your turn, let me suck you or you fuck me. So you say, "give me a little something extra", and you charge them more.' The service most frequently asked for is oral sex followed by 'the full service'. A few clients, however, want to be penetrated. As Chetos said, 'For every ten who fuck, three will want to be fucked.'

All interviewees felt that life on the street was very dangerous. Gerardo explained that 'In the name of decency and concern about security, there has been an increase in police violence with a consequent greater infringement of human rights.' This has affected both *vestidas* and others involved in sex work. Working in large groups is now less common, and sex workers have become less visible. As Almendra explained, 'Recently, it's been really scary. It has become very dangerous to go out in the street. I have friends who go out to steal. The clients who have been victimized then pick on any one of us to pay them back. Or sometimes afterwards they refuse to pay, and they leave you in the lurch. I don't like going out in the street, everything has become very heavy.'

The case of Francesca illustrates well the indirect risks to which *travestis* are exposed.

> Not that long ago I was out working and I got shot, and now I'm quite frightened. Some guys assaulted a client I was with and I got three bullet wounds, two in the lung and one in the arm. Before that I was really daring, I used to go to Garibaldi,[3] to the centre, everywhere alone, and I didn't care. I'd take some drugs, and nothing mattered. Now, sometimes I go out and I don't know whether men come up to talk to me just to see how much I charge, or what. The first thing that goes through my head is 'This guy's got a bad face', and it's best to go. You'd never believe it, the street isn't what it used to be.

Gerardo expanded on his theme:

> In addition to the clients, there are real risks from the police and from no-gooders. You have to be very brave. If you are in the street, it's not for pleasure but out of necessity ... *vestidas* are much more vulnerable to extortion than are their female counterparts. People nowadays don't know how to behave properly. It's easy to see it. There's too much aggression and violence.

The police not infrequently demand money from sex workers for not arresting them. Alternatively, they may force them into some kind of shady deal. They often turn up when a *travesti* is with a client and threaten to tell the client's family unless he pays them money. Other policemen try to get *travestis* to provide sexual services for free. As Francesca put it, 'There are some really bad police, as soon as they see you they are really awful, they're always after your body. Sometimes they also ask for money.' Gerardo said that with recent increases in police repression and intolerance, more *travestis* are being taken to the police station, where they are beaten up and forced to provide oral sex.

One of the few ways in which *travestis* can reduce their fears is by taking drugs. Anti-depressants such as Rohinol or Roche[4] produce disinhibition and can lessen fear. As Chetos said, 'Many people take coke or dope, but above all Roche is best for work. I know. When I go out to work, I always take one because it switches me on.' This same drug makes those *vestidas* who assault their clients braver about doing so. As Chetos explained:

> There are lots of *vestidas* who will mug you. 'Give me what you've got', but if they can rob you in a more underhand way, that's fine. If you're half out of it on drugs, you don't care if they notice or not. With drugs you think you're brilliant. You're Pancho Villa with a gun and they'd better not say anything or else they've had it.

The reasons for becoming involved in petty crime and sex work are distinct, and not all *vestidas* assault their clients. Nevertheless, because such events sometimes happen, *travestis* convey the impression of being dangerous. As Gerardo explained:

> Because of extortion, they have to get more money in less time, and they have to get it where they can. If they stopped [robbing] they wouldn't be able to get enough money through prostitution [alone]. They prefer the trouble of robbing a client to the hassle they might get from the police if they were taken to the station.[5]

It has been very difficult for The National AIDS Council (CONASIDA) and other non-governmental organizations to undertake HIV prevention programmes with *travestis*. As Gerardo explained:

> Women tend to stick together with a pimp or a madame who controls them. Although *vestidas* stick together to be less vulnerable and defend themselves, the great majority work independently. This makes it more difficult to control male prostitution, and there have been very few effective programmes to reduce petty delinquency among male sex workers. These programmes are unusual. We managed one of them, but it is very difficult for someone who doesn't know the game to become part of the scene or to provide any kind of leadership. Moreover, because of prejudice it has been difficult to use the techniques and principles that have worked well in female sex

work, like for example when the person in charge [of pimping] comes to an agreement with the authorities so as to avoid prosecution. The authorities have always blocked this kind of initiative. It is them [the authorities] who make things difficult, and this is always done in the interest of money. There is a lot of cash involved in the world of prostitution. I've tried to get things organized for a long time, and you can see the effect I've had. The worst of it is, though, I've had to take a year of free vacations [in jail].

Travestis' clients come from all backgrounds, but the majority are married with children. As Chetos put it, 'The truth is, a lot of married men like a bit of cock.' Various interviewees said that their married neighbours not infrequently asked them for sex, and paid them for it. Francesca said:

Sometimes, I've had it with clients here in this street. To be honest, it makes me a bit worried [when I do it] with people I know. Two neighbours have had sex with me, and paid me and everything. They are married. Not three houses away from where I live there's a married man with two sons. He's fat and ugly, and he roams around Zaragoza. He was a client. He gave me some money and was very discreet. But last time I saw him, he said 'Get into the car and I'll pay you as much as you want,' I replied 'There are limits, and the limit has now been reached!'

All *travestis* interviewed said they were afraid of AIDS, but responses to questions about whether they used condoms varied. Almendra said, 'I sometimes use condoms. But if I know the customer, then I'll do it without a condom. The men I meet in the street, they have to use a condom.' Francesca said:

I'll be honest with you. When there are some around, I'll use them. Sometimes I find the time to go and get them. It's for my own safety. Lately so many people have been infected. When I don't have any condoms though, I don't use any. When a client wants to fuck me, we go to one of the hotels. Here in the health centre they sell condoms from the health ministry for three pesos each. But even though they only cost that little, I don't buy them. When I have oral sex, I rarely use a condom, for the stupid 20 pesos you're charging, you must be mad to spend some of it on a condom. You say to yourself, no, it isn't worth it [laughter].

The idea of having or 'not having condoms' will be returned to later when we discuss prevention implications.

Within friendship groups, the capacity to be violent and to fight maintains hierarchy. Gerardo said:

To the extent that I show I have the capacity to be violent, I can prevent others being aggressive towards me. It's a kind of defence mechanism. People get used to being violent and it becomes part of life. It's also a kind of game. In their own way intellectuals do the same thing. They are always measuring up to each other to see who is better and who knows most. When we meet socially to have fun, there are various ways of seeing who is stronger, but violence is above all a defence mechanism. Some are better equipped to take their place at the top of the pyramid.

Indeed, on the last occasion the first author visited the group of *travestis* interviewed, she met Josefina with whom she had been friends for nearly five years. She had recently had to have surgery after a rival group had beaten her so violently that a cheek bone had been broken. Nevertheless, alongside the constant violence and difficulty of going out on the street, a playful atmosphere and some enjoyment prevails. As Francesca put it, '*Vestidas* have good fun, we are more open and sincere than those who are straight.'

Those who work in Ciudad Nezahualcóyotl said that the economic crisis in Mexico had affected them seriously and money was short. Nevertheless, Chetos said:

We always pick someone up, every single day. If you are in the street and someone attractive passes by, but he has no money, you screw with him just for the pleasure of it. Only of course if he is a real hunk, if he has a little moustache, and he has strong legs, and is dark skinned and if he has a [insinuates a big penis], or even if he doesn't have one, but if I like him because of his moustache, I'll have sex with him, and I won't charge him.

But street life takes its toll. The constant danger and the physical exhaustion of the schedule makes many a *travesti* think of changing her work. A number of those interviewed had beauty shops and left sex work for relatively long periods of time to work there, or in a friend's place. As Francesca said:

Before, when I started I liked it a lot. I wanted to have sex with everybody. Now things have changed, it is only as a result of necessity. I'd like to find some other kind of work, in an office for example. Recently, there have been so many people at night that try to fool you. I have known a lot of people who, when they get carried away they promise you the sky, the moon and the stars. They've said to me, for example, 'I'll give you a job, you look great as a woman, you carry it off well. My offices are in such and such a place. I'll come and call for you at home. Whatever you say . . .' But first of all I charge, and then maybe with a bit of luck I might get work in an office. My hope never dies, but when will that day come? Never.

Masajistas: It's not for Pleasure

Throughout Mexico City there are many public bath houses, which derive from the fact that many lower-class neighbourhoods have no regular water supply. The low cost of these public baths, which sometimes include saunas, means that they offered a useful service. In the past there were a very large number of these places but more recently, as public water supplies have been extended across the city, and as economic crisis has made it more difficult to pay, many bath houses have closed their doors. According to Mata (1997) there were 450 public baths in Mexico City in 1980, but 10 years later there were about 250, and by 1995 the number had decreased to 150.

In addition to their regular services, some public bath houses provide attractive alternatives for sexual activities. Some heterosexual couples, for example, find the private rooms available in the baths more accessible and cheaper than hotels for having sex. In various baths, the general sauna areas have become a haven for homosexual activity, including group sex. In several bath houses, clients are offered a range of other services, including shoe shining, hairdressing, refreshments and massage. In at least 10 of them, massages are in reality a hidden form of sex work arranged by the bath house manager (Hernández, 1997).

The price paid varies from one site to another. In some, a combined service is offered. Men enter the general area first, then if they don't pick someone up there, they pay for sex. Sometimes paid sex takes place in the public areas, and sometimes it occurs more discreetly in private rooms. The bath house where interviews took place was of this latter type, and one of the most expensive on the market. At the entrance near where you pay the person in charge, there was usually a group of very attractive young men. Some of them have very good bodies and are into physical fitness. Others, who are also very attractive, have less well developed bodies. As Juan Jacobo Hernández says 'The city boys are the ones you can most easily identify because their bodies are very well defined, but there are others that are obviously from the rural areas. There are many *morenos*, for example, of the kind you find in rural areas.'

One of the *masajistas* takes the client to the bath that has been assigned. He carries his soap to the massage bench, along with towels. The client is then asked if he would like a massage. If, in reality, he wants nothing more than a massage, it is probable that he will accept this from the first person who offers, since the client has the option of choosing whom he receives the massage from. If, on the other hand, he would like to have sex, he can either accept the first young man who offers it, or indicate who he would like to do this. Ricardo explained the procedure: 'The clients they know what to do. After you've asked "Do you want a massage?" they choose someone, maybe the person who gave them the ticket, or the one with the white shirt. Or the client might say "You give it to me." ' If the client does not select anyone, different young men will knock on the door in order to see if they can offer him something. As

Nicolás says 'We sit there at the entrance. Generally, they prefer someone new. However there are some [clients] who always like [to have] the same one.' If the *masajistas* do not know a particular client, they first need to find out whether he is looking for sex, but the majority of young men working in this particular sauna consider that most clients came there with that purpose. Ricardo explained what he does. 'I massage them face down, so then I put my cock in their hand; if I see that they try to fondle it, I realize, yes. If they take their hand away, I give them a normal massage.'

INTERVIEWER: Do you take off your clothes when you're providing massages then?
RESPONDENT: Yes. When I know someone wants a normal massage I wear a towel. But if it is the 'complete service' I strip completely.
INTERVIEWER: And what do the clients like most?
RESPONDENT: The majority want the special service.

All the young men interviewed said they were heterosexual, and did the work only out of economic necessity. They explained that there were some sexual practices they would participate in, and others they would not. When a client arrives, and once it has become clear that sex is on the agenda, a price is negotiated. As José explained:

> When the client arrives you need to negotiate with him to avoid problems later. Because half-way through they might say to you 'I really want to kiss your arse' What a thing [to say], and if you don't like that sort of thing what will happen? It's better if the client knows what you do, and you come to some kind of arrangement beforehand, like I say 'Well, I like this, and this and this, but I don't do that.' Before being asked what you like to do, it's best to say 'I don't like being fucked and I don't like sucking [you] either.'

The 'full service' costs from 100 to 150 pesos.

Interviewees agreed that clients most frequently asked to be fucked. The sexual service provided, be it penetration, fellatio or masturbation, costs the same. If, however, while having sex, the client asks the *masajista* to ejaculate, the price is re-negotiated and can end up almost double that initially agreed. The *masajista* is paid before the client leaves the room.

Masajistas learn how to control themselves so as to avoid ejaculation, and the service finishes when the client comes. When Jorge was asked if he ejaculated, he replied, 'If I'm working in the morning I may give a massage, and then another later. And . . . usually I come with the last [client].'

INTERVIEWS: You can manage all day?
RESPONDENT: Yes, it's a matter of concentration. What happens is, if I'm enjoying it and I feel I'm going to come, I think about other things.

Others ejaculated with their first client in order to manage the rest of the day. *Masajistas* interviewed were initially insistent that they were the ones who penetrated and who were fellated, never the reverse. When asked if they had clients who wanted to fuck them, they replied yes, and some might offer them more money for it, but they said they never accepted. All agreed that in this particular sauna that was the norm. Juan Jacobo Hernández, who has conducted HIV prevention work in Mexico City's bath houses for many years now, agreed that this was the general picture. His colleague Anuar said, 'What they're also selling is an attitude.' *Masajistas* build the fantasy for the client that he is with a very macho man, with a *chacal*.[6] In response to the question 'Have you ever been penetrated?', only José said yes. He said 'The truth is yes ... but I'll tell you something, afterwards I cried. I cried bitter tears. But this experience taught me something, because what would it have meant if I had liked it?'

When a client insists that he is the one to penetrate, interviewees reported passing him on to someone else who would provide this service. After talking further, however, it became clear that of the 10 young men working a particular shift, two or three might allow themselves to be penetrated. However, none of those interviewed admitted to being one of these. All spoke at length about their heterosexual partners. José, who was 29 years old, had had a girlfriend for about a year and a half, and wanted to marry her. He had worked in the bath house for three years and had left it for a period of six years. He told us, 'I used to sell meat and things were going well but unfortunately business got worse and worse, and the owner was forced to close. I was planning to get married and this ruined all my plans. So I came here because I lost my job.' None of the interviewees reported having told his girlfriend about the work. José continued:

> About work, I'm having her on. She knows what I'm like, she wants me under her thumb. I must get a job. Sometimes I ask my customers to help. Like I say to them, can I give your telephone number to my girlfriend so she can speak to you and you can tell her I work for you. Is that ok? That calms her down, because lately when I'm with her, she has been asking, 'What do you do? Where do you get the money from?' and she has begun to think I'm thieving.

A small number of men worked regularly in the baths, but it was more common for them to come and go depending on financial needs. As Juan Jacobo Hernández explained 'People come and go. For example, the other day I met a boy called Juan from Acapulco who had worked for one and a half, maybe two years in the baths, and who had [then] gone away. He went to open a modest restaurant in Cuernavaca, but then he came back because things went badly.' It must be remembered that these men can earn in one day's work in the sauna as much money as they might get for a week's work elsewhere. Seen in this light, it is easier to understand the attraction sauna work holds, and to appreciate why, once involved, the baths offer a safety net which can be returned to as necessary. All of those interviewed said that the principal reason that they were involved in this kind of work was financial. As Nicolás put it, 'The truth is, I have to work. I have to give money to my mother [who lives in Pachuca] because my father died. Only recently I got together with a chick.' Javier, who was 22 years old and came from Jalapa, used to sell clothes. He explained how a friend of his had introduced him to sauna work, and what he needed to do '[He said to me] "You just have to fuck them and that's it. Easy money."'

In order to work in the bath houses, it is necessary to be introduced. Sometimes introductions are effected by friends or relatives. A number of recruitment networks exist in different parts of the country. As Juan Jacobo Hernández explained:

Some come from Pachuca, others come from the area around San Martín Tezmelucan, from different fruit-growing communities near Puebla, some come from Veracruz, others from Acapulco, others from Michoacán. Some of the boys from Puebla came specifically to work in the baths, but normally they come when there's no work at home, when they're not planting or picking fruit.

José comes from Michoacán and arrived with a friend. Ricardo was brought by his brother, who had worked in the bath house for nine years before emigrating to the United States. He has now been there for three years and is not thinking about retiring yet. He recently brought two of his cousins, Raúl and Nicolás, country boys who look very different from him. All of them come from Pachuca in Hidalgo, and migrated to Mexico City at different times. Raúl used to work for a printer, earning the minimum wage. He explained, 'I began this out of necessity. There was no work for me there, so I came here.' Nicolás used to work in heavy engineering and as a waiter. He said, 'In the factory I used to earn 300 pesos a week and as a waiter between 100–120 a day, but that kind of work was fairly irregular.'

There is an important contrast between the young men who worked regularly in the sauna and those who did so more occasionally. Raúl, who had been there for five months, and Nicolás, who had only arrived a few weeks earlier, gave the appearance of being rather shy, and their insecurity was evident. Raúl also said that the work made him feel ashamed and much of the time he regretted being there. He wanted to find some different kind of work. He said, 'Once I've got my papers together, I am going to try to find some work with Corona.'[7] When asked if he did not think with time he might become accustomed to the work, he replied, 'Yes, now it's not the same as the first time, but I don't like it and now once I marry, I'll like it even less.'

Nicolás said, 'It's really disgusting here. I don't like having sex with other men.' Both spoke of the difficulties adapting to their new occupation. Raúl described the first time he had sex with a client.

RESPONDENT: The client was very nice.
INTERVIEWER: Did you tell him he was your first?
RESPONDENT: Yes, later afterwards I explained.
INTERVIEWER: What did he want you to do?
RESPONDENT: To fuck him.
INTERVIEWER: Did he help you get aroused?
RESPONDENT: Yes, he told me to relax and everything and that I should imagine that I was with a woman. I thought that it was going to be more difficult, but it wasn't.

Nicolás, who had arrived more recently, was having a harder time. We asked him whether he had had sex with men before coming to the bath house and he replied, 'No, never.'

INTERVIEWER: And what's it like now?
RESPONDENT: No ... it makes me anxious.
INTERVIEWER: And your first time, what was that like?
RESPONDENT: No, no, I couldn't. I was too worried, so I just gave him a regular massage.
INTERVIEWER: Did he ask for anything else?
RESPONDENT: Yes, of course, but I couldn't, passed him on to someone else.
INTERVIEWER: And when did you do it the first time?
RESPONDENT: To be honest, I still can't do it really well.
INTERVIEWER: Didn't it help to look at pornographic magazines and things like that?
RESPONDENT: Yes, looking at women in pornographic magazines. Yes, I get turned on right away, but once I'm here, I lose it.

Those who had worked at the sauna for some time said that they did not have problems with their work and gave the impression of being secure in themselves. They felt that they were professional and devoted to their work. As Juan explained, 'Most of the clients really like my body ... it's what guarantees my living, it's something in my favour.'[8] Ricardo, on the other hand, only worked one day a week and said that for him it was a good kind of work, because 'for me it isn't difficult'.

Some *masajistas* enjoyed their work and gained pleasure from their relationships with clients. When we asked Jorge if he had had difficulty getting used to the work, he said, 'No I didn't, because I liked it from the start. If they give me a good blow job. The truth is I like it, I really like this work.' There is an important paradox here. These men interviewed were not forced to participate in sexual practices they did not like. They were not humiliated or maltreated. Their work was relatively secure and the police did not harass them or clients. Moreover, they had a good income. Nevertheless, they lived in a situation of unquestionable exploitation. They only earned money when they gave massages or provided sexual services. They received no income for simply being at work in spite of the fact that they carried out everyday duties necessary for the functioning of the establishment. They looked after the soap and the towels, they were involved in the cleaning of the bath house as well as the room(s) in which services are provided and, when clients so wished, they cleaned shoes (a service for which payment is given directly to the manager of the bath house). As well as all this, they were required to give 20 per cent of what they earned from each client to the bath house manager. Since this was the only money that passed directly to them from the client, when they can, they try to cheat the manager, although in general there is a minimum charge made per client.

When it comes to deciding whether to restrict their sexual activities with clients to the workplace or continue them elsewhere, different strategies were adopted. José, for example, only worked at the bath house on Tuesdays.[9] His strategy was to use relationships at work to meet clients, or friends of clients, outside. In contrast, Ricardo said that he would not work outside the bath house for anything. He said:

RESPONDENT: I've never liked to do it. I've had lots of invitations, but me, never, never, never.

INTERVIEWER: Why?

RESPONDENT: I don't know. It doesn't feel good to do that sort of thing. Sometimes I feel that if I go somewhere or to a hotel with a client, anything could happen to me, or I could end up getting done by the police.

Raúl's response was even more emphatic: 'No, no, no [with great emphasis]. It would make me feel ashamed. I could never imagine being seen doing that.'

In Juan Jacobo Hernández's opinion, as well as providing anonymity, meeting men in the sauna has other benefits: 'There are older people who don't want to waste time picking someone up . . . or people who don't want the hassle. They know what they want and they pay. They know what's on offer in the bath house.' Raúl expresses astonishment at the fact that married men come to the baths. 'I don't know what they come for if they have wives, although some of them even come with their wives.'

A small number of clients are couples, and all *masajistas* reported occasionally providing services in this way. Ricardo explained that he has two couples who are regular clients:

INTERVIEWER: About how often do they come?

RESPONDENT: They come about once a week.

INTERVIEWER: And what do they want you to do?

RESPONDENT: The guy wants to watch while I give her a massage and afterwards while I fuck her. He likes watching. He just masturbates. The other couple come for the same kind of service, the 'complete service', both of them.

Raúl, who has more recently arrived, has provided services to only three couples, but in conversation with us he said, 'There are some [men] who just want to watch, and others who want you to fuck both of them.' Curiously, when sexual services are provided to couples the price is less if only the woman is fucked. According to Raúl the cost for this kind of service is typically 50 to 80 pesos.

Several of the *masajistas* used drugs to help them work and sometimes they were offered these by clients. José explained, 'The truth is, I really like marijuana, I also like coca[ine], and pills, but I've stopped taking them. Lots of people like them and they help the work. I go to a self-help group for drug users that has helped me to stop drinking. I still drink, but they've taught me moderation. But the pills I stopped, because if I take one, I want more. I react badly. When it's only one or two . . . , but you start getting turned on and you start doing really stupid things.'

All interviewees where asked whether or not they used condoms, and all with the exception of Fabián, said they used them when having penetrative sex with clients. For fellatio, sometimes they used condoms and sometimes not, depending on the client. Fabián is probably atypical, however. He was a slightly older *masajista* than the others, with a face that shows the scars of many a fight, and he was not always well-balanced. He spoke relatively incoherently, saying that he wanted to die and did not believe in AIDS. For him, it was all the same whether he used a condom or not. He also talked about the drugs he had taken, pure alcohol, crack cocaine, and 'sometimes [I] inject, maybe 15 times I've injected, crystal, cocaine and sometimes heroin.'

Masajistas said that sometimes the sauna manager provides condoms for free, or sells them cheap. If none were around when needed, someone went to get them. We asked Ricardo when he used a condom.

INTERVIEWER: I've always used condoms.
RESPONDENT: How do you get them?
INTERVIEWER: I bring them with me. If at the moment of truth you have to go to get one, another guy can come and you can lose the score.

According to Ricardo, some clients wanted to have sex without condoms, but he always refused them.

INTERVIEWER: Do you always use a condom?
RESPONDENT: Always, always.
INTERVIEWER: Including when they suck you?
RESPONDENT: Without a condom sometimes, but for penetration always.

Ricardo had been taught how to use a condom by his brother. Other *masajistas* said that they already knew how to protect themselves in this way. The manager of the bath house said that he taught some of the more inexperienced young men to use condoms when they first arrived. This is part of the process by which they learn how to massage and what the 'complete service' involves. Much emphasis, he said, was placed on the regular use of condoms.

Conclusions

As stated earlier, relatively few educational interventions have taken place in Mexico with men involved in sex work. An additional problem arises from the fact that much AIDS activism in Mexico has its origins in the gay movement, which has a somewhat ambivalent attitude towards *travestis* in particular. As Juan Jacobo Hernández says, '*Vestidas* have ideologically divided the gay movement. They are considered the buffoons of the system, products and accomplices of machismo, who reinforce all the worst feminine stereotypes. Because of that, *travestis* end up facing a double discrimination, both as homosexuals and as women.' It was not until the early 1970s that a gay group undertook any work with *travestis* in Mexico.

Both of the groups of men described in this chapter tend to come from the lower socio-economic classes, but have very different identities, work conditions, risk practices, sexual behaviours and HIV prevention needs. *Masajistas* in general tend to have come relatively recently from the countryside. Many of their families remain in the country and while links remain, the former do not generally know about the work the young men do. In contrast to *travestis*, the profile identity and behaviour of *masajistas* is similar to those of many Mexican men from the same social background (Liguori, González Block with Aggleton, 1996). Since their behaviour does not transgress cultural norms, *masajistas* can move into and out of sex work at minimal cost. Moreover, because their work generally takes place during the day, those who want to, can maintain a regular family life.

The background of the *travestis* interviewed was generally urban. For them, however, the consequences of making so profound a personal transformation were far-reaching. While *travestis* live marginal lives, they do not question the social norms governing everyday life in Mexico today in the same way as, for example, the gay movement. Nevertheless, their lives are full of daily confrontations and difficulties.

The income likely to be generated by sex work is always unpredictable. *Travestis* working in middle-class areas of the city charge more for their services than *masajistas* (and obviously more than other *travestis* in more working-class neighbourhoods). Nevertheless, they are much more likely to be exposed to danger and violence. In general, however, travestis are not exploited by others in the same way that *masajistas* are exploited by sauna owners and managers.

In relation to the types of sexual service provided, *travestis* indicated that they provided a wide range of services. As Chetos explained, 'Many men have very dull sex lives and occasionally want something different, like their cock sucked, or their balls sucked, or they like their buttocks to be grabbed. When they are married, their wives are very conservative or don't like to do those things. Such men go out to buy what they can't get at home.' He also claimed that clients often preferred *travestis* to female sex workers. As he put it:

> To go out with [a] *travesti* is more fun than with a woman because if a man wants to have 'that' [implying his penis] or his arse scratched, well a queen will go right ahead and do it. Many men want you to kiss their arse holes. They can't ask for these things from their wives, and very few women sex workers will do them either. But *vestidas* are wilder, and so they do it. That's why men like *vestidas*. When they know it is a *vestida*, they say, they have nice arses, tits, a prick, and a lot more attitude.

With respect to preventive behaviour, the response in the baths was much more uniform. Here, condoms were reported as being consistently used for penetrative sex with clients, both out of personal conviction and because of bath house policy. With fellatio, *masajistas* said they did not care and left it up to the client whether or not to use condoms. Among *travestis*, the vast majority of those interviewed said that in general when they have penetrative sex they tried to use condoms, but did not use them if there were none around. For oral sex, practically none reported using condoms. Although the risk of HIV transmission through oral sex is low, a number of other sexually transmitted diseases can be transmitted this way.

Several aspects of the present situation in Mexico give cause for concern. The first is a general absence of a culture of prevention based on condom use. This is probably a consequence of the sustained pressure by conservative forces in the country and the absence of explicit mass media campaigns. Moreover, sufficient work has not been carried out to educate and promote safer sex among different groups of men who have sex with other men. This can be confirmed by even the most cursory observations of the 'back rooms' and 'black houses' that have appeared in Mexico City, where men do not use condoms consistently. A further complicating factor is that it is not unknown for young men detained by the police to be accused of being sex workers if they are carrying condoms at the time.

Related to the above, is the fact that few HIV prevention efforts have aimed to promote a culture of condom buying. This perhaps explains statements such as 'the condoms ran out' or 'there weren't any around at the time'. In reality, of course, condoms do not simply 'run out', they become unavailable when no one has thought about buying them in advance. Ideally, condoms should be freely available, perhaps on a subsidized basis or via social marketing programmes. While in the past, activists with good access to condoms have distributed them in massive giveaways, it remains to be seen whether this is a sustainable HIV prevention strategy, or whether more innovative techniques are needed to make condom buying a part of everyday life. Perhaps the cost of condoms could be included in the price charged for sexual services, or perhaps in the entrance fee paid to saunas and public baths.

In Mexico, as elsewhere, male sex workers continue to be treated as a population that either does not exist, or does not warrant the effort when it comes to HIV prevention. If there is homophobia towards men who have sex with men in Mexico, it is much more marked in the case of male sex workers. Not even activist groups concerned with HIV and AIDS have been able to identify successful ways of working with men selling sex. As Palacios-Martínez *et al.* (1992) put it:

> As a group men who sell sex are heterogeneous and require integrated forms of education and intervention as well counselling, AIDS and STD prevention, drug rehabilitation, vocational education and so on. All of these require the development of special forms of organisation among sex workers and the co-ordinated participation of government and non-governmental organisations.

The issue of sex work is extremely complex, and there are no simple solutions. What is clear, however, is that authoritarian and moralistic strategies which do not take into account the social and psychological factors that lead some to sell sexual services and others to buy them, are destined to fail. Repression and prohibition only drive the buying and selling of sex underground, and increase the physical and health risks faced by all involved. Intolerance does not favour a culture of prevention. For those who seek to promote liberty, for those involved in struggles to achieve sexual and reproductive rights, and for those who work to challenge the heterosexism and homophobia so prevalent in Mexico, life is a constant struggle against the many-headed Hydra. In the absence of a modern-day Hercules, who but we ourselves can cut off the seven heads? For if we fail to do so, no one will.

Notes

1 The Partido Revolucionario Institucional (PRI) has held power in Mexico for more than 60 years.
2 Different kinds of oils are used. This practice is a major health risk and can lead to tissue damage or irreversible damage to vital organs such as the liver.
3 Garibaldi is a downtown park where people go to hear *Mariachis* (traditional music bands) play.
4 Named after Roche, the company that manufactures Rohinol.
5 Here Gerardo is speaking figuratively, since he is no longer directly involved in sex work himself.

6 *Chacales* are strong rough guys, from working-class backgrounds – construction workers, market porters, mechanics.
7 He is referring here to a beer factory. Corona is a well known Mexican beer.
8 When Juan was interviewed he took off his shirt. Later when the first author had gained his confidence he said, 'Yes I was hot, but the reason I took off my shirt was for you to see the merchandise.' By the end of the interview he was beginning to behave quite suggestively, implying that he would like to offer his services.
9 The baths concerned have been managed by the same man for many years. On his day off, they are managed by his assistant. This is important because the men who work there have the choice of working six days a week or one, since the manager is not happy for *masajistas* to come and go as they wish. On Tuesdays, his day off, the assistant accepts those who just want to work there for one day.

References

CARRIER, J. (1995) *De los Otros. Intimacy and homosexuality among Mexican men*, New York: Columbia University Press.

GÓMEZJARA, F. and BARRERA, E. (1978) *Sociología de la prostitución*, Mexico: Editorial Fontamara.

GUTMANN, M. (1996) *The meanings of Macho, Being a man in Mexico City*, Berkeley: University of California.

HERNÁNDEZ, J.J. (1997) Personal communication.

LA JORNADA (1995), 27 June.

LIGUORI, A.L. and ORTEGA, G. (1989) 'Vestidas y alborotadas', *Nexos*, **139**, pp. 55–6.

LIGUORI, A.L. and GONZÁLEZ BLOCK, M., with AGGLETON, P. (1996) 'Culture and sexual practices of construction workers in Mexico', in P. AGGLETON (Ed.) *Bisexualities and AIDS*, London: Taylor & Francis.

MATA (1997) Personal communication.

NAVARRO, J.C. (1993) 'Justicia sólo justicia', *Del Otro Lado*, 6, May, pp. 25–6.

PALACIOS-MARTÍNEZ, M., LUNA, M., RAMIREZ, O., RAMAH, M., VALDESPINO-GOMEZ, J.L. and SEPULVEDA-AMOR, J. (1992) 'Prostitución masculina en la ciudad de México', paper presented at the VII International Conference on AIDS, Amsterdam.

PRIEUR, A. (1994a) 'Power and pleasure: male homosexuality and the construction of masculinity in Mexico', paper presented at the 48th International Congress of Americanists, Uppsala, Sweden.

PRIEUR, A. (1994b) 'I am my own special creation: Mexican homosexual transvestites' construction of femininity', *Young-Nordic Journal of Youth Research*, **2**, 2, p. 16.

RONQUILLO, V. (1994) *La muerte viste de rosa*, Mexico: Ediciones Roca.

VALDESPINO, J.L., GARCIA-GARCIA, M.L., DEL RIO-ZOLEZZI, A., LOO-

MENDEZ, E., MAGIS-RODRIGUEZ, C. and SALCEDO-ALVAREZ, R.A. (1995) 'Epidemiología del SIDA/VIH en México; de 1983 a marzo de 1995', *Salud Pública de México*, **37**, 6, pp. 556–71.

ZAPATA, L. (1979) *El Vampiro de la Colonia Roma*, Mexico: Grijalbo.

Chapter 7

Three Decades of Male Sex Work in Santo Domingo

E. Antonio de Moya and Rafael García

This chapter examines changes in the social construction of male sex work in Santo Domingo over the past three decades. During this period, the population of the capital city of the Dominican Republic has grown from half a million to more than two million people. Vertical mobility and social anonymity have increased dramatically as a result of modernization, and poverty and unemployment have grown enormously. These factors, together with more lenient sexual attitudes, have created a favourable milieu for the development of male sex work. In this chapter we will look at the impact of HIV/AIDS on male sex work in Santo Domingo.

Social Context

The average age for sexual initiation among Dominican men is 13 years old, with a decreasing trend over time. On average, initiating partners are nine years older, regardless of gender (García *et al.*, 1992). By European cultural standards, many Dominican adolescents' sexual interactions with adults would probably be defined as sexual abuse, but this ethnocentric interpretation would be misleading. In Dominican culture, there is room for asymmetric age relations, as attested by the popular expression 'love has no age'.

De Moya and García (1996) have postulated the joint operation of phallicism and homophobia, which attract and repel men to and from each other in an approach–avoidance conflict. In the Dominican Republic, boys and teenagers have constantly to compete with each other to show who is more 'masculine'. This occurs mostly through comparisons of penis size, displays of courage and daring to break rules. This social construction of masculinity seems both to rank-order and seduce Dominican men.

The conflict between attraction to the phallus and aversion to the anal receptive role, is often resolved in the form of reciprocal oral sex for payment. This practice is less stigmatized, and is not necessarily taken as evidence of a homosexual orientation (Ruiz and Vásquez, 1993). Many young men occasionally engage in paid homosexual relations (for example insertive anal and/ or oral sex, or reciprocal oral sex) with older men. These do not directly threaten their self-definition as masculine, so long as strict role definition is preserved. If clients attempt to transgress this code, sex workers are expected to feel insulted (having been misperceived as 'gay') and to react aggressively.

By the age of 12 to 15, many lower-class and socially marginal boys have learned that for adults, sex has a cost and may be a way of generating income. They have also discovered that virginity and youth have near cult status, and that there is a relatively stable demand among adult men for occasional, non-committed sex (De Moya, 1989). However, while Dominican society seems to be quite tolerant of sex work, it is not so of sex workers (García and Renshaw, 1987).

Male adolescents frequently urge one another to demonstrate that they are not *pendejos* ('jerks' or 'chicken'). As grown-up men, they should be *tígueres* ('tigers') or slick, fearless and daring men. This implies showing an interest in money and not being afraid of other men (De Moya, 1989). The ultimate in *machista* cultural transgression is the *tíguere rapa tíguere* ('a tiger who takes [that is sodomizes] tigers'). Paradoxically, by having sex with receptive 'homosexual' men, some men are able to prove that they are not 'gay'. This culture paves the road for an engagement in homotropic sex work without having to self-identify as being homosexual. Payment becomes sufficient justification to de-stigmatize the behaviour.

Frías and Lara (1987), for example, found that 28 per cent of lower-class and 18 per cent of middle-class 17–28-year-old males in Santo Domingo reported having had sexual intercourse with other males. Two-thirds of them also reported having had intercourse with women. One-third of the lower-class and one-half of the middle-class respondents who had sex with men said they had charged their partners for this.

In contemporary Dominican society, there is a strong emphasis on the distinction between insertive and receptive men who have sex with men. The anal insertor is known as *bugarrón*. This term derives from the French word *bougre* ('bugger' in English), heretics of supposed Bulgarian origin who were said to practice 'sodomy' (see Boswell, 1981). In everyday usage, being a *bugarrón* is almost synonymous with being the insertive partner in paid homosexual relations. The overt, public motivation for this transaction is economic need, not choice or pleasure. Nonetheless, the *bugarrón* may also feel he has to earn his money by providing good quality sex to clients.

Three kinds of insertive sex workers are identifiable in Santo Domingo, although they usually do not look any different from other young lower-class and lower-middle-class men. First, there are the true *bugarrones*, men who are anal insertors with both men and women.[1] Second, there are *hombres normales* (normal men) or *machos*, who are vaginal insertors with women but anal insertors with men. Third, there are *sanky-pankies* (from hanky-pankies or *gigolos*) or young men who sell sex to both male and female tourists in beach towns (De Moya *et al.*, 1992; Tabet *et al.*, 1996).

An anally receptive man is derogatorily called a *pájaro* ('bird', 'queer') or *maricón* ('fag'), the antonym of *bugarrón*. These two words are not exclusive to receptive sex workers, as they are often applied to all men who are homosexual by choice. The latter are often the paying partners in homosexual relations. Many of the characteristics of the *berdache*[2] – or 'two-spirited person' – survive today in Dominican transvestites. De Moya and García (1996) have described two types of modern *berdaches* who sell sex. The first are the urban *travestis*, who are socially 'heterosexual' 'female' street sex workers in a few large cities, or female impersonators in night clubs who travel around the country. The second are the *masissís* ('sissies'), who are Haitian and Dominican–Haitian boys on sugar-cane plantations brought up as social, 'expensive' women, usually born with a 'mystery' and a 'sacred phallus'. Many of these modern *berdaches* are not exclusively receptive as might be expected. This seems to occur mostly because of the fascination that 'phallic women' create, and their readiness to provide satisfaction in either or both gender–sex roles.

Palomos or 'cock-pigeons' are 12–17-year-old homeless street boys, and constitute an in-between group. Most of them self-identify as *normal men*, and are induced by their peers to sell sex. Because of their scant negotiating power, they may be oral and/or anal insertors, receptors, or both, depending on clients' preferences and pay. After the age of 18, many *palomos* become *bugarrones*. From age 24 and over, they may become *maipiolos* (go-betweens) who will procure for younger sex workers (De Moya, 1989; Ruiz and Vásquez, 1993).

Research on Dominican Male Sex Workers

A small number of studies in the Dominican Republic have looked in detail at male sex workers. De Moya (1989) interviewed 30 homeless *palomos* aged 13 to 17 in sex territories (streets, parks, beaches) of Santo Domingo. Respondents were either illiterate or had at most four years of formal education. They generally began sexual intercourse at age 10 to 11 with their male and female peers. When having paid homosexual relations, they exhibit emotional detachment from clients, sharing with peers the financial gains, and spending money on girlfriends and female sex workers. When clients are not present, they may jokingly interact as 'fags' and compete at being 'feminine'. A clear power hierarchy is established between them and clients, based most usually on a masculine/feminine distinction.

Among such men, condom use is not perceived as necessary so long as the client is 'known, clean, and trusted'. Some of the men interviewed did not really understand the logic of using condoms in anal intercourse. They said they always used condoms when playing the insertive role with clients, but failed to do so when playing the receptive role. They believed that the penis 'sucks' HIV in through an assumed 'vacuum' produced at the moment of ejaculation, and did not understand the role of semen in HIV transmission.

A group of *sanky-pankies* who 'escorted' male and female tourists in a small beach-town were interviewed by De Moya, *et al.* (1992). Respondents' median age was 22, slightly older than other groups of sex workers, since tourist women rarely accept partners younger than 18 to 19. Their average schooling was fifth grade. While it was estimated that up to half of sanky-pankies used to have sexual relations with male tourists in the 1980s, by the 1990s the number has decreased to two in ten, largely because of homophobia reinforced by fear of AIDS. Men interviewed reported a median of 20 lifetime female tourist partners. Less than half stated they always used condoms. Reasons for not using condoms included drunkenness, desperation, liking the feeling of skin contact, trust, and 'love'.

Ramah, Pareja and Hasbún (1992) conducted interviews with 188 men who have sex with men, from the ages of 14 to 47 years, in five Dominican cities. Nearly two-thirds of respondents had had sex with women at some time in their lives. Those who had had sex with women also tended to be the insertive partners in their male-to-male behaviour. Forty-three per cent had received payment for sex. Those who had sold sex were predominantly of lower socio-economic status, had lower levels of education, were married, and had had more female partners in the past six months. They classified themselves as men who sold sex, and tended to have older, foreign and higher socio-economic clients.

Ruiz and Vásquez (1993) interviewed 76 *palomos* and *bugarrones* in Santo Domingo. Their median age was 18 years, and most had completed sixth grade at school. Those older than 24 years acted as *maipiolos* for younger ones, because of the reduction in demand with age. All reported having had vaginal intercourse, and 41 per cent had had anal intercourse with women, generally initiating these practices by age 11 to 13. Interviewees reported a median of 24 different female partners per year, 43 per cent had intercourse with female sex workers, and 26 per cent defined themselves as the *chulos* (pimps) of these women. In their last five insertive heterosexual relations, only 19 per cent said they had consistently used condoms, 40 per cent had used them inconsistently, and 41 per cent said they did not use them at all.

Homosexual relations were generally initiated around 14 to 15 years of age, mostly because of economic need (64 per cent). Having receptive anal and/or oral sex for pleasure was seen as a highly stigmatizing practice by nine of every 10 respondents. About a third did not regard these practices as a sexually identifying criterion, provided they got enough cash or gifts from clients. Insertive anal sex with men had been practised by 90 per cent of men interviewed, but only 39 per cent consistently used condoms. Nearly a third admitted they had practised receptive oral and/or anal sex for money, 33 per cent had practised oral sex for pleasure, and 12 per cent had practised receptive anal sex for pleasure. Only 1 per cent lived with a male lover.

The mean number of male clients was 36 per year. Almost all had had sex with foreign gay clients (called *nueves*, or 'nines'), whom they preferred because of the better pay and a sexual relationship regularly less threatening to their masculinity (that is, receptive oral sex and/or insertive anal sex). Half of them had foreign clients who periodically sent money from abroad or brought presents such as clothes, shoes or a Walkman, when coming to Santo Domingo for yearly vacations.

Silvestre, Rijo and Bogaert (1994) studied 412 12–17-year-old street and runaway children of both sexes, involved in sex work in five Dominican cities. The young men involved were unemployed and tended to hang around streets, parks and beaches, catering mostly to male clients. The origin of their involvement in sex work was attributed to extreme poverty. Age of initiation into sex work was 11 to 12 years, with a tendency to be lower in younger recruits. Younger adolescents (12–15-year-olds) tended to attract the oldest male clients. From 65 to 88 per cent of clients were foreign tourists. Only a third used condoms regularly when having sex with men.

Tabet *et al.* (1996) studied sexual behaviour and HIV risk factors in 354 men (13 years and older) who have sex with men in Santo Domingo. Consistent condom use was practised by only 25.6 per cent when having receptive sex, and 30.7 per cent when having insertive sex with men. HIV seroprevalence was 34.4 per cent among *travestis* and 11.7 per cent among 'gays'. HIV seroprevalence ranged from 6.1 to 8.2 per cent in *bugarrones, hombres normales* and *sanky-pankies.* Serologic evidence of syphilis, receptive anal intercourse with more than three partners in the last 12 months, and having visited or worked in local male brothels during the 1980s, were independently associated with HIV infection.

A re-analysis of these data (De Moya *et al.*, 1995) attempted to measure STD and HIV risk among male sex workers. A sub-sample of 254 participants who answered 'yes' to a question about whether they had asked other men for money or gifts in exchange for sex was selected for analysis. Twenty-four (9.5 per cent) self-identified as *travestis*, 48 (19 per cent) as 'gays', 20 (7.8 per cent) as *sanky-pankies*, 31 (12.0 per cent) as *bugarrones* and 131 (51.5 per cent) as *hombres normales.* Thirty-three per cent said they 'always' asked their sex partners for money or gifts, 17 per cent 'sometimes' asked for money or gifts, and 50 per cent never asked for money or gifts. Seventy-eight per cent of *bugarrones*, 75 per cent of *sanky-pankies*, 48 per cent of *hombres normales*, 46 per cent of *travestis* and 27 per cent of 'gays' received rewards of that kind and were defined for the purposes of the study as sex workers.

A significantly higher proportion of sex workers had had intercourse with women (90 per cent) than non-sex workers (78 per cent). Sixty-nine per cent of sex workers and 44 per cent of non-sex workers had penetrated at least one man in the last 12 months. A significantly lower proportion of sex workers engaged in receptive anal sex (13 per cent) than non-sex workers (32 per cent). Condom use at last intercourse was also more frequent among sex workers (57 per cent) than non-sex workers (32 per cent). The two groups did not significantly differ in their serology for syphilis, hepatitis B or HIV.

E. Antonio de Moya and Rafael García

The Evolution of Sex Work in Santo Domingo

Two main factors have impacted on the nature and form of male sex work in Santo Domingo over the last three decades: organized mass gay sex tourism and AIDS. In this section we will analyze some of the major events and responses during this period. The data reported on here were specially collected between October and December 1996 from informal conversations and in-depth interviews with key informants, such as sex workers of different ages and levels of experience, female partners, foreign and Dominican male clients, intermediaries (go-betweens), taxi drivers, employees, managers and neighbours of male brothels.

The First Decade (1970s): Rediscovering America

In the early 1970s, the Dominican Republic was in the process of recovery from a succession of social nightmares including a 31-year-old military dictatorship, civil war and two US military occupations in 50 years. These years saw a continuation of a five-century history of authoritarian rule aimed at forcing people to comply with, and privately accept, cultural patterns that clashed with their own belief systems. The result of this history are forms of social behaviour characterized by the public, verbal acceptance of an ideal set of standards and the private, behavioural transgression of that same ideology.

Historical records from the sixteenth century onwards suggest that bisexual and homosexual behaviour involving adolescent/adult partners was probably relatively common in the Spanish colony of Santo Domingo. Because of homophobia, most of these transgressive relations had to be clandestine, relatively impersonal and publicly denied (see Oviedo/Las Casas, 1988). It is not clear when adult men in the colony started paying poorer adolescent males for sex, but it is likely that up until 1844, when slavery was abolished, some masters used to have sexual relations with enslaved adolescent males. Many other teenage males were the children of enslaved women. Some of these females were the property of nuns' convents and their tasks included helping financially to sustain the whole religious community. One of the socially sanctioned activities such women performed in order to support the convents they worked in, was providing sex to male citizens (Deive, 1988). The enslaved children of these women were probably not infrequently raised in an environment tolerant of, or even promoting, sex for money. When slaves were no longer available, paid adolescent/adult homosexual encounters may then have become common.

The dictatorship of Rafael L. Trujillo (1930–61) did much to encourage widespread homophobia. In the 1970s, adult men were eager to state that there were three wrongs they would never do: kill a person, steal from somebody and have sexual relations with other men. By definition, it was impossible for a man to love another man. If he did, the mere feeling would defile and convert 'him' into a woman. In this sense, two males could have sexual intercourse, but one of them had to be 'the man', the dominant anal insertor, and the other had to be 'the woman', the subordinate anal receptor. There were no conceivable in-betweens. Extreme sex–gender role differences were incompatible, although complementary.

In lower-class sexual culture, such definitions were not only pervasive, but also allowed for teenage/adult sexual interaction. The presence of a 'homosexual' man with some power (political, economic, moral or religious) in a lower-class community not infrequently triggered the 'curiosity' of neighbouring youths. For them, his presence was an opportunity to obtain money or gifts, while proving to peers that they were the dominant 'male' partners in the relationship with a subordinate 'female'. Peer pressure and conformity often made it possible for whole networks of adolescents in a neighbourhood to have sexual relations with the same man. While money was a *sine qua non* condition for the relation, there was frequently some form of social education as well, as in more ancient forms of pederasty.

In the 1970s there were only 10 gay and bisexual zones (four parks and six lower-class, virtually clandestine discothèques) in Santo Domingo. Five of these were shared by *travestis* and *bugarrones*. Two other spots excluded *travestis*, and two excluded *bugarrones*. One excluded both groups. Virtually no foreign homosexual tourist visited these relatively hidden and 'dangerous' lower-class places.

The Second Decade (1980s): Strangers in Paradise

The international image of Santo Domingo as a newly discovered gay paradise was created early in the 1980s. In 1981–82, a small colony of foreign gay residents started opening accommodation and recreation facilities for an increasing number of middle- and older-age gay tourists from North America and Europe. These hotels and apartments were widely advertised at the time in gay magazines and travel guides. Exotic sexual pleasures were offered virtually free in an apparently idyllic environment. In this way, the Dominican Republic started to become a destination for international travel with sexual gratification as the central motivation. In the context of sex tourism, where natural beauty, extreme poverty and alcohol consumption usually coalesce, the dividing line between 'paid' and 'unpaid' sex is often blurred (Herold and van Kerkwijk, 1992).

In the first years of the decade, two three-star gay hotels opened in the commercial area of Colonial Santo Domingo. A few years later, four smaller gay hotels were added to the growing gay sex industry. Geographic proximity among establishments allowed sex workers to move between hotels and to other accessible gay territories in search of clients. In the space of a few years, organized gay sex tourism became quite widespread. The network of gay hotels linked Santo Domingo to two other beach towns in the southern and northern coasts. Port-au-Prince, the capital city of bordering Haiti, offered an additional dimension to the vacation adventure. Three-day round trips by plane to that city were regularly organized.

Groups of tourists escorted by friendly young sex workers travelled frequently to several of the largest Dominican cities. On the whole, interaction was limited to tourists and escorts. There seemed to be little communication between tourists and Dominican gays and *travestis*. The latter had traditionally played the role of 'lover-clients' of *bugarrones*, as they were largely responsible for initiating adolescents in sex work. Payment in this kind of relationship was more symbolic than real, since money served to show who was the 'dominant male' partner. Gays and *travestis* complained about the competition from foreigners, arguing that they 'spoiled' *bugarrones* by paying them more money than was culturally expected as 'help'. Nonetheless, both groups seemed largely to ignore each other, while sharing many gay and bisexual territories. No overt hostility or clash between them was reported.

According to key informants, during the early 1980s most tourists were interested in 12–17-year-old adolescents from poverty-stricken communities. Most of these teenagers used to work on the streets of the city, shining shoes or selling roasted peanuts. They were induced into male sex work mostly by a mixture of poverty and the desire for social recognition. They spoke only Spanish and communicated with most tourists largely by gesture. They stood in front of the existing gay hotels, waiting for clients. When tourists approached the front door, sex workers made non-verbal sexual signals to them. Sometimes there were fights among sex workers over competition for a client.

Payment for sex was understood by both partners as a necessary token of gratitude for the good time spent together, in the context of poverty and true financial need. It could take the form of a shirt, a pair of jeans, tennis shoes, a bottle of perfume, two or three dollars, or a night's entertainment (dining, drinking and dancing). Young sex workers did not usually charge money directly, but showed clients a pawnbroker's receipt, or asked for 'help'. When sex workers played the receptive anal role, payment was higher. Instances of sexual abuse frequently occurred. Some sex workers were also paid for performing in amateur pornographic videos.

In those naïve days, some young men used to introduce foreign clients as friends to their unsuspecting families. Some clients were said to spend fortunes, either on international telephone calls attempting to take teenagers back to their countries, or for the treatment of (sometimes invented) family diseases. A few were successfully adopted in Santo Domingo and taken to North America and Europe as 'lovers'. For many sex workers, the main motivation was migration rather than emotional involvement. These relationships were often difficult to sustain because of the couple's not infrequent asymmetry in age, language, socio-economic status, and lifestyle. Abroad, many remained as 'kept boys', frequently locked up in apartments because of jealousy or fear that they could run away. When they reached young adulthood, many adoptive 'son-lovers' did run away. Most stayed abroad illegally, some were deported and some have returned voluntarily.

The first cases of AIDS in Santo Domingo occurred in 1983. Around 70 per cent of cases between 1983 and 1986 were related to the gay sex industry. Not surprisingly, the first to die were some of the discoverers of the gay paradise. In spite of the initial international impact of AIDS, the gay tourist boom continued to grow until 1985–87. It started to decline around 1987–90, when the Ministry of Tourism closed all gay hotels and organized tours stopped coming to the country.

Despite the threat of AIDS, the apparent bonanza created by sex tourism brought important changes to the infrastructure of the local 'gay environment'. A concomitant boom occurred with transvestism, which became fashionable among those young lower-class gay adolescents who felt they were women. Small groups of seductive young female impersonators made their way through 'heterosexual' show business and television variety shows. An eager and incredulous audience attended their artistic presentations, often being puzzled and sometimes being tantalized. Quarrels between man and wife were frequent at their shows, as many men flirted with the unusually beautiful and mysterious 'phallic women'. Among the lower classes, a new cohort of adolescent *travestis* became visible in most gay discos, usually as impersonators of famous *vedettes* and singers.

At its height, 24 territories (four parks, one beach, three movie-houses, six hotels and 10 discothèques) were predominantly or exclusively occupied by gays and bisexuals in Santo Domingo, 14 more than in the previous decade. Sex workers were regularly present in 21 of these places, evincing how pervasive was their influence. Ten of these facilities were shared by both *travestis* and *bugarrones*. Thirteen additional gay spots included only one or other group: *travestis* were admitted in four, and *bugarrones* in nine.

During the ensuing years, male sex work started to come of age. A relatively large community of young adult sex workers (18–24-years-old, a few older) became the sexual supply for a large Dominican and foreign clientele. Sex workers usually described themselves as 'muscular working-class dark mulattos with large cocks who usually had sex with women'. The androphilic (adult oriented) image of the young black man as a sexual athlete, rather than the hebephilic (adolescent oriented) image of the more delicate adolescent, seemed to become the dominant aesthetics. Now sex workers could be found in every hotel (not only gay), discothèque and drinking place, waiting for the invitation of a gay tourist, rather than on streets. At times, the ratio of sex workers to tourists in gay territories was about two or three to one. Their main motivation for selling sex was money, gifts and the hope of travel and migration.

The growing clientele's age and gender–sex role preferences became more varied. This had implications for the level of risk that clients were willing to take. Sex workers became older, more professional, and were often vilified. Clients frequently demanded group sex and sadomasochistic activities. Some sex workers began to steal from over-confident clients. Although there was enough demand for both young and older sex workers, dominant ones soon started to gain control over foreign clients' access to minors. In this way they attempted to increase their income and to reduce competition from younger workers. In local neighbourhoods, they used to recruit lower- and lower-middle-class more inexperienced adolescent males willing to earn some money from gay tourists. About half of the cash these teenagers got had to be shared with intermediaries. After the age of 24, the chances of attracting clients were quite limited and they usually had to retire from the trade.

The Third Decade (1990s): The Hangover of AIDS

The impact of HIV/AIDS on individuals involved in the gay sex industry in Santo Domingo has been strong throughout the 1990s. Key informants knowledgable about the gay hotels that used to be open, provided information on 31 non-*travesti* sex workers and 13 foreign clients (both residents and tourists) who had died of this disease. Most interviewees believed that the impact had been most severe on sex workers and clients who were anally receptive, or who used to exchange receptive/insertive gender–sex roles. Links between some of the infections was assumed by members of the groups. Several female sexual partners and infants of these male sex workers had also died of AIDS.

Both AIDS and economic crisis have also had an impact on the structure of the gay environment of the city. For some gay residents, AIDS has dramatically changed the urban sex scene. Only about a third of the foreign clients who used to come now return each year. Relatively few foreign tourists visit gay bars and discothèques nowadays. Few young men enter into sex work as a result of fear of AIDS. *Bugarrones* became the focus of suspicion about HIV infection, and there has been a substantial reduction in local clients' demand for their services. Competition among sex workers is now more aggressive, since finding clients is increasingly difficult. The present ratio of sex workers to clients can be seven or eight to one in some gay bars. Muggings, violence associated with crack cocaine consumption, and minors' threats of scandals as a way to extort money from older tourists are frequently reported. Commercial sex in Santo Domingo is less naïve, but more unpredictable and violent.

In the late 1990s there are only 14 gay zones (four parks, one beach, two movie-houses, no hotel, four discothèques and three bars), ten less than in the 1980s. At least three bars and discothèque owners have been harassed in the last two or three years by the police. In parks, the beach and movie-houses, there are fewer gays or sex workers. Three discothèques maintain a relatively large clientele of young gay habitueés. A new upper-middle-class discothèque was opened in mid-1997.

Sex workers are present in 12 of these environments. Six of the spots are shared by both *travestis* and *bugarrones*. Two others only admit *travestis*, and four only admit *bugarrones*. The number of *travestis* has continued to grow, as many lower-class teenagers start cross-dressing at a younger age. They usually sell sex to insertive males over 30 years old, although they seem to prefer younger partners for lovers. Receptive oral sex is much more practised now, perhaps as a substitute for anal sex.

Palomos and lower-middle-class males are also sexually initiated at a young age. Some of these young men, who increasingly self-define as gay, are starting to solicit by 12 or 13 years of age in two or three sex territories. Brief incursions into sex work are occasionally made by a few young men, who are now approached mostly by *travestis*, with little outside competition from tourists. Sex worker/client reciprocal masturbation and oral sex have probably increased as alternatives to anal sex. The absence of a tradition of durable erotic relationships is still apparent. Few new or older *bugarrones* remain in the trade. The illusion of migration through adoption has been shattered. *Hombres normales* apparently keep having sex for money with other men, but usually on a less commercial and more intimate basis. Some restrict this interaction to married clients who are less likely to put strong sexual pressure on them and who provide financial 'help'. *Sanky-pankies* are now much more oriented towards female tourists in their work. There has been a dramatic reduction in the demand for 'casual' sex among Dominican gay and bisexual men, because of fear of HIV infection. With foreign tourists, sadomasochistic practices and group sex has also disappeared. Massage, froteurism, voyeurism and other 'safer sex' practices tend to substitute for anal sex.

Conclusions

Overall, the data described in this chapter suggest that exchanging sex for money or kind is an important part of the social construction of male homo-sexual relations in the Dominican Republic. Homotropic male sex work seems to be linked to local ideologies of masculinity and stereotypical gender-role relationships. Bisexual behaviour is more prevalent among professional and occasional sex workers than among non-sex workers. Continuing to have sexual relations with women helps dispel doubts about the masculinity of the men concerned. Condom use is significantly higher among professional and occasional sex workers than among non-sex workers, possibly because paid relations imply a lesser emotional and affective bond between the partners. Both the rejection of receptive anal sex and the more prevalent use of condoms seem to be strategies to countervail HIV infection.

In sum, the last three decades' changes in male sex work in Santo Domingo are suggestive of the continuance of a more ancient culture of paid male-to-male clandestine sexual relations, characterized by asymmetry in partners' age, social class and sexual preference. This pattern seems to be an adaptive social response of a phallicist and homophobic bisexual orientation to the challenges of a traditionally repressive society. The gay sex industry's successive expansion with sex tourism and constriction with the impact of HIV/AIDS appear to evince how pervasive is this mostly 'underground' culture, and how speedily it may react to environmental threats. In the meantime, perhaps as a consequence of AIDS, a more open sexual culture is perhaps arising.

Acknowledgement

We thank José Ernesto Vega for conducting many of the interviews described in this chapter.

Notes

1 Heterosexual anal intercourse is relatively rare and highly stigmatized in Dominican society. It is socially perceived as a sadomasochistic practice which is seen as evidence of a homosexual orientation on the part of the male partner.
2 'Kept boy' or 'male prostitute'.

References

BOSWELL, J. (1981) *Christianity, Social Tolerance, and Homosexuality*, Chicago: University of Chicago Press.
DEIVE, C.E. (1988) *La Mala Vida. Delincuencia y Picaresca en la Colonia Española de Santo Domingo*, Santo Domingo: Fundación Cultural Dominicana.
FRÍAS, M.M. and LARA, S.S. (1987) 'Actitudes y comportamiento sexual en hombres de 18–27 años en Santo Domingo', unpublished BA Thesis, Psychology Department, Universidad Autónoma de Santo Domingo.
GARCÍA, R. and RENSHAW, D. (1987) 'A contemporary prostitution accepting culture', *British Journal of Sexual Medicine*, **14**, 3, pp. 72–5.
GARCÍA, R., FADUL, R., DE MOYA, E.A., GÓMEZ, E. and HEROLD, E. (1992) *Conducta Sexual del Adolescente Dominicano*, Santo Domingo: Instituto de Sexualidad Humana, Universidad Autónoma de Santo Domingo.
HEROLD, E.S. and VAN KERKWIJK, C. (1992) 'AIDS and sex tourism', *AIDS and Society*, **4**, 1, pp. 1–11, October–November.
DE MOYA, E.A. (1989) 'La Alfombra de Guazábara o el Reino de los Desterrados', paper presented at the First Dominican Congress on Homeless Children, Santo Domingo.
DE MOYA, E.A. and GARCÍA, R. (1996) 'AIDS and the enigma of bisexuality in the Dominican Republic', in P. AGGLETON (Ed.) *Bisexualities and AIDS: International Perspectives*, London: Taylor & Francis.

DE MOYA, E.A., GARCÍA, R., FADUL, R. and HEROLD, E. (1992) 'Sosúa's sanky-pankies and female sex workers', unpublished manuscript, Instituto de Sexualidad Humana, Universidad Autónoma de Santo Domingo.

DE MOYA, E.A., TABET, S.R., KRONE, M.S., GARRIS, I. and ROSARIO, S. (1995) 'Catamitas y exoletos modernos en la República Dominicana', paper presented at the First Dominican Congress of Sex Workers, Santo Domingo.

OVIEDO/LAS CASAS (1988) *Crónicas Escogidas*, Santo Domingo: Ediciones de la Fundación Corripio.

RAMAH, M., PAREJA, R. and HASBÚN, J. (1992) *Dominican Republic: Lifestyles and Sexual Practices. Results of KABP Research Conducted Among Homosexual and Bisexual Men*, Santo Domingo: USAID/AIDSCAP.

RUIZ, C. and VÁSQUEZ, R.E. (1993) 'Características psicosociales y motivación para la prevención del SIDA en trabajadores sexuales homotrópicos', BA Thesis, Department of Psychology, Universidad Autónoma de Santo Domingo.

SILVESTRE, E., RIJO, J. and BOGAERT, H. (1994) *La neo-prostitución infantil en República Dominicana*, Santo Domingo: UNICEF/ONAPLAN.

TABET, S.R., DE MOYA, E.A., HOLMES, K.K., KRONE, M.R., ROSADO, M., BUTLER, M., GARRIS, I., THORMAN, M., CASTELLANOS, C., SWENSON, P.D. and RYAN, C.A. (1996) 'Sexual behaviors and risk factors for HIV infection among men who have sex with men in the Dominican Republic', *AIDS*, **10**, pp. 201–6.

Chapter 8

Cacherismo in a San José Brothel – Aspects of Male Sex Work in Costa Rica

Jacobo Schifter and Peter Aggleton[1]

Male sex work has a history as long as female sex work, and there is evidence of male Sumerians and Greeks selling sex to other men (Dover, 1978). However, female sex work has received more attention from researchers; so much so that as an institution, sex work is often viewed as a female occupation. In patriarchal societies, where service labour is largely undertaken by women, men who provide services to other men are often seen as doing female tasks (Carrier, 1985). Indeed, one of the characteristics most associated with femininity in Costa Rica is that of sexually servicing the man (Kashak and Sharrat, 1985). This is one reason why it is important to analyze the nature of male sex work, particularly that undertaken by men who see themselves as 'men' and who beyond the sex work context are largely heterosexual. This chapter focuses upon a group of such men working in a *casa* or brothel in San José, the capital city of Costa Rica. The aim is to offer insight into the self-understandings and social practices of such men, and the kinds of sexual culture that emerge in these conditions.

The focus here is on one form of male sex work, as practised in the mid-1990s in a specific setting. It should not be assumed that all male sex work in Costa Rica, or indeed even the majority of it, takes this form. A variety of different kinds of male sex work currently coexist within the country, and there is some fluidity between them. They include street-based work, work in public parks, the provision of sexual services through formal and informal networks and agencies, and the transgendered sex work undertaken by *travestis* who cater for a primarily heterosexual male clientele. Also important is the provision of sexual services by men to local women and to female tourists. None of these forms of sex work will be the focus in this chapter. Instead, we report on findings from recent fieldwork conducted as a prelude to a sexual health promotion intervention among young men working in a *casa* in an outlying neighbourhood of San José.

Methodology

A total of 25 young men aged from 15 to 17 were interviewed.[2] All worked in the same *casa* and most only went there at night to find clients. Two interviewers, both members of the Latin American Institute for Prevention and Health

Education (ILPES), conducted the interviews over a three-month period between January and March 1997. Each interview lasted about one hour and was conducted in private. Each participant was paid 5000 colones (about US$20) for their time. An open-question interview schedule was used. Questions focused on sexual initiation, self-definition, sexual orientation, love, drug use, sex work, family rules, and relationships with men and women. All the interviews were recorded, transcribed and coded so as to anonymize interviewees and the location. Analysis took place using a specialist database developed by ILPES.

Access was gained through the owner of the *casa* as part of work leading to the development of an HIV prevention and sexual health promotion project based in the brothel. In view of the fact that pandering is a serious crime in Costa Rica, and that many of the young men interviewed were under 18 years of age (the legal age for sexual consent), total confidentiality was promised and the names of interviewees have been changed.

Both interviewers were gay men, one of whom was a friend of the owner of the *casa*. The other was introduced as a gay researcher interested in writing an article on male sex work. The only condition requested by the owner was that interviews should be held in private. The fact that interviews were carried out by gay men should be taken into account when examining the responses. Had the interviewers been heterosexual men or women, it is possible that the respondents might have provided rather different answers to some of the questions asked.

The Importance of Profit

Research on male sex work in England, and elsewhere, has established that money is the main reason why some predominantly heterosexual men sell sex to other men (West, 1993). This was the dominant explanation given by the majority of the young men interviewed, although as we will see later, other factors can influence the decision to become involved in sex work. A charge ranging from 2000 colones (US$10) to 5000 colones (US$20) was made per act of sexual intercourse (depending on whether or not penetration occurs). Since the number of clients can vary between two and eight per day, the monthly income delivered by this kind of work varies from 80 000 to over half a million colones. Most possibly earn around 150 000 colones a month, a salary which is significantly higher than that of a university professor. Because most young men have not received much formal education, a clerical job such as that they might be likely to obtain, would provide only a quarter or a tenth of this.

Cacherismo

As in other contexts in Costa Rica, homosexual behaviour in the *casa* does not affect the sex worker's inherent heterosexuality, since men from the lower classes do not generally see homosexual behaviour as determining sexual orientation or identity (Schifter and Madrigal, 1996). Much more important are distinctions between activity and passivity, and between masculinity and femininity. For them, 'homosexuals' are those men who show the characteristics of the opposite gender, and who show their desire for other men. Male sex workers in the *casa* see themselves as *cacheros*[3] or 'men' whose public liaisons are with women and who display all the characteristics appropriate to their gender. Noé does not consider himself a homosexual because 'I am not attracted by men', Eric defines himself as '100 per cent for the vagina' and Julio feels heterosexual because he only feels attracted to women. Mario considers himself bisexual, but he defines this as being a man who likes to penetrate both men and women; for him, 'it is the same, having sex with a woman or with a man ... the bottom is what I like.'

According to Tío, being gay is 'feeling like a woman'. There are different degrees of gayness. The most extreme is the *loca* ('queen' in English) who is 'obsessed with being a woman', but for Tío being gay is not synonymous with being effeminate. What makes him different from gay men, however, is that he does not 'like other men': 'I do not turn to see them in the street, as others do.' Tomás agrees that cruising other men and rejecting women is what determines homosexuality.

These different perceptions of homosexuality are symptomatic of a particular gender dynamic. People are defined by a behaviour we will call *cacherismo* rather than by internal personalities or sexual practices. Being recognized as a *cachero* demands a power hierarchy in which, symbolically at least, the male sex worker remains in control. For such sex workers, homosexual practices do not make them gay, homosexual or bisexual, and although they use these words, the meanings they give them differ from those more commonly used.[4] As long as sexual desire continues to be shown towards the opposite sex and behaviour is masculine at all times, one is still a man.

The *casa* is located in a marginal area of San José where other sources of employment are scarce, and most adult men are unemployed. In this context, selling your body is one of the few ways of earning money and gaining the social prestige that comes with this. So long as gender conventions are preserved, male sex workers are largely accepted by the communities in which they live, where gender is defined primarily through strength and physicality rather than through supposedly different psychologies.

Male sex workers such as those described here are masculine, they play male sports like pool and soccer, they get married and they have children. They do not openly question the gender system. In this respect, it is interesting to observe how other customers of the pool halls nearby, aware of the fact that these youths work in the *casa*, do not discriminate against them or reject them as friends. This is not the same for the owner of the brothel, who is seen as a *loca* for being an exclusive and effeminate homosexual. He has not left his home for about seven years, and never talks to neighbours.

In order for *cacheros* not to be seen as homosexual or bisexual, they must differentiate themselves from their clients. This is achieved through dichotomizing sexual behaviours and life projects. If the *cachero* is character-ized by his youthfulness, focality (concentrating on a specific geographical or institutional area when working), masculinity, heterosexuality and dominance, the latter is typified by his passivity, homosexuality, old age, multifocality (going back and forth between gay and straight places), and submission to the *cachero*'s desires. These oppositions are not neutral: one has higher value than the other. *Cacheros*, according to the dominant discourse, are worth more than homosexuals.

Materialism

A young *cachero* has sex for money. José tells us that 'money is my only interest'. He is not interested in emotional relationships with men since, as his friend Arnoldo states, 'women are for that'. Neither would have sex with men if 'payment was not involved', a view also shared by Mono. None claimed to feel sexual attraction towards a man, even during their childhood. All of them had their first sexual experiences with women, and enjoy sexual relationships with them, not with other men. Clients, on the contrary, 'want to be told that they are interesting and attractive, but I do not care about them', says Alberto.

Focality versus Multifocality

Cacheros are unlikely to participate in the Costa Rican gay community. They stay away from homosexual bars, clubs, activities, organizations or gay gather-ing places for fear of being recognized or thought gay. José, for example, emphatically denies 'having put one foot in a gay bar'. Julio does not like to 'greet, recognize or meet clients outside the brothel'. If he is walking on the street and recognizes a client, he tries to ignore him. Vernol explains that he 'never greet[s] a *loca* in the street'. Miguel thinks that it is best not to be seen in any homosexual place because 'they themselves [gay men] begin gossiping with others'. Leo told us that when he sees a client, he 'crosses the street and pretends not to see him'. For those interviewed, socializing outside the brothel means homosexualizing themselves. 'My mother knows that I work in the *casa*', says Rodrigo, 'but she does not like me to go to gay parties because I will become like them.' Nevertheless, some of the men do visit private apartments or houses. Once the client has given a phone number, they can make dates, but only if the visit is to a private place and in the context of sex work.

Temporality

The type of *cacherismo* displayed by the young men interviewed is an activity of youth, and is usually short-lived. Once the individual gets married, has children or leaves sex work, few would label him bisexual or homosexual.

There are no male sex workers over the age of 25 in the *casa* and it is expected that only a few years will be spent in sex work. Thousands of now mature men may therefore have been involved earlier in this kind of sex work without anyone having the slightest idea. Mono feels that 'at 25, I am already considered a veteran'. Arnoldo thinks that his work 'is temporary. One can never be old and a prostitute.' Carlos knows many men who used to work in the house, but who have now totally 'abandoned this work'.

As if to demonstrate the transitory nature of their work, many of the young men have girlfriends, have lived with a woman or are already married. Most have more than one child. Only one of them admitted to not having an ongoing relationship with a woman, though he too has occasional sexual relationships with women. Many of their female partners know about the work they do, or at least suspect it. Noé admits having told his wife what he does to avoid 'somebody else coming and telling her'. Rodrigo's mother knows her son is a *cachero*, and she laughs about it, although she wants him to marry. Mono's girlfriend waits for him in the pool hall next to the brothel. As he explains, 'She knows that I do this for money and that I am not being unfaithful.' Whether women know about the activity or not, *cacheros* make it clear that they have female partners. 'I cuddle my girlfriend near the pool so that my friends see me and know that I am not gay', says Tomás.

Indifference

When they walk into the brothel, *cacheros* sit down and talk, and casually greet the customers. An understood behaviour is not to show a preference for any of them. When Tío was asked if he was attracted to any particular client he answered with a definite 'No.' Erick told us that the client is the one who chooses, 'I do not choose.' Rodrigo thinks the same: having sex with 'old, fat, bald, or ugly clients, does not matter to me'. Noé likes to penetrate his clients anally: 'I stick it in anyone who gives his ass to me.' Tomás does not have any problem when having oral sex: 'As long as they don't bite my dick, any sucking is good.' Arnoldo tells us that he does not reject any of the customers: 'Money is money.'

When a preference for a special client is felt, the desire is usually repressed. Julio tells us that there are times when 'I like a client more than another . . . but I try to avoid this'. When he was asked why, he said 'I was afraid of liking him.' The same thing is true of Miguel, who confesses that he has never liked men, but with this kind of life he is afraid of 'homosexualizing myself' since sex work becomes habitual and 'one could get to like it'.

Older Men

Most of the interviewees admit to preferring men over 40 years of age. In principle, this may be logical since these are the ones with more money, and many of them have the greatest need to pay for sex. While some younger gay and bisexual men visit the brothel, workers reported rejecting them. Jorge told us 'I don't like youngsters, I could not have sex with them.' Vernol said that 'The young guys that come here are too effeminate; they are young *locas* that demand too much and want to be treated as women.' Sex workers feel that by having sex with men of their own age they are 'homosexualizing' themselves. Although the young client also pays, his youthfulness blurs the boundary between sex work and homosexuality. In order to be a *cachero*, there has to be a hierarchy with visible power differences. An older man has less power because he has lost his youth and 'has to pay', says Herson. Between two young men, this kind of difference does not exist.

Sexual Practices

There was no consensus among interviewees regarding the practices that were possible, and those that were not. Most claimed that they never allow themselves to be fucked, and that this is what differentiates them from their clients. Vernol stated he had 'a huge dick' and that clients would 'die' for him to fuck them, or 'let them suck me'. 'Few of them can take me, and sometimes I spend half an hour trying to shove it in. But when I get it in, they cry with happiness ... They need to be very *macho* to endure such a big dick. I couldn't.' Tomás also considers that he is a man because 'I don't give my butt to any gay. If they want a dick, they can get it all. It is gross for me to suck, and I would never let them fuck me.' Mono thinks in a similar way. 'Homosexuals', he says 'like anal sex. Not me, never.'

Another illustration of power differentials in the sex work context links to violence and cruelty. Some workers said they enjoyed hitting and hurting clients, humiliating them in many ways. Vernol likes to slap his clients when he fucks them. Bryan makes his customers suck him, scratches their backs, and when least expected, 'I hit them with a whip'. Rodrigo forces customers to beg him to touch them.

Cacheros rarely admit to participating in oral sex. Most of them say that it is their clients' desire to fellate them that helps them have an erection. The *casa*'s owner said that in his experience what 'hooks' some otherwise heterosexual men on male sex work is the quality of oral sex that clients provide. 'Women do not know how to suck, and the youngsters go crazy with the clients' expertise on this field', he said.

Kissing is out of the question. Noé says that he 'feels like vomiting when he has to kiss a client'. Miguel says he never kisses a client on the mouth. 'I let them kiss my neck or my legs, but never my mouth.' Herson says the same: 'I'm not the kind who likes kissing a man.' Semen, however, is less of a problem. Since masturbation is a very common practice, sex workers do not worry about getting semen on their hands, or wiping away a client's semen. Neither does it bother them to ejaculate in a client's mouth. Interviewees reported generally using condoms with their clients. Most said that they would never have penetrative sex without one. This was not the case with female partners or wives. 'I never use the condom with my wife. She does not know what I do in the street, and it would worry her', says Marco. The same thing is true for Mono: 'My lover is very hot, and so am I. Sometimes I come from fucking three men and she wants sex. She does not like me to stick it with the condom. She says she likes the shape of my dick.'

There are other differences, too, when having sex with women. With a girl, says Miguel, 'one is more tender and delicate'. Noé feels that women 'only want men to fuck them in the vagina, and they do not like anything else'. Vernol agreed: 'Only once did I fuck my girlfriend up the ass. She said that she wanted to know how homosexuals had sex. But she never let me do it again . . . she said it was not natural.' Arnoldo had asked his girlfriend to let him do it, 'but she said it is not normal'.

Oral sex was not very common with women either. Few of the interviewees said that their female partners fellated them. 'Women do not know how to suck', said Miguel. Rodrigo agreed that women do not 'have experience'. Yet, the *cacheros* did not have any problem giving oral sex to their female partners. Julio says that he likes to suck his girlfriend's cunt and 'to lick it all'. He would never do this with a client. The same was true of Vernol, who uses his tongue 'before sticking my cock in. When she screams that she wants it . . . then the whole thing goes in.'

It was not only sexual practices that differentiate relations with clients from relations with girlfriends and wives. Language (or lack of it) is also important. Paid sex normally occurs in silence. 'I do not like to talk because I lose concentration', said Augusto. César believed that if clients ask him to say nice things to them, his erection will 'go down' immediately. Vernol does not want 'to hear anything from the client'. This is especially true if the client 'is effeminate because [then] I feel I am with a woman'. Tomás finds that he likes to tell 'dirty things' to women, but 'not to my clients'. Rodrigo confesses that he prefers 'not to say a single word after agreeing the price'. For a *cachero*, talking with clients while having sex is either an obstacle to fantasizing about women, or an intolerable emotional bond.

Contradictions

A series of factors work against *cacherismo*. These threaten the self-definition of *cacheros*, and the social relations that distinguish sex workers and clients.

Pleasure

Theoretically, sex workers seek only money in their relations with clients. In order to have an erection with a man, most of them said that they closed their eyes and fantasized about having sex with a woman. Herson says he imagines he is with a woman and concentrates on this. Otherwise 'everything is a disaster'. In spite of these difficulties, some have learned to enjoy sex with men and to change their way of thinking. One of these was Noé, an attractive bricklayer and soccer referee. He says that he began because 'a friend invited me to come to the *casa.*' Never before had he 'even thought of making it with a man'. Although the first time he had sex with a man he felt 'dirty and ashamed', little by little he has changed his way of thinking. 'I have to be honest with you. There is nothing so delicious as to stick your dick into a butt. When women lubricate, they open so much that you don't feel anything, while a butt gets tighter and it feels more.' Mono agreed with this by saying that in some ways homosexual sex is more enjoyable. 'Women are like an endless hole, while there are men that are so closed that one can come much better.' Carlos believed the same: 'I do not feel any attraction towards men, but it is true that one feels better, physically speaking, fucking a man than a woman.'

Oral sex is also a source of enjoyment. The fact that girlfriends, wives or lovers do not want to practise it, make some sex workers enjoy it more with their clients. Some of them feel so randy that when no clients show up, as was the case for Marco, 'I jerk off thinking about the way this client usually sucks.' Others reported sometimes fellating one another when no customers show up, because 'you begin to miss it'.

Pleasure therefore poses a major threat to a predominantly heterosexual identity. Rodrigo stated that he has come to like sex with some clients so much that he is becoming homosexual. Carlos also admitted to something of a crisis because now he does not enjoy sex with his wife as he did before. Tomás has cut down having sex with women since he got into 'orgies with men. Imagine having someone sucking you in the front and in the back, and another one pinching you all over your body.' And Miguel thinks that sex work has made 'the gay [that all] men have inside' come out.

Vernol's relations with men had put him into situations where the line between heterosexuality and homosexuality was blurred. He described having been invited back by one gay man, and to his surprise, the man had also invited a lesbian friend and her partner. The 'more feminine' lesbian took off her bra and jumped into bed. His client asked Vernol to fuck her while the more masculine lesbian 'wanted to fuck me with a vibrator'. 'I refused this', he said 'but I had to fuck the prettiest dyke first and then the other one let me do it to her too. I took turns with one or the other while the guy was waiting for me to fuck him, and only come in him.' Vernol recalled having had 'a great time, it was crazy sex that night. I don't even know who was taking me.' 'I hope this does not mean that I will become gay', he concluded. But these orgies 'confuse me'.

Money and Drugs

Another factor that threatens *cacherismo* is an over-dependence on the money that sex work can bring. Many young men confessed that they did not know what they spent their money on, and that it was like a drug for them. Ricardo said 'I get sexually excited just by thinking about the five-thousand colones bill that I will earn.' Julio said that he never thinks a man with money is ugly, the 'money makes them look more attractive'. Mono admits that he earns hundreds of thousands of colones, but he loses it as quickly on gambling, which is one of his weaknesses. Arnoldo confesses that he never has enough money to buy the things he likes, and buying those things is 'as delicious or more delicious than sex. When I buy a shirt I like, it's really pleasurable.' Noé did not know where he had spent all the money he had earned: 'It's like water, it goes out of my hands without my even realizing it.'

Money can also be used to buy alcohol and other drugs. Only one interviewee stated that he had never taken crack. Most smoked marijuana and drank a lot of alcohol. Arnoldo admitted having sold his mother's clothes in order to buy crack. Mono said that the first thing that came to his mind when he was paid for the interview was to go and 'smoke the money'. Noé said the same, and added that he cannot quit. He took the food away from his children 'to buy drugs'. Herson believed that he was not totally hooked by crack, though he knows he 'cannot quit'. Rodrigo believed that he 'was not going to be trapped', but 'I am already into it'.

The need to buy drugs can result in *cacheros* providing sexual services that run contrary to their self-identities. Noé is aware that because of drugs, 'he has given his butt and [even] lived with a man'. Augusto admitted the same thing: '[sometimes] I need drugs so much, that I do whatever is necessary, even suck and let myself be fucked by a man.' Arnoldo said he has not gone into that yet, but he knows that 'many of them give their butts in order to buy drugs'. Mono laughed about one of his workmates who got involved with a client that only likes to penetrate. He got 'ten thousand colones he would not have earned if he didn't let the guy fuck him'.

Some *cacheros* establish relationships with gay men in order to have a better life or to buy drugs. Tomás said that he once went to live with a man in order to have the luxury he wanted. 'People began to call me gay, and to say that I had become a *loca*, but as they are not giving me any economic support, I do not care.' Rodrigo felt the same: 'I want to stop being poor and I want to have what I desire. If a guy comes and gives that to me, I am willing to go and live with him.'

A need for money and drugs therefore changes the sexual geography of *cacherismo* and its temporality. Some young men begin to work in gay saunas to earn more money; others go to parks and even to gay bars to hook someone. A few establish more lasting relationships with regular clients, and some may divorce and abandon their children.

Romantic Love

The dividing line between homosexuality and *cacherismo* is romantic love. *Cacheros* should not love their clients, nor should they establish emotional relationships with them. Relationships should be seen, by clients and friends, as a business in which one party sells and the other one buys. Yet, there is evidence that popular sector discourses of sex and sexuality are becoming more flexible in their treatment of love between men.

In popular and marginal sectors in Costa Rica, love is generally expressed by the things that one person is willing to do for another. The idea that two people in love have some kind of psychological bond or more 'profound communication' belongs to the middle rather than the lower classes. The belief that men and women are psychologically different is also more common among the middle classes. For poorer people, men and women simply *do* different things at home and at work, they do not have different psychological 'mentalities'. Both have to find ways to survive in a world of scarcity, and that is why their bodies, not their minds, have to find ways to do so. Love is expressed through the care they show for each other (Schifter, 1989).

But love is also something of a drug, justifying anything that is done on its behalf, including choosing the wrong gender (Scott, 1978). Jorge considers that love is 'the most wonderful thing on earth', a 'crazy thing where you lose control and do not care who you get involved with'. When he is asked about how he realizes that he loves another person, he says that he feels 'passion', 'obsession' and that he 'cannot stop thinking about her and doing things for her'. Alberto agrees that love erases any 'loneliness' and 'forgives' any failure. Arnoldo believes that when one is in love, one 'does things that one would not do otherwise'. Mono believes that love 'overcomes any obstacle', and forgives 'any fall'. When one loves, he says, 'one forgives anything and one can even fall in love with another man'.

When respondents were asked how they express their love, the answer was clear: through the things they *did* for the other person. Arnoldo buys chocolates for his girlfriend. Noé cuddles and caresses his wife. José cleans the house to show his lover that he loves her. Augusto goes to the supermarket 'every once in a while'. Pedro brings his wife a cup of coffee. Vernol does it through sex: 'I show her that I love her with good sex.'

When passion is over, a relationship begins. Passion is substituted by caring for each other (Johnson, 1983). In the case of the *cacheros* who are used to experiencing love through the care that two people give one another, and less through communication about intimate issues or traumas, Hollywood style, it is not difficult to fall in love with another man for whom they do not feel any passion.

Tomás is aware of this when he told us that the man who supports him treated him 'so well and with so much tenderness' that he is 'enchanted' by this relationship. The same happened to Rodrigo who felt like 'dying' when a client who supported him abandoned him to go with another man. Noé has lived with another man for seven years, and when he was asked if he loved this man, he said 'Yes.' Jeffrey confessed that he could fall in love with a man 'that would be willing to give me good clothing and other kinds of things'.

Because *cacheros* belong to a social class in which love is not character-ized by psychological complementarity, they are more vulnerable to falling in love with someone who helps them survive and cope with the 'burden of life', as Marco put it, whether this person is a man or a woman. When a client appears who can establish a relationship with one of these men, this is when *cacherismo* receives its worse threat, and this is when the dividing line between sex as a business and homosexuality vanishes completely.

AIDS

Cacheros are very aware of AIDS. When they were asked about sources of transmission, they all replied that anal sex without a condom posed the great-est risk. They also showed sophistication in pointing to the lack of consensus among scientists about the dangers of oral sex, and of passivity versus activity in anal sex. Greater awareness about AIDS was shared by clients, some of whom have changed their 'likes', as Noé says. As a result, active anal sex seemed less in demand: 'Most clients only want us to "jack them off"', accord-ing to Arnoldo.

One of the impacts of AIDS has been an apparent homogenization of sexual practice between *cacheros* and clients. 'Nowadays, with all this mastur-bation it is not possible to tell who is active or passive', says Luis. 'Before, the *cachero*', says Noé, 'was the one who fucked a gay man, but now, . . . I don't know.' A few *cacheros* feel that their active role is evaporating: 'I like to fuck, but I do not do it here very often because I am afraid of transmitting a disease to my wife', says Marco. 'The truth is that you do not know who is active and who is passive anymore', he concludes. There is generally less demand for anal sex, but the decrease in demand has been greater with regard to passive (receptive) than active (insertive) sex (because clients think the latter is safer), and some clients try to take sex workers away from the brothel to live with them so as 'to have only one person fucking them', says Vernol. A few clients are willing to pay more in order to have the 'safety of having a loyal partner', he says. They ask for AIDS tests, or for the man to go and live with them, in order to 'be safe', says Tomás. The chance of finding an older man who will pay for their studies, support them, give them lodging and friendship has increased. José described a friend, Esteban, who met an American who 'took him to Miami and now he comes back with a lot of money and [is] living a great life'. Augusto was economically supported by a 'gay' who gave him a 'life of a king' in exchange for sex: 'My partner does not care if I have sex with my girlfriend, he just prohibits me from having sex with other men.'

This new demand for more permanent relationships has a great impact on the *cacheros*. Some try to fool their neighbours by saying, as Alberto did, 'I live with my uncle.' Others continued to live with women in order to hide their male lovers. Most problematic of all is the fact that their relationships with men take them out of their communities, expose them to be seen by others, involve them in the gay community and turn them into 'homosexuals', the *cachero*'s most feared stigma.

Lila

One of the most important actors in the *casa* is its owner, an effeminate gay man of about 50 years of age, who has been in jail for prostitution. Lila, as he is known in the brothel, lives off prostitution. For every sexual relation in the *casa*, he charges 1000 to 2000 colones for the room. For years, his business has been to recruit young men from the streets, pool halls, parks, toilets and amusement parks. Now he does not go out, and young men are brought by their friends or by clients needing a place to have sex.

Recruitment is based on physical beauty. Lila does not look for any signal that the boy is interested in sex work. He invites him to the *casa* (or the boy is brought by others) and 'tests' him to see what shape he is in. Clients prefer youngsters with big penises, but this is not the only criterion for acceptance. Some are extremely beautiful and this is enough. Recruitment takes place primarily from areas where the population has more Spanish than *mestizo* characteristics since, in Lila's view, boys from very marginal areas, with many Central American immigrants, are not attractive to his clients. Young men are recruited at varying ages. Tomás, for example, was taken to the brothel by a friend when he was only 10 years old. Lila taught him oral sex and kept him doing this until he turned 14, when he began to penetrate his clients. Mono arrived there at 14 years, and has stayed for almost seven years. Others work part-time while they are still living with their parents and other relatives. There are some mothers, like Rodrigo's, who take the boys to the brothel, and there are also brothers who recruit one another.

The young boy arrives without really knowing what will happen. The first sexual experience with a man may be shocking, but none of them said that it had been a trauma. In many cases, the reason given for this was their prior heterosexual initiation. When asked to talk about their first sexual experience, most reported it as having been with a much older woman. Mono, for example, was seduced by a cousin who was 20 years older than him. The same thing had happened to Noé, whose first experience was with a female friend of his mother. He was only 13, and the woman invited him to have some coffee, and after some time, 'she took off the dress and asked me to go down on her and suck her'. Herson was initiated at the age of 11 by a 15-year-old. She invited him to her house and 'took off her clothes'. For him, the experience was a surprise because 'I did not know what a vagina was.' Nevertheless, they had sex and continued to do so for several years. Carlos was initiated by a sex worker who was much older than he was. His friends took him to see her practically by force when he was 12 years old.

If we compare these sexual experiences with those Lila promotes, we do not see a great difference, apart from the gender of the initiators. Many of these young men, according to some 'modern' criteria, were sexually abused, both by men and women. They were initiated into sex at a very early age by tricks and false means. However, from the interviews, it cannot be inferred that there is any lasting hostility towards the men or the women who abused them. The fear they felt, and even their shock at seeing sexual organs they had never seen before, is recognized. Yet, there is no personal recognition of abuse. When past events were talked about, they were related in such a way as to suggest that respondents were recalling the best times of their lives.

This could explain why so few show any resentment about Lila having introduced them to sex work. Contrary to expectation, there were no feelings of revulsion towards him. Instead, there was much apparent gratitude because of the protection offered, the fact that he lends them money and allows them to stay in his house when they are kicked out of their homes. 'For me, Lila is like a mother', said Mono. 'I did not have anywhere to live, and Lila gave me a home for seven years.' Herson feels the same: 'I never knew my parents because I was raised by my grandparents. Lila has been my father and my mother.' Others who have never lived with Lila also feel love for him: 'That *loca* is the only person I can count on when I need help.' The young men were also aware that Lila does not like them to do drugs. He does not provide them and only tolerates them because 'I cannot do anything to stop them.'

Since Lila is like a father-mother for those *cacheros* who do not have support at home and/or who come from poor families, some start to see homosexuality in a favourable way. A few, like Noé, see homosexuals as hard-working and creative. Mono does not like *locas*, but feels accepting towards more masculine gays, and he considers them 'my friends'. Rodrigo says that he cannot stand people mocking gays: 'I tell them that one should not talk bad about anyone because one never knows what could be his punishment.' The relatively cordial environment of the *casa* facilitates a degree of intimacy between *cacheros* and clients. In contrast to saunas in Costa Rica where sex workers rarely talk to their clients before or after sex, Lila's house is a place where jokes are told and where both minorities share their common problems. 'I have been impressed by hearing what gays have to undergo just because they were effeminate when they were children. I never imagined such a big pressure', states Mono. The living room in the brothel, in contrast to the rooms where sexual relations are held, is a space for conversation and relaxation within the prevailing culture of *cacherismo*.

Compartmentalization

One of the things that immediately attracts attention on entering the *casa* is its dirtiness. Lila breeds dogs, and as he does not have a backyard the smell and the excrement are too strong to ignore. The *cacheros* are aware that the place is not attractive and that as a result they lose clients. Yet, they step on the excrement as if it does not exist. This may lead us to think that the boys are dirty, but they are not; they are both well-dressed and attractive. Their indifference towards the excrement is a symptom of something beyond carelessness, which we will call compartmentalization.

When the interview transcripts were read, and what the boys said was compared with what they did, it was tempting to conclude that they were lying. There is evidence, for example, that their sexual practices are very different from those dictated by the dominant discourse of *cacherismo*. A substantial number of respondents practised both insertive and receptive sex. Very few said they enjoyed the latter, but those who were more honest recognized that only a few who work in the *casa* 'do not give their butt'. That is why the statement that *cacheros* are only active is untrue. The need for money, drugs or even love, leads to all kinds of practices and risks.

It is evident that condoms are not always used in the brothel. Lila does not provide the boys with condoms, and use is inconsistent. Few condoms were evident in the rooms or in the garbage cans. Some interviewees said they used them, but others did not. Others admitted that either they, or their clients, do not like to use them.

Some of the sex workers also had serious problems with crack use. It was not accurate, as some said, that they can control their drug consumption and that they do not steal or commit crimes. When the information Lila provided was compared with that from *cacheros* themselves, it became clear that many of the latter had already had problems with the law, and some had been in jail.

These, and many other narratives, could be considered 'lies'. José tells us that he has only had sex with three men in all his life, whereas Lila says that this is his daily score. Mono told us that he was 23 years old one day, 25 the next and 27 the next. Noé says he has never been penetrated, but other clients say he has. Instead of analyzing these narratives as 'lies', it is better to see them as compartmentalizations, that is, different ways of viewing things that are established when there is no possibility of living otherwise with conflicts and contradicting pressures.

Cacheros such as those described here, have learned a discourse that protects them, in theory, from being stigmatized as homosexuals. The rules of the game in this discourse are known and supported by them. But social pressures often sabotage these norms. The line that divides sexual commerce from homosexuality is very thin. That is why, in order to remain perceived as *cacheros*, they have to separate off the contradictions and exceptions to the rules. This is what compartmentalization achieves, a set of mental 'compartments' that do not link easily to one another.

The young men know very well that when they go through the door of the brothel they 'are transformed into another thing', says Arnoldo. This means that they have to be very different in the street from what they are in the *casa*. In the brothel, they are men who have sex with men; in the street, they are lovers, boyfriends, and fathers. Jorge feels that 'I have several personalities; there are many Jorges out there.' Miguel does not understand 'why I am one thing in my home, and another in the street'. Carlos knows that 'nobody really knows who I am, not even my wife'.

The effects of compartmentalization are also reflected in language. *Cacheros* talk one language in the brothel, and another one outside. Rodrigo says that inside, they speak in a 'more feminine' way. This means that they can talk about emotional things that they would never discuss in the pool hall. They like to imitate Lila, and 'move' like *locas*. In the street, says Vernol, 'one walks more like a *macho*, speaks tougher, does not accept anything from anybody'.

Cacherismo and Compartmentalization

While it is impossible to know where *cacherismo* originated, it has long existed in Costa Rica. It still exists in jails and agricultural zones where women are largely absent, and almost certainly predates urbanization and industrialization. Lila is over 50 years old and remembers that he had relationships with *cacheros* when he was a boy. Prior to the Second World War, Costa Rica was a small, agricultural and poor country. Men had to marry and support their families and women were supposed to be virgins until they got married. It took time to achieve the independence from home to get married. Marital postponement could have been one factor motivating sexual practice among men. The *cachero* institution may have emerged so that men could have sexual experiences with other men without being perceived as homosexual. Nevertheless, factors such as the ones described in the interviews are beginning to challenge the dominance of this discourse. Increasingly, the *cacheros* are facing an identity crisis.

HIV Prevention

The young men interviewed have good knowledge of AIDS prevention and safer sex. All were aware of the dangers of AIDS and the need to use condoms. Some also knew friends who had died of AIDS. Nevertheless, condoms are not always used and AIDS remained a distant threat. 'There are [more everyday] problems of survival that concern me', said Miguel, and 'AIDS is not the major one. I need to eat first.' It was not Lila's worst fear either: 'I am always afraid of the police and of spending my last days in prison.' When asked why he did not provide condoms, he replied: 'Well, clients do not like them. If they did, they would bring them. I only charge for the room and cannot afford to lose clients over this.'

As a non-governmental organization working in the field of sexual and reproductive health, ILPES had a moral responsibility to do something about HIV infection. One possibility might have been to inform the police. This would have had little impact since there are several other *casas* in San José where these young men could go. Even if all of these could be closed, many young men would turn to the streets and disappear from sight.

Since we were not going to wait for Lila or the young men to change their minds about the use of condoms, ILPES opted to provide them for free. Lila agreed to give one to each worker each time he had sex with a client. Condoms started being used more frequently. 'If there is a condom available, I insist on using it with everyone', said Enrique. 'Now that Lila gives me a condom, I use it when I fuck a client', said Luis. Notwithstanding this success, not all *cacheros* protect themselves. Mono recognizes that some clients do not like them and that it takes too much time to convince them. 'I can negotiate, but many of the young boys here can hardly talk', he said.

Several factors are directly relevant to the use of condoms in the *casa*. Crack and alcohol use is one of them. Some *cacheros* lose their capacity to communicate and negotiate when they are under the influence. 'Yesterday I smoked so much crack that I don't remember anything I did. I could have had sex with four clients but I don't recall anything', says Mario. Mono recognizes that he will now do 'anything for 5000 colones to buy crack'. Another barrier to condom use is intimacy. *Cacheros* distinguish between paid and romantic sex by whether or not a condom is used. Some men are willing to protect themselves with clients, but not with male or female lovers. 'When I am in love with a woman, I never use a condom. I must express I trust her', Enrique told us. 'If a man supports me and loves me, I show him my love and confidence. He expects me to protect him by having sex only with him', argues David. Love is then expressed through trust, fidelity and lack of protection.

Lack of solidarity is a further obstacle. *Cacheros* do not see each other as members of an organized community. 'Here everyone is on his own,' remarked Luis. Mono thinks that everyone is a potential competitor. Carlos believes that 'If there were not those who would give in to having sex without a condom, we could force clients to use them. But I get very upset when I know that such and such gave in to being fucked without a condom.' Arnoldo also thinks that those sex workers who have sex without a condom 'force us to do the same'.

Compartmentalization also affects the capacity to practize safer sex. The fact that some of the boys live in different 'worlds' which demand contradictory behaviours makes them especially vulnerable to the unintended effects of some national AIDS efforts. The national AIDS campaign in Costa Rica, for example, has targeted mainly heterosexuals by promoting fidelity and marriage. The gay community's campaign, on the other hand, has emphasized condom use. No one has addressed issues of prevention in the context of male sex work. When these young men learn about AIDS, they do so in the context of *either* heterosexuality or homosexuality, and not from a *cachero* perspective. As a result, they use different messages in different contexts. Mario, for example, uses condoms when having sex with men, but when engaging in heterosexual relations 'I don't use condoms. I follow the message of fidelity.' Carlos does the same: 'I am faithful to my girlfriend. I don't have sex with other women. I don't need to protect myself.' Preventive behaviour obeys the same compartmentalization that rules their lives.

One possible solution to these challenges lies in breaking down some of the mental 'compartments' through which *cacheros* live their lives. Perhaps this can be achieved through the kind of community-building strategy that is now underway. With the support of the Embassy of the Netherlands in Costa Rica, ILPES is working to establish a local pool hall for *cacheros* to meet in, hang out, and learn more about health issues. It is intended to recruit old *cacheros* as role models to talk about AIDS and drug prevention. Educational videos will be also be shown and more individually oriented prevention programmes started. Evaluation will show whether these relatively innovative efforts contribute to the kinds of harm reduction that it is hoped to achieve.

Notes

1 The study described here was conducted by Jacobo Schifter and colleagues at ILPES in Costa Rica. The chapter was prepared by Jacobo Schifter and Peter Aggleton.
2 The fieldwork associated with this study was conducted in collaboration with Antonio Bustamante, a researcher with much experience working with *cacherismo* in Central American prisons. Bustamante made the initial contacts and prepared the way for the fieldwork reported here.
3 *Cachero* is a word that does not have a clear translation into English. The closest counterpart would be 'top-man'. *Cacheros* are not considered homosexuals or bisexuals, but heterosexuals who have sex with other men because of money or lack of women.
4 For example, for *cacheros* 'sodomy' is not anal penetration, but masturbation. Likewise a 'gay' is not a homosexual man who has come out of the closet, but a *loca* or 'queen'.

References

CARRIER, J.M. (1985) 'Mexican male bisexuality', in F. KLEIN and T. WOLF (Eds) *Two Lives to Lead. Bisexuality in Men and Women*, New York: Harrington Park Press.

DOVER, K.J.D. (1978) *Greek Homosexuality*, Cambridge, Mass.: Harvard University Press.

JOHNSON, A. R. (1983) *Understanding the Psychology of Romantic Love*, San Francisco: Harper and Row.

KASHAK, E. and SHARRAT S. (1985) 'Los roles sexuales comparados: sorpresas en Costa Rica', *Rumbo Centroamericano*, 11–17 July.

SCHIFTER, J. (1989) *La Formación de una Contracultura. Homosexualismo y SIDA en Costa Rica*, San José: Editorial Guayacán.

SCHIFTER, J. and MADRIGAL J. (1996) *Las Gavetas Sexuales del Costarricense*, San José: Editorial IMEDIEX.
SCOTT, P. (1978) *The Road Less Travelled*, New York: Touchstone.
WEST, D.J. (1993) *Male Prostitution*, New York: Harrington Park Press.

Chapter 9

Natural Born Targets: Male Hustlers and AIDS Prevention in Urban Brazil

Patrick Larvie

This chapter examines the challenges of preventing HIV and other sexually transmissible infections among male sex workers in Rio de Janeiro, Brazil. Based on a 1992 evaluation study of an AIDS/STD prevention programme for male sex workers in Rio de Janeiro, the analysis looks at the ideological determinants of this segment of the sex industry, the logics that inform understandings of risk, and the overall strategy of health care provision to male sex workers in place at that time. In particular, it focuses on the role of homophobia as both a structuring component of one segment of the male sex trade (*michês*) and as one of the chief obstacles to the effective provision of health care – including AIDS prevention services – to this population.

The arrival of AIDS in Brazil in the early 1980s was accompanied by general panic in the press, fuelled both by dire predictions of impending catastrophe and by the lurid curiosity of media consumers eager for details about the new 'plague' and its 'victims'. Official and unofficial health authorities purveyed confusing and often bizarre advice on avoiding infection: the purchase of individual manicure kits, the avoidance of suspect hairdressers, abstention from 'promiscuous' sexual relationships, and the segregation of those known to be infected. These recommendations circulated in both the popular and scientific media, making it difficult to distinguish fact from fiction and routes of viral infection from mechanisms of moral contagion. There was, however, one common denominator to most representations of AIDS and advice on how to avoid it: it was a disease of sexual, moral or social others, of people represented as separate and distant from the so-called general population.

This lack of clarity over exactly what separated the 'risk groups' from the 'general public' prompted efforts to establish more clearly demarcated boundaries between social and sexual sub-populations as a way to contain the epidemic and calm the public (Galvão, 1992). As in other regions of the world, sex workers were quickly identified as potential 'vectors' or 'reservoirs' of infection and as a threat to the 'general population', and Brazilian health authorities acted quickly to warn of the dangers of commercial sex. Federally sponsored prevention campaigns warned television viewers to avoid 'promiscuous' sex, while showing stylized scenes of urban red-light districts

(Hildebrand, 1995). In the late 1980s, male sex work was singled out as a 'bridge' across which HIV was said to move from the once neatly circumscribed 'risk groups' to the 'general population' (Cortes, 1989; Parker, 1987, 1988). Male sex workers were said to have commercial sex with homosexual males and non-commercial sex with females, thus 'explaining' the spread of HIV to those outside the risk groups. At this point in the history of the epidemic in Brazil, numerous 'bridges' were theorized in an effort to explain why HIV infection was not limited to the previously defined risk groups. The strategy of targeting prevention initiatives at male sex workers proved to be ambiguous. On the one hand, it recognized this group as being in need of specialized AIDS and STD prevention services, a positive change from previous policies which seemed to deny the very existence of male sex work. And, importantly, the federal AIDS programme attempted to utilize community-based prevention techniques among male sex workers, a tacit recognition of the government's lack of expertise in working with this group. On the other hand, this strategy performed an important and at times homophobic dislocation. By identifying male sex workers as the 'bridge' through which HIV moves from groups with higher seroprevalence rates to groups with relatively lower rates of infection, this strategy imagined homoerotic desire, bisexuality and risk of HIV infection as being contained within a relatively small group, separate and distinct in important ways from the 'general population'. The risks associated with HIV infection, like the symbolic risks associated with manifestations of homoerotic desire, would be contained within an imagined population of male prostitutes – identifiable and controllable through appropriate public health measures. In this way, risk for HIV infection and homoerotic desire were not ascribed to the bodies or minds of Brazilian men in general, despite growing evidence that AIDS was moving beyond the so-called 'risk groups'.

This chapter focuses on the challenges related to preventing AIDS among male sex workers, from the establishment of the conceptual foundations for controlling the epidemic to the formulation of guidelines for research and service delivery. Findings from a 1992 evaluation study of an AIDS prevention programme for male sex workers in Rio de Janeiro are analyzed. As I will argue, the group of male sex workers interviewed as part of the study were indistinguishable in many ways from the so-called general population. At the same time, their knowledge about the risks associated with HIV infection and about prevention were substantially better than that of the general population as surveyed by the Brazilian National AIDS Programme. Both of these facts suggest that the concept of community-based prevention initiatives may have to be reformulated for this group.

While the Brazilian National Programmes on Sexually Transmissible Diseases and AIDS has made many important and positive changes since the early 1990s – the time at which this research was conducted – many lessons can be learned from early attempts to control the epidemic through the management of male sex workers' bodies. An examination of these early attempts to define male sex workers as a distinct group and to target them for AIDS prevention services may provide important clues as to how to more effectively provide the health care services needed to control HIV infection among marginalized groups. Male sex workers in Brazil, like other sexually marginalized groups throughout the world, frequently are members of multiple communities, only some of which may relate to their participation in a stigmatized form of sex. The most effective means for providing prevention services may well require the targeting of communities based not on epidemiological studies but, rather, on research which shows where and how members of marginalized groups obtain information related to health.

Male Sex Workers in Urban Brazil

When male hustlers (*michês* in Portuguese) in Brazilian cities were identified in the late 1980s and early 1990s as posing a threat of AIDS to the 'general population', it was not the first time that they had been singled out as a uniquely dangerous group. Popular and academic accounts of *michês* had portrayed them as important actors in an urban underworld marked by violence (Perlongher, 1987). Yet despite the relative abundance of media representations of *michês* as dangerous (and, significantly, alluring), male sex workers are difficult to define as a group for the purposes of targeting AIDS prevention services. AIDS-era academic studies have described *michês* as lacking a cohesive identity based on sexual practices or as professionals in a particular segment of the sex trade (Perlongher, 1987; Parker, 1988). In other words, they may not self-identify as gay, bisexual or even as sex workers. These same studies indicate that many *michês* work only sporadically and in spaces which are geographically distant from their places of residence. For these reasons, they may not be reached by programmes targeting homosexually active men or sex workers. But *michês* in Brazil do share characteristics which are significant for the purposes of planning and carrying out health-related interventions. For example, researchers have described them as having little or no access to health-related services specifically designed to detect and treat sexually transmissible diseases (Longo, 1990). In part, this may be due to the fact that many *michês* are from the lower working classes of urban Brazil, often from the periphery of large cities, where access to virtually all public services is scarce. But it may also be due to their reluctance to use specialized STD clinics, often located in the centres of cities like Rio de Janeiro or São Paulo and frequented by sex workers. Lastly, it is also important to point out that some gay activists have identified *michês* as dangerous, claiming that their resistance to self-identify as homosexual or bisexual may be related to the frequency with which they are recognized as aggressors in cases of violence against gay men (Brazilian Ministry of Health, 1996a). While it would be a mistake to assume that homophobic aggression is a characteristic common to all *michês* in urban Brazil, this link identified by gay activists may provide an important clue about the reluctance of some of them to use services targeted at either homosexually active gay men or at sex workers.

While the provision of HIV/AIDS prevention services to *michês* is the focus of this chapter, this is not the only type of male sex work in Brazil. In broad terms, male sex workers can be divided into two basic groups, the first being the hyper-masculine *michês* and the second the ultra-feminine *travestis* (very roughly, transvestites or drag queens). *Michês* most frequently display, in exaggerated form, the signs of stereotypical straight male identities, with the appropriate mannerisms and bodily transformations. Often, their masculinity is produced with a level of theatricality that forces the observer to see it as an artifact, as a production mediated through the exaggeration of conventional symbols of masculinity. *Travestis* engage in a complex simulation of femininity rather than a mere imitation of it (Braiterman, 1996). Their clients seek them out because of their gender performance and their ability to perform 'male' acts while simulating femininity. *Travestis* do not compete with biological female sex workers for the same client base; their simulation of femininity is marked by a unique gender performance.

In order to understand the practice of male sex work in Brazilian urban centres like Rio de Janeiro, it is important to understand the cultural and social contexts in which it occurs. As de Zalduondo (1991) has argued in relation to female sex work, apparently similar practices may acquire strikingly different meanings across cultural contexts. And even though male sex work is a familiar phenomenon in many countries, it has important specificities in Brazil. One of these has to do with the important and structuring role of homophobia on the practice of male sex work in Brazilian cities. *Michês* clients are often publicly straight men who wish to live out their homoerotic fantasies in a way which insulates them from the stigma associated with homosexuality. And this stigma is not slight: the Grupo Gay da Bahia estimates that one homosexual is murdered every three days in Brazil. Research done by this group shows that when murder victims are homosexual, the police tend to have greater difficulty in bringing the aggressors to justice (Grupo Gay da Bahia, 1996). There are many other reasons why apparently heterosexual Brazilian men might want to divorce their homosexual experiences from their everyday lives. Among the most obvious are the possibility of rejection by their families, the threat of violence on the street and discrimination in the labour market. While homophobic violence and discrimination are not unique to Brazil, the relative lack of social support for homosexuals, including effective legal protections, works to ensure that they remain powerful influences in everyday life.

In very broad terms, much of this segment of the male sex trade depends on what I have termed an erotics of the closet. This logic is especially apparent in instances in which the client is a married man in search of a clandestine encounter with another man. Here, the *michê* is called upon to be the guardian of a secret and a repository of stigma. That is, the *michê* participates in a stigmatized urban subculture so that his clients do not have to. Further, the social differences which often structure the *michê*/client relationship work to heighten the erotic appeal of the encounter. *Michês* tend to be socially distant from their customers: darker skinned, less educated, and from a lower social class. In many instances, they may be runaways and lack access to the resources afforded by acceptance into one's biological family. In a society which is extremely hierarchical and unequal, this form of sex work serves to provide opportunities for cross-class and cross-race sexual contact. Significantly, it also serves to guarantee that the client remains distant both from the 'underworld' of sex work and from those publicly marked as having unacceptable sexual identities or practices. The peculiarities of *michê*/client interaction, occurring within the context of a stigmatized urban subculture, make male sex work a viable means of socializing sexual desires which are considered intolerable in many segments of Brazilian society.

Clearly, this logic is not the only one which might structure the contexts in which male sex work occurs. And, in fact, there is some reasonable degree of diversity in this segment of the sex industry in Brazilian cities. There are male sex workers who consider themselves to be professionals, and there are lesbian and gay people who manage to thrive, despite the adversities of everyday life. However, for the vast majority of male sex workers, homophobia continues to be an important structuring component of their work. This is true with respect to their clients – who continue to seek them out so that they do not have to suffer the negative consequences that non-clandestine homosexual activity might imply, and with respect to their working conditions – sex work continues to be confined to the 'red-light' districts of urban areas, where sex workers are often the victims of police and customer aggression. For male sex work to function as a service – much as other legal commercial services operate – the symbolic and material inequalities between client and provider would have to be mitigated in some form, either through real improvements in the providers' socio-economic status and the diminution of stigma associated with homosexuality, or through access to state-sponsored mechanisms for conflict resolution. It is important to note that, according to the Brazilian Penal Code, sex work is not a crime. Nonetheless, sex workers of all sexes are frequently the victims of police violence and seldom benefit from the same protections afforded to other workers. Clearly, sex workers are treated as second-class citizens by the institutions of law enforcement and justice in Brazil.

AIDS Outreach with *Michês* in Rio de Janeiro

Despite the preponderance of negative images of male sex workers, *michês* constitute an important attraction for residents and tourists in search of nocturnal diversions in the 'red-light' districts of large Brazilian cities. Brazil's tourist industry promotes the country as one which offers sexual attractions as part of the nation's natural and cultural resources. Rio de Janeiro occupies a key position within Brazil as the centre – whether real or imagined – of the nation's sex industry. Whether deserved or not, the city is notorious both nationally and internationally for being a centre of sex work and sex tourism. The prevention programme which was the focus of the evaluation study provided its services in two Rio neighbourhoods. The first of these, Copacabana, is a middle- to upper-middle-class district on the south side of the city. A mixed residential and commercial area, the neighbourhood is also a destination for domestic and international tourists. The second, essentially a commercial area adjacent to Rio's financial district, is located downtown. As the site of a major commuter train station, this latter neighbourhood is also a transit point between the city centre and the outlying working- and lower-class suburbs.

One of the Rio's most famous neighbourhoods, Copacabana is the site of a beach which is one of the city's most important tourist destinations. Separating the neighbourhood's most chic apartment buildings and hotels from the beach, Avenida Atlântica is both a spectacular avenue and, at night, an important centre for sex work. The neighbourhood was also the site of a beach-front bar where outreach workers could make contact with *michês*. Copacabana is socio-economically mixed, but the ostentatious apartments along the avenue and the presence of luxury hotels and foreign tourists along the beach give the impression that the neighbourhood is much wealthier than it really is. While tourists comprise a significant number of sex workers' clients in this area (and perhaps provide a disproportionate share of their earnings), the majority of clients are Brazilian, even at the peak of the tourist season. Though sex work in this neighbourhood has strong links to tourism, both foreign and national, it is not entirely dependent upon it. Many of the clients who purchase the services of the sex workers are residents of the city, and many of them reside in the middle- and upper-middle-class neighbourhoods located along the beach front on the city's south side. There is, however, a notable increase in the number of *michês* who work during peak tourist seasons, especially summer and Carnaval. When hustlers find clients, the *programas* (as sex-for-money transactions are called) most often take place in the hotels or residences of clients. Occasionally, clients will rent rooms in inexpensive hotels in the area which cater for sex workers and their customers.

The evaluation study also interviewed hustlers working in the Central do Brasil train station, which is located in the centre of the city and is an important transit point for workers going to and from the city's suburbs. While the suburbs are socio-economically mixed, they are significantly poorer than the beach neighbourhoods of the *Zona Sul* (Copacabana and Ipanema, for instance). The *michês* who work at the central train station cater to clients with comparatively little disposable income, or at least to clients who are unwilling to spend much money on sex work; the price of a *programa* is considerably lower here than in Copacabana. They find clients by waiting on the sidewalk in front of the train station or by walking through a nearby park. The *michês* working at the central train station take their clients to the inexpensive hotels or *hospedarias* located nearby which are intended for such use. It is important to note that this location was considered hierarchically inferior to other locations in the city where male sex work occurs, including Copacabana. In this sense, the Central was a lower-end venue for sex work, not only in terms of the clients' ability to pay, but also in terms of the self-evaluation of the *michês* working there. At both sites, educators from the outreach project, called Programa Pegação at the time, worked by distributing condoms and information directly on the street or at tables in nearby bars and luncheonettes. The outreach team included six part-time staff and a co-ordinator.

Health-related Knowledge and Practices among *Michês* in Rio de Janeiro

Over the course of the six-month evaluation study, we interviewed 45 of the *michês* served by Programa Pegação at the two locations described above. Follow-up interviews were also conducted with 18 of these hustlers approximately 60 days after initial contact with the evaluation team. Results of this study were published in the form of a technical report for the World Health Organization's then Global Programme on AIDS (Parker, Larvie and Cardoso, 1992). The analysis here focuses on the fit between the prevention project and the group it intended to serve. The project, based loosely on principles of 'peer education' and community outreach, defined *michês* as a group sufficiently distinct from others to warrant a specialized approach to prevention. It is important to remember that these sex workers were defined as a group only because they shared a common contact with the outreach programme, and not because they formed a cohesive, self-defined group. Nonetheless, as I will argue, many of the *michês* who participated in the study did share important characteristics. While perhaps insufficient to distinguish these men as a group from the so-called 'general population', these attributes are an important indicator that *michês* have a somewhat different relationship to information on AIDS and AIDS prevention than does the population at large.

Demographic Characteristics

The 45 *michês* interviewed ranged in age from 15 to 38, although most were between the ages of 17 and 25. The relationship status of the interviewees is indicative of their relative youth: 32 of them said that they were neither married nor living within a consensual union of some other type. The educational status of the *michês* was more difficult to ascertain. There was a strong sense of shame about illiteracy and about having an insufficient mastery of 'high-brow' spoken Portuguese, especially in Copacabana. We observed that *michês* who claimed to have completed grade school or even high school often had difficulties reading the instructions provided by the outreach workers on how to use condoms and lubricants. For this reason, instructions on how to use these items or how to access health related services were not universally comprehensible. In part, this was due to difficulties with reading printed text, but other significant obstacles included the lack of familiarity with certain regions of the city, such as the location of the specialized STD clinic to which outreach workers made referrals.

Very few of the *michês* interviewed in Copacabana were native to the city of Rio de Janeiro. Most were either from the state of Rio de Janeiro (excluding the city) or from neighbouring states. Of the 29 *michês* interviewed in Copacabana, 14 lived in rooming houses or shared apartments (often with many other sex workers) located in the *Zona Sul* or downtown. Although many of the *michês* we interviewed were reluctant to comment in detail on their families, it was apparent that a significant number had left home on unfavourable terms; they may have run away from an intolerable domestic life or have been expelled from their homes for reasons relating to their sexual activities. Some *michês* reported living in rooming houses where, in exchange for the privilege of paying their rents on a day-to-day basis, they paid two to three times the cost of sharing an apartment with one or two other people. Not all of those interviewed in Copacabana lived in such precarious conditions. As one might expect, given their relative youth and relationship status, many (nine) lived with their parents or relatives in outlying areas of the city. It is also important to point out that seven of the hustlers we interviewed described themselves as being 'in transit' from one city to another. Given that the first round of interviews was conducted just before Carnaval, this fact lends support to the idea that sex work may be an activity that some young males engage in only occasionally, especially during the tourist season. The housing situation of the *michês* interviewed at the central station is indicative of their relative lack of access to material resources of any kind. Almost one-third of the 16 men interviewed at that location said that they were living on the street, and that they had no fixed residence of any kind. Of those who did have regular housing, most lived in outlying areas of the city accessible by the trains that go to and from the train station. Half of the respondents who said that they had a place to live were staying temporarily in homes of parents or relatives.

Paid and Non-paid Sexual Activity

The *michês* we met during the evaluation study worked hard and got little in return. One of the most striking aspects of the data from the study was just how few *programas* they had had in the seven days prior to the interview. Twenty-four of the 45 respondents reported that they had not had a single *programa* in the seven days prior to the interview. The number of *programas* was low regardless of interview site, and the sex-for-money transactions were unevenly divided among the *michês*. Just seven respondents accounted for almost two-thirds of all such reported transactions. We expected there to be an over-reporting of paid sex transactions and, indeed, the one respondent who claimed to have had 10 different *programas* in the seven days prior to the interview may have been exaggerating. Still, it seems rather clear that the *michê* business, at least that sector of it that operated on the streets through the course of the evaluation study, is not a particularly lucrative one. For most of the interviewees, sex work offers little in the way of either sex or money.

But these data also suggest that, at least among the population served by the outreach programmes, there are two groups of *michês*. The first and most numerous is comprised of those who only occasionally are able to earn money from sex, but nonetheless continue to frequent the spaces in which clients and *michês* meet. Our observations suggested that this group includes those who live at home and do not depend entirely on the money derived from sex work for survival, and those who live and work on the street full-time. For the latter, hustling is but one of many possible ways to earn money. Although we did not inquire directly about income earned from illegal activity, our observations indicated that those living on the street often engage in petty theft and, less frequently, the drug trade as a means of earning money. The second group includes those who regularly make money from sex work, and who might well be more likely to think of themselves as professional sex workers. It is important to note that these hustlers seem to direct themselves towards clients who might reject sex workers with an unkempt, dishevelled appearance. In this way, the capital necessary to make a living as a commercial sex worker becomes apparent: those with the means to maintain their appearances and to have access to things like telephone lines and a permanent mailing address are much more likely to make money as sex workers.

Nevertheless, the mere lack of economic opportunity did not keep the vast majority of *michês* away from the streets or bars. Many had visited the central station or the bar in Copacabana each day of the week before the interview; the vast majority had been there at least twice. Twenty-four of the 45 reported making at least four visits to the locale in the seven days prior to their interviews. And some of them had been at it for a very long time, especially at the Central. Two-thirds of the *michês* interviewed at the train station had been working there for at least three years. Those interviewed at the bar in Copacabana were somewhat newer to the area; half of them said that they had been frequenting the bar for a year or less. Sex work was not considered to be a year-round job or the sole source of income by the majority of interviewees. Many said that they had been frequenting either the bar in Copacabana or the central station off and on since they began selling sex.

It is also important to note that some of the *michês* we interviewed objected to the section of the questionnaire in which we asked questions about involvement in sex work. Frequently, the interviewees denied that they were prostitutes or that they were in the interview locales for the purposes of soliciting clients for paid sex. Comments such as 'Of course I'm not a prostitute. But I expect the man to pay for my expenses', or 'I'm not here to pick up any one, but if a man propositions me, I might not turn him down', were typical of those who objected to being classified as sex workers. Others had no problem telling us how long they had been 'in the life', as well as how business had been recently. Once again, these data suggest that there is a core group of professionals and another group, significantly larger, of 'amateurs' or 'part-timers' who do not identify as sex workers and who may think of hustling as a way to find sexual contact with men. For the latter, money is not the principal focus of their activities on the street. It is, rather, the idea that they will be paid or compensated in some way for their sexual relations with other men that makes it possible for them to put themselves in a position to be propositioned. The idea of sex for money provides the context – but does not constitute the principal objective – for sexual relations between many of the *michês* we interviewed and other men. In this way, sex work operates as an institution that provides a ritualized exchange (material or symbolic payment) that justifies otherwise stigmatizing sex acts.

The *michês* we interviewed had surprisingly little sex, even when non-commercial sex is taken into account. As mentioned, most had a very hard time finding even one paying client during the seven days prior to their interviews. We also asked if they had any non-paying, non-regular partners (7 said that they had), and whether they had had sex with any regular non-paying partners (6 said yes). So the majority of the *michês* had not had sex with any regular partners, or any casual sex, and only about half were able to find someone willing to pay for their sexual services. These findings cast serious doubt on the suggestion that male sex workers may act as 'bridges' between 'risk groups' and the 'general population'. Particularly for those who do not derive income solely from selling sex, male sex work would appear to be more of a context for sexual experimentation or perhaps a pretext for engaging in a stigmatized form of sex. For those already living on the street, selling sex may serve as one of many ways to earn money. As one truck driver from a faraway state told us, 'I'm not really here to earn money. But I only get to Rio once a year and this is one of the few places I know where I can meet other men.' In this sense, for many males the act of 'prostitution' may actually be more akin to a ritualized form of sexual transgression than the kind of sex-for-money transaction that occurs commonly among female and transvestite sex workers.

Knowledge, Attitudes, and Beliefs about HIV/AIDS

We asked *michês* to rate their own knowledge of safe sex, or of their ability to prevent HIV infection or the acquisition of other STDs. We also asked them to estimate their own risks for HIV infection. A third evaluation of knowledge related to prevention was provided by the evaluation team. We scored the *michês* on their knowledge about routes of transmission, means of prevention and the actual techniques of condom and lubricant use.

Self-evaluations of risk and knowledge did not always, or even often, agree. Many interviewees gave themselves high ratings for both knowledge about safer sex and risk for HIV infection. For these *michês*, fear of infection seemed to outweigh their own sense of self-efficacy; many did not seem to believe that their knowledge could have an impact on their actual risks for HIV infection. Others seemed to believe that their risk for infection did not depend on their knowledge, but articulated this idea in a different way: they gave themselves low risk ratings without knowing very much about HIV transmission or its prevention. *Michês* who claimed that they were really 'straight' and only took the role of the insertor in sexual encounters frequently reported that they felt they were not at risk for infection regardless of their levels of knowledge.

According to the ratings of the evaluation team, two-thirds of the interviewees had serious difficulties in explaining how to use a condom. The majority of *michês* interviewed were unaware that oil-based (such as petroleum jelly) lubricants destroy latex condoms. Since penetrative sex is, at least theoretically, an important part of their repertoire, such knowledge is essential. Many *michês* reported having used oil-based lubricants in the recent past. This was a serious problem, since water-based lubricants were both difficult to find in Rio de Janeiro and extremely expensive. In addition to the significant burden of looking for and purchasing high-priced, water-based lubricants, the packaging of commercial brands of lubricants made them extremely inconvenient to carry on one's person. We also felt that difficulties related to the reading or the comprehension of instructions about how to use lubricants posed a serious problem for *michês*. These instructions presumed that they were aware of the chemical composition of many of the substances commonly used as lubricants; they were not aware, and they frequently had difficulty identifying 'off-limits', oil-based lubricants. Fortunately, virtually all *michês* were aware how to acquire and use the condoms correctly up until the point at which the use of lubricants becomes necessary.

The evaluation team also posed a series of questions, requiring 'agree' or 'disagree' responses, as an additional way of understanding the ways in which *michês* perceived their risks for HIV and AIDS. Thirty-six *michês* agreed with the statement that 'there are some neighbourhoods in this city where the risk of HIV infection is higher'. When asked which neighbourhoods they felt were most risky, most *michês* indicated the neighbourhoods in which they lived. Twenty-seven agreed that 'people who have only one [sex] partner are not at risk for HIV infection'. As a general rule, sense of risk seemed to be related to participation in a specific and highly stigmatized sector of the sex industry, that linked with multiple homosexual encounters. The perception of risk suggested here was not unlike that found in the section of the interview in which we asked them to rate their knowledge of safe sex and their chance of becoming infected with HIV. In both cases, risk seems to be a quality that adheres to stigma, which they cannot escape unless they are willing and able to identify themselves as 'straight'.

The perceived risk of a sexual encounter seemed to be determined by self-ascribed identity, by the type of sexual relationship and by the type of sexual act. The perception of risk was sometimes, but not usually, reduced by self-perception of adequate knowledge of safe sex techniques. In theory, there should be no neighbourhoods that are more dangerous than others for HIV infection. If one is able to protect oneself, that protection should be universal. Perception of risk seemed to be consistently related to the interviewees' identification with the concept of 'risk groups': to the extent that they saw themselves as either homosexual or as sex workers, to that degree they identified their own risk for HIV infection. Conversely, those who said that they were 'straight' or who denied that they habitually engaged in sex for money always rated their risks as low. These attitudes are not unlike those of the population at large. In a 1991 survey, for example, the Brazilian Ministry of Health found that 85 per cent of the adult population surveyed believed that it was 'impossible to "catch AIDS" through "normal" [*sic*] sex' (Brazilian Ministry of Health, 1991). Further, and perhaps as a corollary to this statistic, 49 per cent of the population estimated that their risk of 'catching AIDS' was close to zero (Brazilian Ministry of Health, 1991).

Knowledge about HIV transmission and AIDS is an issue that is quite separate from perceptions of risk. Almost none of the interviewees could distinguish between infection with HIV and AIDS. This, combined with the idea that the number and type of partner determine risk, led some to believe that they could 'choose their partners better' by having sex with only those they thought of as being unlikely to be ill. In practical terms, this meant choosing partners who *appeared* unlikely to be 'gay' or 'promiscuous'. Again, the perception of risk and illness seems to be most closely related to ideas of social stigmatization; knowledge of safer sex techniques seemed to offer little comfort to those we interviewed. Knowing that a person can be infected with HIV and show no signs of illness also seemed to matter little; to identify a client as 'homosexual' or as 'promiscuous' was virtually equivalent to a diagnosis of AIDS.

It is worth pointing out that the model of health promotion that connects knowledge of safe sex techniques with risk reduction assumes that *michês* actually have the power to negotiate the safe sex practices with their clients. Given power imbalances between sex workers and clients, this is not a safe presumption. While few of the *michês* we interviewed reported unsafe or dangerous working conditions or reported having encountered violent clients, we heard many more stories of violence and abuse outside the context of these interviews. In general, there was a tendency to deny any involvement in sex acts which might suggest a risk that the *michê* was infected with HIV, with the exception of penetrative sex with girlfriends and spouses.

Implications for AIDS Prevention

It is important to remember that Programa Pegação was targeting *michês* using a methodology loosely based on principles of 'peer-education' and 'community outreach'. These methods have proven to be successful elsewhere, especially among female sex workers and homosexually identified men whose access to public or private health services is precarious at best. In part, these strategies work because these groups have an internal level of cohesion that is sufficient to support peer education within a context of a 'community', usually defined by a shared minority status in relation to the larger society. In thinking about the usefulness of this strategy among *michês* in Rio de Janeiro, it is important to take into account the specificities of male sex work·as a culturally inscribed institution in urban Brazil. Its meanings are multiple and diverse, differing in important ways from the sex-for-money transactions involving female or transvestite sex workers in Brazilian cities. The results of the evaluation study and my own observations over the course of nine months of fieldwork indicate that the institution of male sex work in Rio de Janeiro might be understood as including three key domains of meaning and practice.

First, sex work is sometimes a commercially oriented segment of the sex industry catering to closeted men, tourists and a limited number of self-identified homosexual males. This kind of sex work occurs both on the street and in closed environments. Men involved in this domain of male sex work are more likely to think of themselves as professional sex workers.

Second, sex work often serves as an institution in which sexual contact between men is permitted and not subject to the usual sanctions which would apply outside this highly circumscribed context. In this case, the payment of money for sex is not the chief objective, but its symbolic value is of extreme importance. The payment insulates the client from the social world of the sex worker and the stigma attached to an underworld of prostitution and homoerotic desire. For the *michê*, the payment provides symbolic insulation from the homosexual desires of his client and the attendant loss of a 'straight' identity.

Third, sex work is also a context in which various forms of exploitation may occur. Runaway youths, sometimes referred to as 'street children', may turn to sex work as a way of making money. They may steal from their clients or engage in other illicit practices to supplement their earnings. Unscrupulous customers may prey on those who appear to have no means of support. In both instances, these practices are forms of abuse which take place under the guise of sex work.

In all three domains of meaning, homophobia operates as an important and structuring factor. The continued existence of homophobia ensures that clients will continue to seek out sex workers in order to avoid the stigma and persecution which often accompany the public disclosure of a homosexual or bisexual identity. Hustling as a commercial segment of the sex industry depends in part on the customers' desire to isolate their homosexual activity from other realms of their daily lives. In the second domain, homophobia appears as both the stigma that must be avoided through the sex-for-money transaction and as the lack of alternatives to sex work for socializing homoerotic desires. The enormous stigma associated with homosexuality in Brazilian society, as well as the very real threat of homophobic violence, work to perpetuate the lack of options for young men who feel sexual attraction for other men. In the third and final domain of meaning, homophobia appears as a factor which silences victims and curtails their access to state-sponsored mechanisms of conflict mediation and justice. Clients seeking homosexual encounters may be seen as 'easy marks' for thieves because they may be unwilling to make their homosexuality public through a complaint to the police. Conversely, adolescent males with relatively little access to material or social support are easy victims for unscrupulous adults intent on sexual exploitation. It should be stressed that these are not the only logics that structure this segment of the sex industry in urban Brazil, though I believe them to be dominant. There is nothing inherently homophobic about male sex work. The homophobia to which I refer lies in the broader social and cultural context in which male sex work occurs.

With respect to the efforts of the outreach programme, the results of the study show largely positive effects. On the whole, the perception of risk for HIV/STDs among those we interviewed was similar to that observed in survey studies of the Brazilian population; significantly, their knowledge of prevention techniques appeared to be considerably better (Brazilian Ministry of Health, 1991). The perception of risk that appeared in open-ended questions seemed to be tied to the stigma of 'abnormal' or 'unclean' sexualities or sexual practices. In this sense, risk and disease were seen as properties of abnormal or unclean acts or persons. Nonetheless, most *michês* were familiar with the rules of condom usage, possessed a condom at the time of the interview, and were able to identify common misperceptions with regard to HIV transmission. As evidenced by these findings, the outreach programmes could be considered effective. The *michês* interviewed not only had superior knowledge of prevention techniques when compared to the 'general population', but they also had relatively greater access to the means to use them. Free condoms were made available, referrals were made to specialized health services, and outreach workers counselled hustlers on techniques of negotiating safer sex with their customers. Nonetheless, observations suggest that there may be room for improving the way prevention services are targeted at those who participate in male sex work by tailoring the services to the domains of meaning ascribed to sex work, whether from the perspective of clients or from the sex workers' own point of view.

Although this programme was directed towards those working on the streets, it actually targeted three different groups: lower- and working-class adolescents in a phase of sexual experimentation (those who were primarily looking for sex); a marginalized population of young males who had been living and working on the street for some time; and, finally, a smaller core group of sex workers who depended upon, and were able to derive income from sex work. Partly as a function of the homophobic logics of the National Programme on Sexually Transmissible Diseases and AIDS prior to 1993, AIDS prevention services for *michês* in Brazil have tended to configure this group as targets of the initiatives rather than as co-formulators, as has proven to be effective in community-based interventions with other populations. In this sense, the general direction of Programa Pegação's outreach initiative represented significant progress. Nonetheless, funding agencies tended to imagine sex work and sex workers as being distinct and separate from the 'general population'. To be fair, such a characterization is accurate to the extent that most Brazilian men do not sell sexual services or procure the services of sex workers. Still, the *michês* served by the outreach programme did not constitute a cohesive group or 'community', and there were important differences among those targeted by the outreach programme which defy easy definition of *michês* as a single, undifferentiated group. More interesting possibilities for serving those men who engage in sex for money may lie precisely in the connections between them and the so-called 'general population', rather than in the differences between these two theoretical groups. To this end, changes on three distinct levels would be extremely helpful, as outlined below.

Changes at the Level of Brazilian Society

Important issues include the extension of civil rights to sexual minorities in Brazil and the reformulation of institutions of police and justice to ensure that the rights such minorities presently enjoy in theory are guaranteed in practice. As the Grupo Gay da Bahia[1] has documented, violence against homosexuals in Brazil is rampant and the perpetrators enjoy an intolerable level of impunity. Police forces throughout the country need to be trained to respond in an appropriate manner to homophobic violence, and judicial authorities need to ensure that violence against homosexuals is treated as a crime. Among other important macro-level changes needed to safeguard sex workers from the threat of violence is the decriminalization of certain activities related to the sex trade. Current legislation does not define prostitution as a crime, but anti-pimping laws prohibit the formation of collectives of sex workers. Changes in this legislation would help to make the work environments of professional sex workers safer. Further, the profession is not currently organized under Brazilian labour law and sex workers are unable to collect social security benefits normally allotted to other categories of labourers – even though sex workers' earnings are taxable under the law.

Intermediate-level Social Supports

Perhaps most apparent is the need for support for lesbian and gay groups and organizations in Brazil. Although there are more than 60 such organizations throughout the country, that number is still small for a nation of over 150 million inhabitants. These groups assist in providing alternatives to sex work for young men with homoerotic desires by providing safe environments in which to meet. In addition, these groups are uniquely capable of providing social support for lesbians, gays and transgendered persons in a largely homophobic society. As in the case of the Grupo Gay da Bahia, organized groups of homosexuals have been instrumental in denouncing violence and prejudice against sexual minorities.

There is also considerable need for social assistance to runaway youths, who often turn to sex work as a means of surviving on the street. Over the course of the evaluation study, many of the *michês* reported that they had been expelled from the homes of their biological families following the discovery of their homosexual activity. As in other countries, lesbian, gay and transgendered youth make up a significant portion of runaways. These youths are at significantly higher risk for health problems of all kinds, and are exposed to situations in which they may easily be psychologically and physically abused. It is important for AIDS prevention programmes targeting *michês* to be aware of the number of runaway (or 'throwaway') youths who work as *michês*, and of the unique needs of this group.

More Effectively Targeting AIDS/STD Prevention Programmes

Programa Pegação proved to be instrumental in raising awareness of the risks of HIV and STDs, and in providing the means necessary to prevent and treat sexually transmissible infections for many of the sex workers it served. Similar programmes, targeting spaces where sex work is known to occur, might be implemented in other areas of the city as well as in other regions of Brazil. New interventions might also target the intersections between *michês* and the so-called 'general population'. This would mean reinforcing prevention programmes for self-identified gay men, for young people in and out of school and, significantly, making information about STDs and AIDS – as well as condoms and lubricant – available and convenient to the 'general population'. Rather than targeting *michês* as a discrete community based on sexual practices, new interventions might address the multiple functions and meanings of male sex work in urban Brazil. Such a re-focusing of prevention efforts might help to destigmatize both *michês* and the provision of targeted AIDS-related services. All too often, such services are seen as being provided to and needed by groups or persons who *are the risk* for AIDS, rather than for groups or persons who are *at risk* for HIV and other sexually transmissible infections.

In prior years, much of the rhetoric around AIDS in Brazil tended to label sex workers in general, and *michês* more specifically, as 'threats' to the health of the nation or as 'bridges' across which HIV could move into the 'general population'. The *michês* interviewed as part of the evaluation study were very sensitive to the fact that they had been unfairly singled out as a public health threat. They were perceived to *be the risk* rather than to *be at increased risk* for AIDS and other sexually transmissible infections. Improvements in the provision of health-related services to male sex workers must begin with the premise that they are not merely strategic targets for prevention programmes but, rather, a group whose needs – including but not limited to health needs – have been severely under-served. Rather than comprising a group distinct and separate from the general population, *michês* come from and participate in multiple segments of Brazilian society. As a culturally inscribed institution with multiple meanings, male sex work is a context in which a diverse array of actors and interests converge. A fundamental step in addressing the problems of AIDS prevention in Brazil – and among sex workers more specifically – is the recognition of the ways in which those once perceived to comprise 'risk groups' are connected to, rather than separate from, the so-called 'general population'. AIDS prevention services may be provided that are focused on these links, rather than on barriers or frontiers. Whether as self-identified sex professionals, runaway youths or sexually curious adolescents, *michês* clearly needed and appreciated the services they were offered. If the provision of these services – and their acceptance by sex workers – were less symbolically loaded with stigma, they would certainly be more effective.

Acknowledgements

The evaluation study described here was conducted in 1992, together with Ranulfo Cardoso Jr and Richard Parker at the Institute for Social Medicine at the State University of Rio de Janeiro. Meurig Horton and Peter Aggleton served as consultants from the World Health Organization's Global Programme on AIDS. I am grateful to the clients of Programa Pegação for agreeing to participate in the study and to the programme's staff, especially Silvio de Oliveira and Paulo Longo. Without their collaboration, the evaluation project would have been impossible. I am also grateful to Jared Braiterman, Andrew Boxer, Bertram Cohler and Gilbert Herdt for their input on this work.

Note

1 This group has recently produced a series of pamphlets for homosexuals with tips for self-protection, including advice on how to avoid being a victim

of police violence. They have also produced a pamphlet which the police forces in some Brazilian cities are circulating in an effort to reduce the levels of homophobic violence.

References

BRAITERMAN, J. (1996) 'Beat it: an anthropology oddity', unpublished doctoral dissertation, Stanford University.

BRAZILIAN MINISTRY OF HEALTH (1991) *Pesquisa de opinião pública sobre a campanha 'Se você não se cuidar'*, Secretaria de Assistência à Saúde, Programa Nacional de Doenças Sexualmente Transmissíveis e AIDS, Brasilia.

BRAZILIAN MINISTRY OF HEALTH (1996a) *Manual do Multiplicador: Homossexuais*, Secretaria de Assistência à Saúde, Programas Nacional de Doenças Sexualmente Transmissíveis e AIDS, Brasilia.

BRAZILIAN MINISTRY OF HEALTH (1996b) *Manual do Multiplicador: Profissionais do Sexo*, Secretaria de Assistência à Saúde, Programa Nacional de Doenças Sexualmente Transmissíveis e AIDS, Brasilia.

CORTES, E. *et al.* (1989) 'HIV-1, HIV-2, and HTLV-I infection in high-risk groups in Brazil', *New England Journal of Medicine*, **320**, pp. 953–8.

GALVÃO, J. (1992) 'AIDS e imprensa: um estudo de antropologia social', unpublished Master's dissertation, Programas de Pos-graduação em Antropologia Social (Museu Nacional), Universidade Federal do Rio de Janeiro.

GRUPO GAY DE BAHIA (1998) *Boletim do Grupo Gay de Bahia*, **37**, January–February.

HILDEBRAND, L.I. (1995) 'Comunicação oficial brasileira sobre a AIDS: um percurso pelas linhas e entrelinhas da telinha da tevê', unpublished doctoral dissertation, Escola de Comunicação da Universidade de São Paulo.

LONGO, P. (1990) 'Projeto Pegação', project proposal for an AIDS outreach programme with male sex workers in Rio de Janeiro.

LONGO, P. (1991) 'Programa Pegação: an outreach for male prostitutes in Rio de Janeiro', mimeo.

PARKER, R. (1987) 'Acquired immunodeficiency syndrome in Brazil', *Medical Anthropology Quarterly*, NS **1**, 2, pp. 155–75.

PARKER, R. (1988) 'Sexual culture and AIDS education in urban Brazil', in R. KULSTAD (Ed.) *AIDS 1988: AAAS symposia papers*, Washington, DC: American Association for the Advancement of Science.

PARKER, R., LARVIE, P. and CARDOSO, R. (1992) 'Programa Pegação: an evaluation of an AIDS outreach programmes for hustlers in Rio de Janeiro', Technical Report submitted to the Global Programme on AIDS at the World Health Organization.

PERLONGHER, N. (1987) *O Negacio do Michê: A Prostituição Viril*, São Paulo: Editora Brasiliense.

DE ZALDUONDO, B. (1991) 'Prostitution viewed cross-culturally: toward recontextualizing sex work in AIDS intervention research', *Journal of Sex Research*, **28**, pp. 223–48.

Chapter 10

Fletes in Parque Kennedy: Sexual Cultures among Young Men Who Sell Sex to Other Men in Lima

Carlos F. Cáceres and Oscar G. Jiménez

In most societies, sex is a commodity that can be sold with varying degrees of commercialization. In the majority of cases, the sex trade not only occupies an important place in social life, but also carries with it complex webs of meaning and practice regarding sexuality, gender, social class, social mobility, power and morality. The population of men who have sex with other men in Lima, Peru, does not seem to be an exception in this respect.

Activos/Mostaceros and the Working-class Male as Sexual Object

Overwhelming anecdotal evidence suggests that sex between feminine, gay-identified men (or their equivalents) and straight young men aged from 16 to 25, particularly those from working-class backgrounds, is fairly common in certain areas of Peru. These sexual interactions are supposed to be role-based. In these relationships, straight men are supposed to engage only in penile-insertive activities, that usually (or desirably) result in the exchange of sex for goods. The straight man expects to be offered beer or to receive money or a present. Diverse social and behavioural patterns of self-presentation and interaction among men who have sex with other men in Lima have been described elsewhere (Cáceres, 1996a).

What seems to be legitimate bisexual behaviour (or homosexual behaviour following the insertive *activo* pattern), however, is not exempt from conflict and social pressures. At least until recently, the fundamental proofs of maleness seem to have been linked to freeing oneself from the implication of homosexuality (Cáceres, 1996b). This subject seems to figure centrally among men's day-to-day concerns, although the men do not usually feel comfortable enough to comment on this topic outside the relatively safe context of jokes. Dominant representations of the kinds of men who seek out sex with other men point to the concern raised by 'passing' homosexual men because of potential complications in social interaction. For example, if a man's homosexual interests are not evident from the beginning of an interaction, such interaction may take a course that becomes 'dangerous' due to its potential overlap with male heterosexual bonding.

The exchange of homosexual sex for money or goods seems to be a fairly common experience among working-class men. Many have heard about it and give information to their friends and acquaintances (*pasarse el dato*) on where to go if they need money. These locations include certain bars or parks in Lima where pick-ups are common, or private parties where it is possible to meet men potentially interested in homoerotic interaction. In a recent study of 1218 working- and middle-class young adults in Lima, 28 per cent of men who had had sexual experiences with other men reported having exchanged sex for money or goods at least once (Cáceres, 1996b). Since the proportion of males who reported having had at least one homosexual experience was unexpectedly high at 14.5 per cent, the actual proportion of men who had exchanged homosexual sex for goods constituted approximately 5 per cent of all male respondents, and thus does not seem to be a rare practice among young men in Lima today.

The most traditional representations of homosexual men among young people in this sample depict them as people whose principal desire is for submissive sex with macho men, and who cannot get sex unless they pay for it. Consequently, homosexual men work basically to get the means to pay for sex. These ideas contrast with other respondents' reported experiences of friendship with young men who self-present as gay. Such respondents may even visit gay discothèques and bars, and often display more general liberal attitudes and beliefs.

The above-mentioned study also suggested that being paid for sex is acquiring increasing legitimacy among men. It is increasingly recognized that young men are sexually solicited by older women or men (that is *tías* and *tíos*, literally 'aunts' and 'uncles') and that, at a time of economic crisis (or in the assumed economic difficulties of lower-middle-class adolescence), it may be fair to take advantage of sex appeal to obtain money, a present or even a glass of beer in exchange for company, petting or actual sex. Female suitors are regarded as being more legitimate, since they are women after all, and representations of older women as sexually sophisticated prevail. However, they are recognized as being less common than male suitors. In the latter case, an ideology of pragmatic homosexual possibility enters into play. Some young men will see their bodies as a commodity from which they can take temporary benefit from men who must be assumed to be homosexual. Since the hegemonic representation of a homosexual is still that of a man who desires to be 'possessed' by another man, homosexual interaction with him is not desirable, but can be acceptable as a resource for needed sexual relief, or as an informal source of income or other benefits in kind. Warnings about the never-absent risk of being 'taken' or 'possessed' by the other man are, however, increasingly heard in the form of jokes in men's gatherings, particularly as the hegemonic view of the homosexual man becomes increasingly less stereotypically feminine.

Fleteo

Fleteo, or the activity performed by *fletes*, is a more professionalized way of selling homosexual sex. *Fletes* are usually young men who frequent parks, particular street locations and other settings with the purpose of selling sex. There are close links between this form of behaviour and a more prevalent pattern of socio-sexual interaction – the *mostacero* pattern. The latter involves responding positively to the supposedly unexpected advances of another man in exchange for goods or money. Certain seductive prolegomena are usually necessary. *Mostaceros* are supposed to need to be convinced by their suitors (usually with the help of generous amounts of beer) to continue an interaction with them that may end up as sexual play. Informality in that exchange is essential, as may be a certain degree of friendship between the actors, related to residence in the same neighbourhood, or to having common acquaintances. *Mostacero* exchanges are casual, and would not be considered formal transactions around the provision of specific services. *Fleteo* and the *mostacero* pattern are, however, not mutually exclusive, and many *fletes* may act as *mostaceros* in their own neighbourhoods.

Fleteo is seen largely as a job, albeit seen as a temporary or complementary source of income. It requires a young man's (usually 16 to 24 years old) presence in venues where he can be picked up by clients, generally well known parks or bars. Transactions are usually more formal than they are between the *mostacero* and his partner(s), and more clearly defined 'sexual services' are exchanged for relatively fixed amounts of money. There is much social and sexual diversity among *fletes*. This permits a range of various sexual services to be available, and attracts clients with diverse preferences. The negotiation of sexual practices is therefore an expected step in the interaction between *fletes* and clients.

Parque Kennedy is a plaza in downtown Miraflores, a wealthy, commercial district of Lima. For about 15 years it has been known among gay men and among young working-class men as a place where *fleteo* contacts between clients driving cars and young men sitting on the benches can occur. It forms part of a circuit that is otherwise comprised of nearby bars and discothèques. One of these – Voglia – is a discothèque whose commercial strategy involves encouraging *fletes*, who in turn bring clients to the place. Until recently, when private telephone-operated agencies appeared, along with cell phone-utilizing individual businesses, *fleteo* in the Parque Kennedy was the most popular source of sexual entertainment among middle-class and upper-middle-class gay men who sought commercial sex. Although *fleteo* in the neighbourhood is undergoing marked decline, the Parque Kennedy seems likely to continue to be a reference point for male sex work in Lima for some time in the future. The present study sought to explore issues of identification regarding sexuality and sex work, as well as aspects of the sexual cultures structuring the experience of some of the young men who sell sex to other men in this setting.

Methods

In the context of a larger study of the sexual cultures of men who have sex with men and women in Lima, qualitative techniques (focus groups and in-depth interviews) were used to elicit insights and information from a population of young *fletes*. Five young men with bisexual experience were interviewed. Interviewers driving cars approached potential subjects in the typical attitude of a client and, after the initial verbal contact was made, they disclosed their purpose and offered economic compensation of around US$10 for the subject's time in participating in the interview. Interviews were conducted in the cars, and were audio-taped. They lasted approximately 45 minutes. Interviewers explored subjects' sexual histories, their experience in *fleteo*, their sexual identity and their identity as *fletes*, ideas about homosexuality and bisexuality, issues related to their support networks and the degree to which their participation in *fleteo* had been disclosed in those networks, matters of self-esteem, and issues related to AIDS and safer sex.

After individual interviews had been completed, two focus groups were conducted. Subjects were recruited with the aid of a key informant who was a gay-identified *flete* and participated in the first focus group. The sessions lasted around two hours, and were held at the end of the day in a university building in Miraflores (which was free of other activities at that time of the day). Participants also received about US$10 for their time. Focus groups were facilitated by two experienced interviewers. Focus group discussions included an exploration of representations of homosexuality and bisexuality, the elicitation of terms and typologies used in the sex trade, a discussion of their experience in *fleteo*, and AIDS-related concerns. After coding, the data was analyzed thematically in relation to the preceding issues and concerns in the general study on men who have sex with men.

Representations of Gender and Homosexuality

Information regarding this subject came fundamentally from focus group discussions. Although we did not aim to elicit information on gender representations, discussion about the meaning of being homosexual inevitably implied reflection on what it is to be a *man*, in so far as hegemonic representations of masculinity establish a dichotomy between being a man and being homosexual. Two points of view seemed to prevail. The first of these, corresponding to the hegemonic perspective held by the general population, suggested that being a man is not in conflict with having sex with other men, so long as proper masculine roles are preserved. *Pasivos* (sexually 'passive' males – those who are penetrated) and *modernos* (the 'modern' or sexually versatile – those who are insertive and receptive) may remain males (*hombres*), but not men (*varones*). The definition extends to the arena of desire: a man cannot desire another man as a man – yet he could want to penetrate him as a male.

Similarly, it is impossible for two men to have sex together: necessarily one of them, the one who crossed the boundaries in order to make sex possible, loses his status as a man.

> if that person is a man and goes with another man, at the moment they are going to have sex, then that man is not a man anymore . . . , the one who wanted to have sex . . . the one who was passive . . . ; then he becomes a homosexual.
> [And, if one person wants to assume an *activo* role with another male, does he stop to be a man?]
> No, for sure he does not . . . ; it is the one who acts as passive the person who stops to be a man. (Second focus group)

> The (*Mostacero/cacanero*) is the guy who has sex with a faggot . . . , with a gay man . . . a man who likes to have sex with a homosexual is a *cacanero* . . . , that is, he likes to fuck a homosexual, [he likes to fuck with] gays, transvestites, everything . . . except with other *cacaneros*. (Second focus group)

A second point of view, held by gay-identified *fletes* and by some more educated *activos*, described a man as a male who never has sex with someone of the same sex. On the other hand, anybody can be a male – including a gay man. Those men who, following an *activo/mostacero* pattern (see Cáceres, 1996a), have sex with other men in conventionally masculine roles, according to this view would not be symbolically *men*, in spite of the fact that they may pretend to be so.

> For me, a man is a person who does not have sex with other persons of the same sex. (First focus group)

> As soon as you are with another male you are already homosexual, . . . you stop being a man. (First focus group)

Activo and *mostacero* (mutually exchangeable with *cacanero*) are related terms, as are *pasivo, olla* and *moderno*. Clear behavioural boundaries must be adhered to in order to be an *activo*. Practices such as receptive oral and receptive anal sex are not compatible with such status. Giving head (oral sex) is out of the question since it compromises masculinity: touching the genitals of another man can occur, but only if done reluctantly at the partner's request.

> an *activo* cannot give head, that would be illogical . . . that guy would then be an *olla*, a dirty *olla*, of course, that would be a dirty *olla* . . . , an anti-*activo*. (Second focus group)

> he can touch [the genitals], yes, he can touch, just because he felt obliged . . . (Second focus group)

A *pasivo* on the other hand is the person who takes a role equivalent to that of the female in a dual gender ideology. This representation goes beyond penetration and enters into the arena of sexual interaction more generally.

> A *pasivo* is the person . . . who receives, the one who likes to be penetrated . . . but the *pasivo* does not necessarily have to be penetrated; he simply likes to play the female role . . . but he, say, likes to be fucked in eighty per cent of cases. (First focus group)

The terms *olla* and *moderno* refer to sexually versatile (that is insertive/receptive) characters. However, while the *moderno* is honest about his preferences, the *olla* tends to deceive in order to negotiate prestige both in paid and non-paid contexts.

> The *moderno* is the person who says 'Yes, I'm *moderno*.' Conversely, the *olla* is the person who says 'I am *activo*' . . . The *moderno* knows what he is and likes, he accepts his reality. (First focus group)

Accounts offered in individual interviews provided information about value judgements on homosexuality. Perspectives ranged from the very negative to the accepting:

> [Homosexuality is] abnormal, since it is not acceptable that two men have sex with each other. (Interview 5)

> Well, now, it's a normal thing, isn't it? It's nothing strange, and nobody should conceal his being homosexual. One should recognize what he is and that's it. I'm homosexual and recognize it, and am not ashamed of being so . . . we are all homosexuals, from the moment one has sex with a homosexual one is homosexual, too. (Interview 2)

Representations of Bisexuality

Bisexual men were represented in two main ways. The first form corresponded to the *activo*. According to this image, the *activo* participates in homosex under the logic of having fun. His gender identity and heterosexuality thereby remain unaffected.

> The *activo*? That's the guy who . . . they are the guys who want to have fun sometimes . . . they are not necessarily faggots . . . they also like girls . . . (First focus group)

Focus group participants often talked about their images of bisexual men in this way. *Activos* were seen as lacking either a gay or bisexual identity (considering themselves to be 'very *macho*' or 'ultra men'), looking very masculine, and normal. They were seen as most likely to have homosex 'after drinking or after a party'. A second image is that of the *doble cara* (double face). This is usually reserved for the married bisexual man who at certain times shows his more 'feminine' side.

> There are gentlemen who are married and come in their cars with their purses, their coiffes, their rouge, . . . truly handsome men and one says 'Wow!' Once a gentleman came in a brand new Mercedes . . . a nice-looking man who had a wife – a blonde, and a daughter, everything, and he brought me to Camino Real, and, God, he behaved like a sissy, like a woman, fuck, I was so sorry for him . . . Anybody would try to pass, right? But he behaved like a woman. . . (First focus group)

Sexual Experiences and Relationships

All the men interviewed individually reported having had sex with both women and men, and all had experienced erotic attraction towards a woman first. All but one had had their first sexual experience with a woman as well. This first heterosexual experience frequently took place with older girls with whom emotional bonds were weak. The women concerned were not girl-friends, but girls with whom to have a *vacilón* (affair). First homosexual experiences had usually occurred in the context of *fleteo*, but varied in recency from one to six years beforehand.

When asked about their sexual relationships, respondents emphasized the quality and quantity of their heteroerotic experience, assigning to it an importance always higher than, or equal to, their homoerotic experience. Female sexual partners were either women for *vacilones* or casual partners with whom no permanent bond was sought. Elsewhere, Jiménez (1996) has described the distinct expectations and experiences linked to the three different kinds of sexual partners of young working-class men in Lima: relatively close girl-friends (*germas*), female occasional partners (*vacilones*), and homosexual men (*maricones*). In a similar vein, while interviewees in this study reported having had at least two girlfriends, none readily assigned this status to the majority of his female partners. Some of the interviewees did, however, have a girlfriend at the time of the interview.

Study participants expressed their feelings about the differences between sexual interactions with men and those with women. In order to be with a man it was not seen as necessary to seduce him. Indeed, were a seductive approach required, they would not be interested.

> More confidence exists with a guy . . . in the sense that you can speak about anything, you can do everything . . . Conversely, with a woman [it's] not [possible], women are more shy. With a woman, you have to speak to her; you have to seduce her . . . With a guy this isn't necessary. You go straight ahead, there is no need for preparation. (Second focus group)

Respondents with the most homosexual experience described having had a range of partners, always highlighting the latter's passive tendencies and stating their own preference for active penetrative anal sex. In one case, the passage of time was reported as having made things more flexible, so that one respondent now lets himself engage in receptive oral sex: 'After four years, you get to like it a bit' (Interview 3).

Another participant, the only one who acknowledged having had receptive anal sex, stated that he did not enjoy it, although he cannot clearly define whether he prefers men or women. There were only two references to same-sex steady partners. One of them was described as 'more *pasivo* [than *activo*]' (Interview 3). Another interviewee claimed that he would like a male partner who was '*pasivo*, young and wealthy' (Interview 4). Here, a material interest complements the sexual one, as the desired sexual partner could possibly help the participant leave street *fleteo*.

Sexual Identity

Much relevant information about sexual identity came from in-depth interviews. In spite of their behavioural homogeneity, respondents varied widely in terms of their sexual identity.

> Some guys consider themselves to be gay, homosexual, bisexual . . . [I don't think I am] any of these things . . . they don't make any sense to me . . . enough sense to call myself that way. [I consider myself to be] a man, that way . . . Homosexuality comes to be like . . . like they stop a bit to be men, right? . . . To decide to be homosexual, that's your own business. For example, if they do it to me and I want to continue to be a man and to like women, then I can do it . . . but some men do it because they like it, and those are the guys who become homosexual. (Interview 1)

> I consider myself a normal person; I consider myself neither *activo* nor *pasivo* nor *moderno* . . . I am normal, I like women as much as men . . . because there are those who are *de ambiente* [who belong to the gay scene] and they don't like women . . . I do like women, but, honestly, there is more confidence with a guy. (Interview 2)

Sexually, I mean, I just wait for the client to tell me. It doesn't mean, however, that I'm going to do what he wants. I don't let them ... well, I don't enjoy everything ... [I consider myself] bisexual ... because I do it with men and with women ... There is no man who only looks at women. All men look at other men up to 14 or 15 years old. Then their hormones start, and they more or less grow up. But if it's still going on, and they continue to like it, then that's something different. (Interview 5)

Representations of *Fleteo*

Fleteo is largely defined as sex in exchange for money, regardless of whether the *flete* enjoyed the sexual interaction:

The *flete* is the person who charges ... it doesn't matter if he enjoys it, but he always has to charge ... (Second focus group)

According to focus group comments, *fleteo* is a very common activity in neighbourhoods beyond Miraflores.

Yes, there is [*fleteo*] everywhere ... in most neighbourhoods. ... The faggots start to look for boys, ... go by the parks, soccer fields. ... Many [boys] get into the cars, [while] some others chase them off with stones. ... You find this even in wealthy areas. (First focus group)

Although everybody seems to know about this, there is little overt criticism, since everybody has engaged in at least one illegal activity.

They say ... that it's bad that you sell yourself. ... [But] in my neighbourhood everybody has done something illegal ... so, no problem, everybody knows about everybody else. (Second focus group)

Debut in *Fleteo*

Involvement in *fleteo* can occur by a number of routes and for a variety of reasons. Some of those interviewed reported having got into *fleteo* 'knowing nothing'. In other cases, the initial experience was reported as having been unexpected but not entirely alien.

I play professional volleyball and went out and met a guy, and he invited me to dinner. ... I was waiting for him in a restaurant and he didn't come. Suddenly, I heard a horn and somebody else was calling me. ... He told me he always came there, and [at that time] I did not even know that people used to wait around there . . . Then I realized that all those guys who were sitting there got into the cars, and I did the same. (First focus group)

I didn't even suspect it . . . I was walking as usual and someone brought me to that place . . . and told me: 'Let's go for lunch.' I didn't know anything . . . but I wasn't so stupid either, so I said to him: 'You know, nothing in life is free anymore' . . . [And he replied] 'Don't worry, I'll give you a tip.' (First focus group)

Most participants reported having become involved in *fleteo* through friends who had told them about it, and the techniques to use with clients:

I got into this through a friend, who told me there were places . . . where I could get money. . . . He told me: 'We can look for a gay guy', and he aroused my interest . . . , and so I came to the park, I liked the place, it's lively, the way the cars come and go, and so I started to come daily. (Second focus group)

A friend said to me: 'Come on, let's go . . . You know that getting a job is very hard. Let's do it!' . . . , and so I did, as simple as that. I knew nothing, the first time I didn't like it, but, you know why? He smoked . . . I think it was cocaine . . . it was a white powder . . . I don't like those things, he might have had more of that and anything could have happened, and I left . . . But, in spite of that, the guy gave me money . . . (Interview 1)

Identity and Motivation

In general, the men we talked with were reluctant to use the term *flete* to describe their experiences. When the term was employed, however, it was used somewhat ambivalently.

I don't consider myself a *flete* . . . it depends on the person who does it, it depends on why you do it, . . . I don't come here everyday, while this is their [the other guys'] job. (Interview 1)

I don't consider myself *flete* . . . since when a *flete* gets into a car, he straight away negotiates a price. I don't do *fleteo* . . . I don't know why they call it that anyway. But I think that if two people want to have a good time, and if the person gives you a tip, why not? (Interview 2)

In focus group discussions, participants talked about their motivation for involvement in *fleteo*. Two main sets of reasons emerged. On the one hand, *fletes* were seen as people who, even if they have fun, 'always charged'. As a result,

> If you realize he's not going to give you anything, you get out of the car [because] you can't waste your time talking when you are working. (Second focus group)

This line of thought was dominated by the idea that *fleteo* is also a service that deserves payment.

For other men, *fleteo* was seen as offering opportunities for fun, entertainment, the possibility of finding a special person and 'a steady relationship'.

> Sometimes I come [here] because I feel depressed and want to go out, to get into a car . . . or simply to have sex, and look for someone I might be attracted to . . . [So, if] I've had a terrible day, my way of getting relaxation is to come to Miraflores, right? But, with the idea of getting into a car and having fun. (Second focus group)

Another respondent claimed that he was not selling himself, since 'When I am there, it's to meet people, and when I meet them I don't think about whether they will pay me or not . . . If they give me a tip, though, it's very welcome.' Yet another said that his requests for money depended on what the other person wanted to do, so that 'so long as there is an agreement, it's fine'. The kind of sex asked for, together with the looks of the client, are both factors taken into account when establishing a price. They link to issues of homoerotic desire and proximity to the gay scene. *Fletes* who have sex for something other than money (for example a *vacilón*) tended to be those linked most closely to the gay scene. Additionally, however, the logic of demand and supply also operates in *flete/* client relationships. There are opportunities that may be very hard to refuse, particularly if they do not affect one's identity. As one respondent put it,

> If you are [out of money] and go for a haircut, and the hairdresser wants to give you head, are you going to say no? (First focus group)

Experiences with Clients

The predominant image of clients is that of married but behaviourally bisexual men. One of the interviewees asserted that the majority of men with whom he went out were 'older men with a family'. Another participant had previously described a 'nice looking man, with a wife – a blonde', who 'behaved like a woman'. Socially, however, clients came from all social strata.

In focus group discussions, comments were passed about places where not only the demand for services, but the prices paid, were supposed to be higher. Barranco (a neighbouring district) was said to be somewhere where 'they pay much better than in Miraflores'. Another respondent mentioned Rimac as somewhere where working conditions were better than in Miraflores, to the extent that there was said to be 'a club for foreigners only: Germans, North Americans, Italians and Swiss'. Yet another claimed that the Plaza de Armas in downtown Lima was somewhere where 'all the Russians go' who 'give you a tip of fifty dollars or more'.

Another way in which clients were distinguished was in terms of their reasons for seeking out *fletes*. While 'some people come to look for us for sex only', 'others [come] to talk; they take you for dinner or for a drink' (Second focus group). Female clients were seen very much as a thing of the past, but there were women in Lima who 'go to the discothèques, go out with the guys and then pay them'.

Clients' approaches to payment also varied. The view is often expressed that 'those who have the most, bargain the most'. Consequently, it was not seen as strange for a client with 'a gorgeous car' to 'give you 10, 20 or 30 soles',[1] while another with 'an old, small car, might give you up to 30 or 50 dollars'. Learning how to bargain effectively comes both from personal experience and from information shared by friends and acquaintances. With experience, *fletes* are able to tell how much an individual client might be willing to pay, with payment being negotiated 'according to the individual'. While *las apariencias engañan* ('looks deceive'), *fletes* can usually tell if the client has money. 'When he tells you "let's go" from the very beginning', then the person probably knows the price, whereas 'When he doesn't seem to have money, you know nothing is going to happen with that guy' (First focus group).

In any event, respondents emphasized that the amount charged depended very much on their own attitude: 'You have to know how to discuss [these things] with the person', that is, 'to gain their respect; otherwise, they give you peanuts'. Negotiating payment takes place at different times according to the individual concerned, as well as 'according to the client', since 'some people can make a lot of trouble at the time of payment'. Finally, good luck is also involved, as it is always seen as possible to come across a client who pays very well or, conversely, to meet 'someone that gives you very little'.

Experience was seen as an important source of knowledge about how to interact with clients in order for problems to be prevented. One focus group participant recalled that 'I started to realize that I should not come everyday, because if you become too well known everything fails.' Another said that 'It's more likely that you'll be picked up if you are by yourself', so that as a strategy 'Some people wait by themselves and not in groups.' Other *fletes* form relationships with one another while waiting on benches, and go out together to discothèques and parties as a group.

Socialization and Social Support

The kinds of relationships that *fletes* have with the local gay scene and beyond are related to self-image in gender and sexual terms, as well as to the meanings given to *fleteo*. Those who self-identify as 'men' and claim to be involved in *fleteo* only because of material interest assert that there is no need to get involved in the gay scene: the only thing to do is to take advantage of it. Only *maricones* (faggots) would do otherwise.

> On the gay scene you find guys who like men, those who like *vacilón* [having fun]. I go anywhere; but once I've got some money, then I leave. I go for something else [that is money], I don't involve myself with them. I go there by myself, everywhere . . . (First focus group)

Among those who are less integrated into the gay scene and do not consider themselves to be gay, an involvement in *fleteo* may not be widely known about by personal networks and friends. One respondent who was a college student described a conversation he had with friends at school. He gave only partial information to them, telling them that the people who pick him up are women:

> Generally, those of us who do this, do it in a closeted way; it is a secret life, a double life. . . . I told them [that my clients] are [older] women, and that I had met a guy but had not gone with him . . . (Interview 4)

Relationships between non-gay *fletes* and friends not involved in *fleteo* or the gay scene are characterized by a constant effort to manipulate information so that *fleteo* remains secret or is made to appear legitimate. Information may be totally withheld, or *fleteo* may be presented as a heterosexual activity. In more tolerant environments, services to *maricones* may perhaps be talked about, but with a strong emphasis on *activo* roles and economic compensation. Gay-identified *fletes*, on the other hand, tend to be much more involved in the gay scene, either for fun or to get money. According to their perspective, the opportunities for friendship and support that the gay scene provides come first, and financial reward is secondary to this.

> I think that . . . to be in the scene means that we . . . come, first, for a *vacilón*, second, for the enjoyment, and third, for some money. (First focus group)

AIDS and Safer Sex

Participants in the first focus group stated they were scared and frightened by 'various reports [on AIDS] on television'. The idea prevailed that *fletes* constitute a group at a particularly high risk: 'We have to be more careful.' A special risk was seen as existing with certain kinds of clients, especially those who wanted to have sex without condoms: 'those guys are those who have AIDS'. With them it is necessary to be careful since 'those who have AIDS are smarter'. They are those who say: 'I will pay you two or three times [what I was going to give you] if we can have sex without a condom.' Overall, clients' lack of interest in using condoms was seen as an indication of the lack of relevance of protection to that individual, and as an indication that he might be willing to infect others.

Opinions about condoms suggested that while they may be widely accepted, they are seen as unpleasant. Condoms were seen as having two advantages, however. First, 'with a condom you get in faster'; second, they are 'cleaner, more hygienic', so that 'you won't get dirty'.

In contrast to the perspectives generated in focus group discussions, and with one exception, individual interviewees reported not feeling at risk for AIDS. Their sense of safety seemed to stem from their consistent use of condoms for anal sex with clients. Condoms were not consistently used, however, when they had sex with women, particularly girlfriends. The main argument here was that they trusted their girlfriends, and the central risk with them was pregnancy, which was prevented either through withdrawal or by using the contraceptive pill. When asked more about this, one of the interviewees reasoned thus: 'I am careful here [in *fleteo*], and that is the way to take care of my girlfriend.' Another interviewee, however, after contracting an STD from a female partner, had decided to use condoms 'even with girls'.

Conclusions

In this chapter we have attempted to present an overview of elements of the sexual culture of young men who sell sex to other men in Parque Kennedy in Miraflores, Lima. Our insights are derived from an analysis of information given in focus groups and in-depth interviews. In self-descriptions, bisexually active *fletes* emphasize heterosexual experience and their *activo* – if not default heterosexual – identity.

Fleteo is defined primarily by the exchange of sexual services for money. Men identified with the term *flete* to varying extents, depending on the value and the degree of stability they assign to the activity signified by that term. Motivations for involvement in *fleteo* vary, with the centrality of money being relativized by some participants on the basis of emotional and personal interests. *Flete*/client interaction may consequently provide space for otherwise difficult contact between people of different ages, social strata, and sexual identities.

A concern about AIDS seems present in the group. Some *fletes* feel at particularly high risk, although such consciousness is not connected to conscious reflection on the need to have safer sex with non-paying sexual partners. Safer sex with the clients is considered enough. Folk discourse among *fletes*, partially in the form of jokes, suggests that clients who are unwilling to use condoms are most probably those who have AIDS.

Fleteo, and more specifically the *fleteo* circuit existing around Parque

Kennedy, constitutes the locus of a complex sexual culture encompassing elements of the gay scene in the wealthy vicinity, the poor-neighbourhood experience of *mostaceros*, and the inner-city lives of working-class gay men. The confluence of such different groups determines a diversity of sexual identities and sexual practices, views of sexuality and *fleteo*, and personal involvement in *fleteo* and in the gay scene.

Fleteo possibly provides an axis of articulation for different subcultures of homosexually active men across social strata, and in some cases helps legitimize behaviours and establish identities through the provision of services influenced by laws of supply and demand. But it also represents a space (albeit somewhat perverse) in which people from very differing positions in society can meet, enabling the partial redistribution of income and social mobility. It may also lay the foundations for some questioning of homophobia and homosexual prejudice, the safer sex education of younger *fletes* by more educated clients, and other forms of social change.

Acknowledgements

This study was supported by a grant from the Ford Foundation, and by training grant TW 0003–05 to Carlos Cáceres from the Fogarty International Center through the University of California at Berkeley. The research would not have been possible, however, without the participation of the young men who trusted us enough to enable this privileged view of their experience.

Note

1 At the time of writing, US$1 equalled 2.62 soles.

References

CÁCERES, C. (1996a) 'Male bisexuality in Peru and the prevention of AIDS', in P. AGGLETON (Ed.) *Bisexualities and AIDS*, London: Taylor & Francis.

CÁCERES, C. (1996b) 'Sexual cultures and sexual health among young people in Lima in the 1900s', doctoral dissertation, University of California at Berkeley, California.

JIMÉNEZ, O. (1996) 'Entre patas y paltas: parejas sexuales, riesgos sexuales y redes personales entre jóvenes varones de Barrios Altos', in M. CORDERO, O. JIMÉNEZ, M. MENÉNDEZ et al., *Más allá de la intimidad: Cinco estudios en sexualidad, salud sexual y reproductiva*, Lima: Pontificia Universidad Católica del Perú.

Chapter 11

Through a Window Darkly: Men Who Sell Sex to Men in India and Bangladesh

Shivananda Khan

HIV/AIDS has generated many new terms in relation to sex and sexuality. Phrases such as 'men who have sex with men' and 'male sex workers' have entered into everyday usage, whereas older terms such as 'homosexual', 'bisexual' and 'heterosexual' continue to be used to describe sexual behaviours and identities. More often than not these descriptions are meaningless when used cross-culturally, and we should perhaps pay greater attention to sexual practices as they are understood in local cultural terminologies and contexts.

In India and Bangladesh the term 'homosexual' has been used by donor agencies, government and non-governmental organizations to identify men who are anally penetrated by other men, while the word 'heterosexual' is used to define those who practice vaginal sex. But people are not so neatly divided. What about anal sex between men and women, does this define 'heterosexuality' too? And there is a significant amount of evidence to suggest that many men who have anal sex with other men (both penetrated and penetrator) also have sex with women. Sufficient anecdotal evidence exists also to indicate that many men in India and Bangladesh begin sexual activity at the age of 10 and younger. Can the term 'men' encompass their activities and needs?[1]

In India and Bangladesh (as well as in other countries of the south Asia region), there is a high degree of amorphousness in indigenous frameworks of sexuality and identity. Here, identities are mostly based on family and community, as well as to a lesser extent on participation in particular sexual practices, most notably those of penetrator or penetrated. Identity is not based so much on who you are but on what you do, and in what context(s) your social life is constructed.

The term 'sex worker' was largely invented to destigmatize what were once called 'prostitutes', a word that was seen to carry a great deal of shame, dishonour, and stigma. This process of renaming now appears to carry a sense of political correctness. At any AIDS meeting, conference or workshop, the use of the term seems mandatory, whether in London, New York or Calcutta. Does such renaming prostitution really dignify sex work? I remember a conversation I had in a village in Orissa with a small group of women who said they 'did work' with their husbands, meaning that for them sex with their husband was seen as work. By way of contrast, husbands would say they 'did duty' to their wives. What are the local terms for so–called sex work? How do people name themselves in relation to such practices? How do individuals at a local level feel about this? Is the new language being imposed from on high? How do you translate these contemporary terms into vernacular languages? And if prostitution is now renamed sex work, then what of the women in Orissa quoted above?

This new term 'sex work' seems to carry a sense of choice, suggesting that sex work is just another job, something that can be left at any time. It over-simplifies what is a complex issue and dehumanizes the struggles that the vast majority of male and female sex workers go through just to survive. For the vast majority of people, sex work or whatever name you give it, is a survival strategy. For most, it is a practice enforced by poverty, degradation, homeless-ness, hunger and powerlessness, a form of slavery to economic, social and cultural deprivation, stigmatization and marginalization. For most men and women who sell their bodies for cash, for clothing, for food, for shelter, it is their only option.

The term sex work appears to imply some form of equality in economic and negotiating power, a labour contract between the customer and the pro-vider. But can this be true in a city like Calcutta, Mumbai, or Dhaka, or in any city in a developing country where poverty, hunger, homelessness and family deprivation are rife, and where significant numbers of such 'workers' below the age of 14 are primary wage earners for their families? Too often there is no other choice, no power to negotiate labour terms and working conditions.

Alam is a 9-year-old boy living in Dhaka, Bangladesh. Every evening you will find him at a religious shrine where some 150 male sex workers congregate regularly. Their 'customers' are local rickshaw drivers, truck drivers, shop-keepers, worshippers, and other men who also come there for sex. He will charge anything from 20 to 100 taka[2] per customer. On an average evening he will get about five customers. Sex is penetrative and with no condoms. The 'boys'[3] vary in ages from 8 to 60, and call themselves *kothi*.[4] Not all sell sex in this place. Some also come to find *panthis*[5] for 'fun', sex and penetration. Many of those seeking fun and sex also receive small gifts, such as an item of clothing.

Alam wears lipstick, acts in a feminine manner, sways his hips seductively at passing men, and hopes one day to find a *panthi* to take care of him. The money he earns helps feed his family as well as buy his make-up and 'sexy' clothes. His parents do not ask where he gets the money as he tells them he has a job working in a rickshaw repair shop. They need his money to help feed his five brothers and sisters. His father has no work and drinks heavily. His mother is pregnant again.

> I have been coming here for a year now. The first time I came here
> with a friend. He left after a little while and I stayed behind because
> I saw all these 'boys' who had make-up on. A man approached me.
> He offered me 20 taka. I was hungry so I did it. The other *kothis* here
> are all my friends. Yes, I am a *kothi* now. I will find a nice 'husband'

for myself one day. He will look after me and my family and then I will stop this life. But that might be hard because I like all these men.

Zahid is 62 years old and operates in the same place. He has a wife and four children, is known as a *tokai*,[6] and is a pavement dweller. He calls himself a *kothi* too, but only when he is in this place. While he likes to be sexually penetrated, he charges for it to supplement his daily income and to buy food for himself and his family.

I can only ask for perhaps 5 or 10 taka a shot because now I am old. What can I do? Look at me, I only have this old lungi. I can't afford to buy myself another piece. I have my family to feed, look after my wife and children.

For us to use Western constructions of sexuality and of AIDS to understand such behaviours is to lose sight of local realities and languages, local sensibilities and constructions. If we use them, we end up creating frameworks that have nothing to do with the realities of people's lives, how they see the world and themselves, and how they survive.

This chapter is about men who sell sex to other men in India and Bangladesh. In this context, the term 'sell sex' is used loosely, for while the exchange may well be in cash, it can also be a meal, or shelter, or clothing. It can also be opportunistic. And who is to say that some of us do not submit to the discharge of others for the sake of love and affection as exchange?

The case studies described arise from conversations held with hundreds of men who have sex with other men over the last four years, whether for cash or gifts, or because of 'sexual tension' and the need to 'discharge', or because of same-gender desire. These conversations have taken place in Dhaka, Calcutta, New Delhi, Mumbai,[7] Chennai,[8] and a variety of towns and villages. The sexual histories, explicitly told, were part of discussions reflecting informants' lives, hopes, aspirations and needs, spoken quietly in parks, bus stands, hotel rooms, at lake-sides, in rickshaws and tea shops, in taxis and on the street. Gaining trust and confidence through self-disclosure and friendship, the people I talked with were primarily from lower-income groups – the working classes, the 'labouring classes' and pavement dwellers – speaking in their own languages. They were hotel boys, shoeshine boys, rickshaw drivers, taxi drivers, tea boys, *kothis*, *panthis*, construction site workers, gay-identified men, truck drivers and 'male sex workers'.

Diversity of Background, Variety of Needs

While this chapter focuses primarily on men from lower income groups, this does not mean that male-to-male sexual behaviour and men who sell sex to other men does not exist in other classes/economic groups. Of course they do.

Terminologies may differ, and emergent gay identities may be more common, but similar themes emerge.

Ranjit is a student studying in a college in New Delhi. He is 19 years old, comes from a middle-class family, speaks English fluently, watches MTV, wears Levi jeans and likes Haagen Daz ice cream.

> I started selling sex accidentally. I was in this park in central Delhi one evening, and this man approached me and offered me 200 rupees[9] for sex. I was feeling 'hot' and I thought why not? The last time I had done anything like this with another guy was when I was 16, when over several months, I and my friend would play together. So I did this guy, got the money, and thought what an easy way to get some money. My parents never give me enough pocket money. So perhaps a couple of times a week I will come here. Here there are 'good people' you know, clean, come from my class. No 'dirty' people here. I usually get taken to a local hotel, or sometimes to the guy's home when his wife or family are not in. Sometimes I will also go to nice posh hotels and sit in the lobby. I know some of the staff in these hotels, and they sometimes will arrange a meeting with a particular hotel guest. I have to give them a percentage though. Or sometimes I get invited to parties where I can get a client. Now I have more experience I can charge much more money. Sometimes I get 1000 rupees, sometimes 5000 rupees. I usually spend the money on clothes or music, but I am also saving what I can for my future. My parents don't notice anything anyway. I tell my mother I have a part-time job. My father is not interested.

Sameer is also a student, 21 and from a middle-class family. His father died two years ago, and his mother struggles to get enough money for his family, and for Sameer to finish his college education.

> I have to do this if I want to finish my education, and get a good job afterwards. My mother tries in her job, but it is a real struggle. I tell my mother that I have a part-time job, you know, computer stuff, which explains the money I bring home. If I didn't sell my arse, we wouldn't really have enough money for me to finish my studies. How much do I get in a month? Well perhaps 10000 rupees if I am lucky, but usually between 5000 to 6000. I know this other guy, a top-class model. Sometimes he can get 10000 rupees from a rich businessman or film star. He stays the night with him. This guy is going to introduce me to someone like that soon.

Within these frameworks, privacy, money and other luxuries of the middle-class operate, and the sex workers are less visible than those from the lower income groups. Middle-class male sex workers organize themselves in different ways, through the telephone, through magazine advertisements, through established social/sexual networks and through parties.

Many of the 'park boys' share similar needs: food, shelter, clothing, love, affection, acceptance. 'I want a husband, a real man who would love me and look after me. I would make him a good wife', was a constant refrain among *kothis* working the parks. 'I only like "real men"' was another. But 'real men' do not touch the genitalia of their partners. They just penetrate or receive oral sex. To touch is to show that you are not a real man. To receive or give anally or orally is the measure of one's identity. They had their own language, a *kothi* language, and they named themselves *kothi*. The word *panthi* or *giriya* (a word used in New Delhi) is their term for a 'real man', someone who is sexually active with them.

But for many others, no sexual identity appeared to be operating. Says Salem, a housekeeping boy working in a hotel in Dhaka:

> It's very hard to find a girl who will give you sex here. Everybody watches what a girl will do, who she is with and so on. I have been having sex with my friend since we were 13. We had been sharing a bed in my home in our village, and he started holding my cock. Well, it was nice, so we did. Then I came to Dhaka to go to a school here and the boys in the hostel were all doing sex with each other. We would watch a blue film, get hot and then start to play. Sometimes we would save up some money and go to a woman prostitute – a clean girl, but very costly. Girls here don't give you sex. You can kiss them, you can 'breast pump' them . . . but getting it inside? Very hard and difficult with no privacy. Then I started working here at this hotel and this hotel guest offered me 100 taka for a massage. Well, money is money. So after my duty shift I did it. The man was only wearing his under-shorts when I came in. I started the massage and he got hard very quickly. He offered me more to shake him. So I said whatever, and did. I got 200 taka from him. Now I get perhaps three or four hotel guests a month. Sometimes they want to fuck me, sometimes I fuck them. Sometimes its thigh sex. It's great. I get regular fun and extra money.

In parks, bus and railway stations, and many other sites there are often social networks among men who sell sex. The 'guru' or focal point is usually the oldest person, who can be of any age. South Asian cultures centre on respect for age. The older male is called Uncle, but in the parks (s)he will often be called Aunty. In one park in Delhi the oldest person was 42 and was still selling receptive sex. In fact the majority of sex for sale in these environments was receptive anal sex. The social networks among men who use parks in this way are strongly framed. Whenever a new person comes into the park there is pressure to join the network. Strong but informal rules govern what you can do, what you can charge, who to avoid. Often the park *darwan*,[10] the local police and other important dignatories can have sex for free, or for a lower rate. In this kind of setting, violence and harassment are part of everyday life, from customers who refuse to pay, to local rowdies who come in groups and beat up the 'boys' before having sex with them, to the local police who may take their money as well as have sex with them.

It takes some time to build up trust with the men interviewed. As an example, consider a group of shoeshine boys in a park in Delhi where a lot of foreigners go to sit and gaze after a tiring walk around the gift shops. After a couple of initial visits to make friendships, it was easy enough for the boys to talk about their sexual encounters with local girls, with 'female sex workers' or with some of the foreign women. But it took two years visiting these young men aged from 14 to 25, before several of them would talk about their sexual activities with other men, both local and foreign. With foreign men they would charge something like US$20 a time. With the local men, sex was more a matter of discharge, it was the pleasure of sexual release, it was *maasti*.[11]

Similarly, after two years of getting to know the young cycle rickshaw drivers in Calcutta, whose homes are their rickshaws and the streets, they began to use the term *jiggery dost*[12] to describe sexual activities amongst themselves. They began to speak of having sex with certain customers who used their rickshaws, and how they sometimes would get cash (on average 50 rupees a time, equivalent to US$1.50). Prior to this, however, they had only talked of sexual encounters with local 'female sex workers'.

Some Life Stories

The accounts that follow are just a few that highlight what I would term the frameworks within which 'male sex work' occurs in India and Bangladesh. Four stories are from India, two from Bangladesh. Given the space available, I have had to restrict the frameworks somewhat. 'Boys' sell sex in a wide variety of locations, situations and life conditions, from the seven-year-old boy at a railway station earning his food and shelter for the night, to the 20-year-old room-service boy in a hotel trying to supplement his meagre salary. From the 14-year-old boy working in a tea-shop who must give his body to the tea-shop owner to keep his job, to the boy in a park who defines himself as a *kothi* and sells sex to keep his family free from hunger. From the rickshaw boy who can get a new shirt or a few rupees more once in a while, to the full-time worker who relies totally on the income earned through sex.

Kamal, Dhaka, Bangladesh

Kamal is 21 years old, lives in Dhaka and works as a lift boy in one of the larger hotels. He goes to the park three or four times a week, where he averages five clients an evening. He has many friends in the park, all of whom sell sex. Like the other boys in this park, he has been taking oral contraceptives so that he can develop his breasts, which are now quite enlarged. He states that the men like him to have big breasts because they like to squeeze them when they fuck him. They do the same to girls, he stated.

I suppose the first time I did sex was when I was eight years old. My uncle had visited our home when I was with my family in C, which is a village close to Barisal. We were very poor, and had only two rooms for our whole family. So my uncle shared the floor space with me. That night, he pushed his cock between my thighs and came. Only for a couple of minutes really. It felt nice, and he was a nice uncle, so I never said anything. He gave me five taka the next morning. Not that my family would have believed me, and what could I say.

This went on for several years, every time his uncle came to visit. After a couple of years, when they were alone in the fields, his uncle fucked him for the first time. It was painful, but after several times Kamal got used to it. There were also a couple of older boys in the village who used to fuck him.

I went to live in Dhaka with another uncle where I worked in his cycle rickshaw garage. I was 13, and there were two other boys of the same age as me, a couple of older boys about 17 or 18, and my uncle. He and his wife and children lived behind the garage, and I slept with the boys inside the garage. After the garage was closed, the older boys used to fuck us younger boys at least once a week. Sometimes they may buy us younger boys a shirt or a lungi[13] as a gift.

I was 14 when I started coming to this park. The first time I came here it was early evening. It is close to my home and I had come to see a friend. Usually I would come in the afternoons. As I walked through the park, I saw several boys, you know, walking in that way. Some of them were even wearing lipstick. I was interested, so I sat down on a bench. Then I noticed a man go to one of these boys, talk for a few minutes and then go into the bushes, there. Then just after that, when I was wondering what was happening behind the bushes, one of these boys came and sat next to me. We started talking, and he told me what was going on. He took my hand, looked at me and said that I could make money like this. He described himself as a *kothi* and the men as *panthis*. He said he would help me. I forgot about meeting my friend and that evening I had my first client. My new *kothi* friend explained to me the prices, how to do in the park, who the *panthis* were. I got to know the other *kothis* selling sex. There are about 50 of them here every night. Between us we do about 300 men every night. I also get to see the other *kothis*, the ones that do not charge. They have their own section of the park, though, and we don't mix too much. They are all from higher up, you know students, shopkeepers and so on. They wear jeans and shirts, live in nice homes. Not like us . . .

I have also had offers in the hotel. Sometimes I take a hotel guest in my lift and if we are alone they will invite me into their rooms. This is difficult, since I am not allowed into any guest's room. But usually I can get 15 or so minutes after my duty shift, when I can say I am in the toilet or whatever. Then I go to the guest's room. I can make quite a lot of money that way.

Khobir, Dhaka, Bangladesh

Khobir is 14 years old and works as a table boy in a small tea-shop/restaurant in Shantinagar, Dhaka. He has been working in the shop since he was eight years old. He came to Dhaka with his oldest brother, who is a rickshaw driver. Khobir lives in the tea-shop with the other boys who work there. There is an age hierarchy, the young boys cleaning the tables and those older serving the tables. There are several boys who are in their late teens and early twenties. None of the boys working in the tea-shop are married, except for the owner who also sleeps in the tea-shop.

My brother first fucked me when I was five years old. I was the youngest and he was the second oldest at 15. He would do this about twice a month. It was my oldest brother who took me to Dhaka. He had already been in Dhaka for several years and worked as a rickshaw driver. He had a friend who worked in this tea-shop and that is how I got this job. I earn about 500 taka a month and I send 400 taka a month to my family. When I first came here to the tea-shop and my brother left me, I was scared but I had a duty to my family, so that was that. After a couple of months, one of the older boys called me over to him when we were going to sleep, and asked me to sleep with him. This wasn't unusual, as several of the boys slept together under their blankets. When I got under the blanket with him, he started to pull my *lungi* up. I resisted, but he whispered that if I didn't obey him he would tell the owner I was a bad boy and I would lose my job. So I stopped resisting. I knew what to expect because of my brother, so when he started fucking me, I didn't make a noise. It was over in a few minutes and he turned around and went to sleep. This boy would fuck me three or four times a month. Some of the other boys would also fuck me. The owner has done it several times too.

When I was 14 my thing grew large and I started fucking the younger boys in the shop. Sometimes, a customer comes in who likes me and gives me a tip, maybe 5 or 10 taka. They usually ask my name and then go on to ask me to meet them outside later. If they are nice I do, and then we go somewhere and he fucks me. Usually he will give me another 10 or 20 taka for this. This money I save and send to my family every month also. My family are very poor. They are farm labourers, and have no land of their own. . . . One of my sisters is already married, but with the other two we have to collect enough money for dowries. And that is a lot of money, easily 50 000 taka.

I would like another job which pays more money. I ask some of the customers quietly, especially the ones I do sex with, if they can give me a job. I want to earn more money. Here I get very little time to myself. I work seven days a week, usually from early morning to late night. I get some time to go to mosque, which is when I get a chance to meet some of the customers who want sex with me. I also want to save for my marriage when I get older, perhaps when I am 25. I have never had sex with a girl, because there is no chance to. Where can I meet girls? And I can't afford a prostitute. So all my sex at the moment is with the boys in the shop or with some shop customer.

Rajesh, New Delhi, India

I suppose I must have been about seven years old when I first had sex with another boy. I was the youngest of six brothers and sisters, and I lived in a small hut in a slum colony in Calcutta with them and my mother and father. Everyone worked. I used to go rag-picking and maybe I would earn about 20 rupees a day if I was lucky. That evening, my family had gone to visit my mother's sister's husband, and I was left alone with Suresh. He was my eldest sister's husband's brother and he had come to stay with us from his village while looking for work. He was 21 years old. He had come home and he had brought a bottle of beer with him and a sexy magazine. Then he started drinking the beer and looking at the magazine, and all the time his hand would go down there, you know, rubbing it against his jeans. I was looking at a picture book, can't remember what it was, and then he called me over to him. The magazine was on his lap and I could see these naked men and women, all foreigners. I asked him where he got it from. He said from a friend, and did I like the pictures. I had never seen naked women and men before. It was interesting. Then he put his arm around my shoulders and said to come and lie on the bed with him so we could look at the magazine together. First he locked the door, then we lay on the bed with the magazine between us. His hand was between his legs, rubbing up and down, and he saw me looking at his hand. He removed it and said 'Look, it is hard.' I didn't understand. 'What is hard?' I said. Then he said, 'I will show you', and he lowered his pants. His thing was standing up surrounded by hair. He then pulled my hand and told me touch it. I was a little bit scared but I touched it. He seemed to shake, and then moving the magazine to one side he hugged me. He pulled my pants off. He touched mine, and told me that one day I will be as big as him. Then he asked me to move my hand up and down on his thing. He showed me what to do, which I did. A few minutes later I could feel his body tense, and he hugged me tight. I felt a wetness between us, and his body shook. Then he moved away, looked at me, smiled, and said don't tell anybody. He then went and washed, told me to wash, and then said go to sleep. About an hour later, the rest of my family came in. Suresh did sex to me several times after that until he moved to New Delhi for work. After Suresh, I did sex with my uncle, a couple of my friends, and some neighbours. Many times it was *gand*.[14] They would call it *maasti*.

When I was 14, my father sent me to his brother in Delhi. There he was living with his wife, his two children, my brother and his wife and their one child. We only had one room and all sleeping in the same room. Sometimes the men would sleep outside. I started working in my brother's shop, cleaning, bringing tea, helping to mend the autorickshaws. I had been in New Delhi for about two months when my uncle took me to this park. It was very large with many trees and bushes. It was about six o'clock in the evening and just growing dark. There were few lights in the park, and there seemed to be many men walking around. I could sometimes see two men go behind a bush, or behind a tree where it was much darker, then after a few minutes they would come out and move away from each other. I didn't know, but I sort of guessed what happened. Then my uncle took me behind this bush and did me. I wanted to do it, but I was very scared. It was outside, and maybe someone would see us. When he finished, we came out and he gave me 20 rupees. It was the first time someone had given me money for doing this. . . .

The boys here have taught me a lot about sex. What to do, what not to do, who is dangerous, who to look our for. With them I have learnt to be *kothi*, which brings me more men for sex and more money. I walk this way, I use my hands that way, my voice I make higher. Sometimes it is hard. Each night, maybe five or six men come and fuck me. They are so fast, and they don't use anything, and sometimes I bleed. I always have problems there. Piles. Yes, I have had these diseases. I go to a friend of mine who gives me something. A few days, or maybe a couple of weeks, it goes away. I have heard about condoms, but many men don't want to use. Anyway, sometimes it is difficult in the park, you know, to take time to put on condom. And who is carrying condom anyway? It is like two lives, one is my park life with my friends, one is my street life with my job. I am like two people, and this gate is the line. Maybe I want to stop, because now I want to find a friend who I can be with as my husband. My other friend here, he has a husband.

Rafiq, Calcutta, India

I think I am 10 years old. I have been staying here at this railway station since maybe for five years. My parents and I, with my sister, came here from a small village, and we used to all live together. They told me we had to come to the city as there was no work in the village. Then first my sister died, and then my parents died. For the last two years I have been on my own. Well not really on my own, as I am with the other boys here. We are a gang. Our gang is about 20 boys and girls, mainly boys. The oldest is 14, and we have one boy who is seven. None of us have families. We live here sleeping near the station. I am always hungry. We all are. We beg here, you know, from the passengers, sometimes we thieve when we can, you know, steal wallets, purses. Passengers rushing around can be so careless. Sometimes we are lucky, some foreigners come here and we can beg lots of money from them. Other times we help passengers with their luggage and they give us a little money, a rupee or maybe two. But all this is never enough. Never enough for food. . . .

I first had sex when I was seven, just after I joined the gang. Ramesh was the leader then, but now he is in some sort of home the police took him to for stealing and other things. He was then 14. We usually all sleep together, and it was cold that night. I was the youngest, and Ramesh chose me to keep him warm. Sometime he woke me up and told me to turn towards him. He put my hand on his 'thing'. It was hard and warm. He told me to move my hand up and down, and almost immediately this warm liquid came into my hand. He told me what it was, that I would one day be able to do the same thing, and then he told me to go to sleep. The next morning we never talked about it. Over time I learned that all the boys were doing it with each other, the older with the younger, and also with the girls, but only the older boys could do it with the girls. It was about one year later that I got paid to do this sex thing with an older boy who was in a different gang. He was about 16, and he gave me five rupees to let him fuck me. I felt a lot of pain, but the money bought me food. Then Ramesh showed me this toilet, where lots of men come for sex with each other. He showed me the railway porters and the local stall people who like to do it. I began to earn money through selling my arse. Sometimes they asked me to use my mouth, sometimes my hand, but mostly it's my arse. Maybe I can make 100 rupees a week, and I use to give some of it to Ramesh. Now I give to Debanuj. He is the leader now that Ramesh is gone. I have done it with a girl. I know I don't have hair, but sometimes my thing gets hard. When it does I go to Ramala and share her blanket, if she isn't with anyone.

Sethya, Chennai, India

I first had sex with another man when I was 18. I had wanted to before, but I was always scared to try. Ever since I was 12 years old, I wanted to. My family is small, only one sister, and my father is dead. I had my own little room. I used to masturbate all the time, thinking on some man who I would see on the street, who would hold me, hug me, kiss me. We are a poor family, and I started working when I was 14 years old.

I met this man on the beach near my home and he asked if I would do oral sex with him and he would give me 50 rupees. He led me to this dark spot against a wall. I did it, my first time. Even though he didn't touch me and there was no kissing and hugging I enjoyed it. It was very quick. The money was good. I didn't earn a lot in my job as an office boy. I am 24 years old now. I have been coming to this beach these last five years and since I lost my job three years ago, every evening. I earn perhaps 200 to 300 rupees in any evening, which I give to my family after I take out what I need for myself. Clothes, cinema, food. I tell my mother I have this office job which explains the money I give her. She doesn't have a job now, and I am also saving for my sister's wedding. I need a lakh rupees [100000] for her husband. . . .

Sometimes there is a 'hot' movie on at the cinema, and I can also find sex in the toilet. There I choose a handsome boy to stand next to and make sure that he knows I am willing to do. Never fails. There I usually do oral sex and perhaps hand sex. I also have regular partners, who I see maybe a couple of times a month. Then I go to their homes and enjoy sex with them. Then there is hugging and kissing, which makes me feel very nice. I like that. I have got to know a lot of the boys on the beach here, and that is where I learned a lot from them, the prices to charge, who to be careful of, who to avoid. Here I learnt about myself as a *danga*.[15] Now I see myself as a *danga*. I make perhaps about 1000 rupees a week. I am looking for a real man who will take me as his partner. I will look after him and be a good wife to him.

Anil, Mumbai, India

I used to live with my family in our village near Almora, which is close to Nainital in Uttar Pradesh. Our family were farmers. My father's second youngest brother had moved to Mumbai and he would send money to his wife every month. When he would come to the village every year for a couple of months to help, he would tell us all wonderful stories about the film stars and the rich city. All of us envied him.

I had sex with my uncle when I was 12 years old on one of his visits. Anita [his wife] was sick with another child, and he had come to visit our hut, talking with my father, his brother. He stayed the night, and we shared my blanket, and things happened. During that stay we had sex together several times. At that time he was 27 years old. I have now been on this beach for about four years. Came here when I was 15. My uncle had suggested that I come here. Told my father he would help me get work in the city. That first night in Mumbai, after my uncle took me around Juhu Beach area so I could see where the famous film stars live, and around the Gateway of India, Taj Hotel, and so many places, we did sex in his room. He told me how I could make lots of money through giving massages and sex to men. Then I could send this money to my family and help them. The next day he took me to this beach, and let me watch. There seemed to be so many boys working here. I could see them bending over this man or that man, kneading their backs, arms, legs. Sometimes I could see their hands moving in the crotch area. A couple of times in the very dim light I could see their faces bending over the middle part of the body. After my sex with my uncle I guessed what they were doing. Seeing this made me hot. Then we went back to my uncle's room: he showed me what to do, how to give massage, how to suck, how to give pleasure, what prices to ask for. I practised on him. Over the next week I would go to the beach with him and just watch. When the police came to clear us out, we would stand by the roadside. There some people would drive past in taxis or their own cars and stop to pick up a boy and then drive off. My uncle said that they would take the boy to a hotel room or their own house and do sex there. The price was always higher.

Then after I had been with my uncle for a few days coming to the beach and just watching, and standing with him on the side of the road, this car stopped. A man, maybe about 30, got out and came to us, and asked me to come with him. I looked at my uncle and he told the man that since I was new in Mumbai we would both come. The man grinned and said OK. That night I did sex with my uncle while the man watched, then the man did sex with both my uncle and myself. He paid us 500 rupees. My uncle gave me 100 rupees and said that was because I was just a beginner.

The next day, with this money, I got myself a towel, oil and a little bag and with my uncle we started out on the beach. After a few minutes we separated and each of us went to work. I earned 200 rupees that night. Sometimes I get fucked. Sometimes I am asked to fuck. Sometimes I suck, other times I get sucked. On the beach it's mainly hand sex and sometimes mouth sex. Anal sex is always in a room. It all changes. I enjoy the sex, although I am careful not to lose too much seed. I sometimes still do sex with my uncle, and I have other friends who I do sex with. Once in a while I go to a female prostitute for sex also. I send my family about 2000 rupees a month, and now I have my own room. My family now are arranging for my marriage. They have arranged it with a local family in the village and next year I will get married. I will still come here to the beach. What other job would give me over 4000 to 5000 rupees a month? I can't read or write, I have no education. This way I can earn a lot of money and enjoy the sex.

Conclusions

There are no estimates as to how many 'boys' sell sex to other men in India or Bangladesh, whether it is for cash, clothing, food or shelter. Nor is it known how many male customers they have. Many of these boys speak of anything from three to 12 sexual partners in an evening. What is clear is that the number is large, and is at least equivalent to the number of female sex workers, if not more.

Classifying men who have sex with men as gay men, homosexuals, or even as male sex workers can be problematic. While there are clear identities such as *kothis*, *panthis*, and even *do-parathas*[16] or *double-deckers*,[17] these identities are spatially as well as behaviourally constructed. They are not clearly delineated. Thus while *panthis* and *kothis* both state that their sexual behaviour is distinctly and always 'one way', evidence suggests that these may just be public statements about what are deemed shameful acts. For a *kothi* to admit that he also penetrates, or for a *panthi* to state that he also gets penetrated, is a potential threat to identity. When two *kothis* have sex with each other it is called *chapati-chapati*, being likened humorously to two sisters having sex with each other.

Significantly, all the *kothis* I have spoken with about 'selling' sex, spoke of their family needs. Getting cash of gifts for sex was a means of sustaining themselves and their family. Not one spoke of keeping all the money for themselves. This does not mean that this does not happen. It means, I believe, that family context and poverty are the two major parameters that shape the sale of sex, while issues of gender segregation, homosociability, homoaffectionalism, male power and lack of social space, as well as male-to-male desires, shape the buying and the doing of sex. There appeared to be few boundaries between these differing dynamics, except perhaps among those evolving gay identities. What boundaries do exist are based on social class, education, economic power and gendered behaviour. *Panthis* and gay men do not socialize with *kothis* except in sexual environments. *Do-parathas* are seen as potential *kothis* by both *panthis* and *kothis*, and as potential gay men by other gay-identified men, and are often more highly stigmatized than either of these other two groups in park socio-sexual networks. These identities, for many of these men, are clearly also separated by time and location. It is not impossible, therefore, for a man to have several identities: a park identity, a street identity, a home identity, a family identity, and of course a marriage identity. A significant number of men who have sex with men, including *kothis*, are married with children, and the vast majority who are not already married take it as given that they will get married at a later date. In both India and Bangladesh, marriage is a cultural, social and religious obligation necessary to sustain family honour and duty.

Implications for HIV Prevention

All the *kothis* interviewed mentioned the speed of anal sex and the rapidity of penetration. Reported levels of condom usage were extremely low, and symptoms of sexually transmitted infections very high. The use of water-based lubricants is non-existent. What lubricants were used varied from motor oil to cooking oil, from Vaseline to saliva. On some occasions I was told of the use of Vick's vapour rub 'because it makes the hole tighter'. The majority of *kothis* selling sex complained of piles. Very few went to doctors for treatment because of shame. *Kothis* will, however, visit a friendly pharmacist or a 'street doctor' and take what is given. They may be lucky enough to personally know of a *kothi/panthi* doctor and go to them for treatment. But many of the *kothis* stated that they would simply use whatever remedies their friends told them about.

The risks of transmission of STDs and HIV are clearly enormous, not only from *kothi* to *panthi*, but also from *panthi* to *kothi*, and from *kothi/panthi* to wives and other female partners. What does this imply for the development of appropriate and effective sexual health promotion strategy for men who sell sex to other men? The above accounts illustrate complex interactions between identity formation (or lack of any specific sexual identity), different naming processes, ubiquitous sexual behaviour, invisibility and denial, multiple partners, risky sexual behaviours, low levels of STD/HIV knowledge and awareness, and low levels of condom use with a lack of appropriate lubricants. Moreover, the socio-cultural dynamics of male-to-male sexual networks are poorly (if at all) understood, with almost no in-country investment in risk and needs assessments, or the development of programmes to provide appropriate sexual health services. Interactions between desire, power hierarchies, economic dislocation and poverty, and the socio-cultural frameworks in which this is embedded, stimulate the emergence of self-definitions that bear little relation to current images of 'sex work', or to the dominant Western sexual ideologies promoted in many HIV/AIDS and sexual health programmes.

High quality and meaningful peer-led research, appropriate and easy access to high quality sexual health products and information, and services that recognize anal sex as an important sexual health issue are just a few of the effective sexual health promotions. It is also fundamental to recognize that future sexual health strategies for men need to look at the impact of men's sexual behaviours and sexual health on women's sexual health. Many of the men described here are married or will be so at some time in the future. This means developing programmes that address the specific concerns of both female and male 'partners'. Men who have sex with men are unlikely to tell their wives or other female partners about their sexual activities. Marriages in India and Bangladesh are not usually based on companionship and friendship, nor for that matter are many male-to-male sexual encounters. Programmes need to be developed, therefore, that enable the female partners of men who have sex with men to address their own sexual health needs without learning about their male partner's sexual behaviours.

The situation is complex, and I am not aware of any current strategy that has evolved, either in the West, or in the so-called 'developing countries', whether government or non-government supported, that can effectively and appropriately deal with such situations. What do exist are small-scale local interventions, which are necessary, but need to be seen in a broader context. They may fail to reach, for example, those men who do not go to parks, toilets, shrines, or hang about on streets, at bus stops, railway stations and bus terminals. They may fail, too, to take on board inter-family, intra-family, neighbourhood, work environment, hotel, tea-shops, and guest house sexual encounters. These are as common, if not more so, than behaviours in public sex environments.

This chapter finishes with more questions than answers. Local work is taking place in New Delhi, Bombay, Calcutta, Dhaka, Salem, Cochin, Lucknow and other cities so as to develop a broader vision. These local strategies are somewhat adventurous, forging a pathway that few have trod. It is too early to evaluate these responses, but we know that effective work requires imagination, flexibility, forbearance and a willingness to experiment. There is no one model to be adopted. There is simply understanding, compassion, empathy and an anger that no people should be denied access to accurate information, the resources to protect themselves and their partner(s), and the opportunity for a future. There is no dignity in ignorance, no dignity in silence, and no dignity where there is no hope.

In the end, we struggle along hiding, slipping between the social and sexual interstices, finding the gaps of allowance. Governments, donors and international agencies must recognize the complexity of the issues, not try to reduce them to simple heterosexual/homosexual dichotomies. Nor should there be constant reference to the claim that 'AIDS is a heterosexual issue in Asia'. This is just another form of denial. Finally, where laws and regulations exist that punish, imprison, and lead to community disavowal, these must be changed so as to provide safe and secure services for male sex workers and other men who have sex with men.

Acknowledgements

My gratitude goes to the boys, young men and others; the *kothis, panthis* and *do-parathas*; the gay-identified men and those with emerging gay identities; the park boys, hotel staff, restaurant and tea boys; the rickshaw and truck drivers; the railway, factory and construction workers; the students, office workers and business men. All of these told me their stories, shared with me their grief and pain, talked of their hopes and convictions, spoke frankly of their desires and needs, and offered a glimpse through the windows of their lives. The sheer capacity for survival of these people is outstanding.

Thanks also go to friends who shared dark nights, cold streets, tea stalls, hotel rooms and lobbies, bus and railway stations, cheap restaurants and other unromantic places, sitting and translating for me. Their patience and forbearance were invaluable. Without their help this chapter could not have been written.

Notes

1 See a range of Naz Foundation reports, including Shivananda Khan, *Contexts – race, culture and sexuality*, 1994; Shivananda Khan, *Making Visible the invisible sexuality and sexual health in South Asia – a focus on male to male sexual behaviours*, 1995. See also Shivananda Khan, 'Under the blanket: bisexualities and AIDS in India', in P. Aggleton, P. Davies and G. Hart (Eds.) *Bisexualities and AIDS: International Perspectives*, London: Taylor & Francis, 1996.

2 Taka are the currency of Bangladesh. At the time of writing (1997), 65 taka were equivalent to UK£1.

3 The term 'boys' in this chapter is used in a south Asian sense which does not specifically refer to biological age.

4 In Dhaka, *kothi* come from all income groups, classes, castes, religions and regions. These boys/men gender themselves through effeminate behaviour in specific spaces. Their exaggerated behaviour makes them visible and is used as a flirtation mechanism. Males in need of sexual discharge irrespective of their sexual choices, may often seek out these feminized males for oral sex, masturbation, and, where space and a measure of privacy permits, anal sex. However, many *kothi* are also married with children. It is not unusual for a *kothi* to speak of having between five and ten sexual partners in one evening, where sexual penetration and ejaculation take between five and ten minutes. *Kothis* claim that they do not have sex with each other.

For them such behaviour is considered shameful. Yet in personal and private discussion, several have admitted that they do so. Condom usage appears to be almost non-existent, since not only is the behaviour spontaneous and opportunistic, but also the penetrators do not want to use condoms. A wide variety of settings are used for such sexual activities: during the daytime, lodges, guest house, hotels, inside shops, behind bushes, derelict locations, cinema toilets, other toilets; at night-time, railway tracks, toilets, cinema halls, derelict ground, construction sites, hotels, inside shops, behind bushes, inside parked buses, trucks, railway carriages.

5 The men who sexually access *kothis* are called *panthis*. These are men who exhibit so-called 'normative' behaviours, and while some may sexually desire other men, for many it is the act of sexual penetration and discharge that is important. The framework appears to be one of 'sexual discharge', that is when the male is sexually 'hot' he visits specific locations where he knows *kothis* are available for sex, whether he has to pay for it or not. Many *panthis* stated that they like anal sex because it is 'tighter' than vaginal sex. Recent anecdotal evidence indicates that many *panthis* see women as vectors of sexual diseases and feel that vaginal sex is more risky than anal sex. The vast majority of these men will be married or will become married. It should be noted that many of these males do not see this sexual behaviour as 'real sex', not even as sex, but rather as *maasti/khel* (which means play, or fun).

6 A *tokai* is a person who lives on the street and earns income from collecting discarded, but useful, rubbish from the streets which he/she can sell.

7 Mumbai is the new name for Bombay, India.

8 Chennai is the new name for Madras, India.

9 Rupees are the currency of India. At the time of writing (1997), there were approximately 50 rupees to UK£1.

10 *Darwan* is the term for the gate or park-keeper.

11 *Maasti* is a Hindi term meaning mischief, or play. It sometimes carries sexual connotation as in sexual play.

12 *Jiggery dost* usually means a close friend whom you go around with. Its sexual connotation signifies sex with one's close friend, and it is often indicated in personal conversations through tone and gesture.

13 A *lungi* is a sarong-like garment used by men in Bangladesh and India. Most men wearing *lungis* in Bangladesh do not wear underpants.

14 *Gand* is a Hindi term which means anus. It is also a slang term for anal sex derived from the phrase *gand marna*.

15 *Danga* is a term used in Chennai and has the same connotations as *kothi*.

16 *Do-parathas* is a *kothi* term meaning a man who does both, gets penetrated and penetrates.

17 *Double-decker*, as *do-paratha*, a term used in Chennai.

Chapter 12

Male Sex Work in Sri Lanka

Nandasena Ratnapala

Sri Lanka is a pear-shaped island at the southern tip of the Indian peninsula. The total land area consists of 65810 square miles and the population is approximately 17885000. The island is inhabited by the Sinhalese (74 per cent), the Sri Lankan and Indian Tamils (18 per cent), the Sri Lankan Moors (7 per cent) and other smaller groups (Department of Census and Statistics, 1991). Buddhism was introduced in the third century BC and since then it has been the dominant religion. Following several invasions, Sri Lankan society has been greatly influenced by India's social, political and cultural values. In the sixteenth century, the Portuguese, the Dutch, and then the British came to the island ostensibly in search of trade, and occupied the maritime provinces by force. In 1815, the entire island was brought under British rule until independence was granted in 1948.

Sinhala and Pali texts from medieval times contain a wealth of information on sex and sex workers. *Pali* is the language in which Buddhist texts of the *Theravada* School of Buddhism, to which Sri Lankan Buddhists belong, were written. These texts are of roughly three types: religious texts (in Pali and Sinhala) brought to or written in Sri Lanka; Sinhala poetry and other forms of literature from medieval times; and folklore containing considerable data on sex and sex workers. Of the mainly Buddhist religious texts, the *Vinaya* texts (Oldenberg, 1883) is a compendium of monastic regulations written in both Pali and Sinhala. It includes material on sexual mores and practices. Of texts written in Pali, the *Samanta-Pasadika* (Takakusu and Nagai, 1938) is an important source of information. This is the commentary written to the Pali disciplinary rules compiled in India. As it was written in Sri Lanka, it contains significant information on Sri Lankan everyday life; particularly sex life. The Sinhala commentaries *Sinkhavalanda* and *Sikhavalanda-Vinisa* survey monastic laws in the Sri Lankan tradition and again contain information on sexual life. The Sinhala poem *Geekavyaya* (Godakumbura, 1958) offers a glimpse into sex and sex workers in medieval times. The *Sandesa Kavyas*, written in the eighteenth and nineteenth centuries, contain considerable information on female sex work. The Sinhala text *Saddhamaratnavaliya* describes sex workers and their activities. The famous Sinhalese chronicle, the *Mahavansa* (Geiger, 1912) mentions how in the twelfth century AD, a king built a pavilion for courtesans near the royal park. Folklore contains data not only on female sex workers, but also on male sex workers. There is, therefore, a substantial older literature on sex workers and sex work in Sri Lanka. This contrasts sharply with the picture in more modern times.

Modern Studies

There have been few recent studies of Sri Lankan sexual behaviour, particularly that of sex workers. A few small-scale studies have been undertaken, and also studies in which a careful methodology has not been adopted. Bond (1980a, 1980b), for example, conducted an 18-day 'tourist study' of child prostitution, but he was largely ignorant of the Sinhala language. His report offers somewhat fantastic descriptions of child sex work, and the data is often recycled with scant attention to the veracity of his sources. Thereafter, an estimate of 30000 child sex workers has been given, both in official government publications and also in international reports (Department of National Planning 1991; Save the Children Overseas Department, 1993). No reliable source for this estimate of 30000 cases has ever been given.

Various NGOs in Sri Lanka have also published reports on sex work, particularly child sex work, as part of their own programmes advocating its abolition. These papers have largely been written with 'advocacy' in mind, hence the absence of precise data and careful analysis. Moreover, the research techniques necessary to deal with an intimate, personal and secretive subject such as sex, have been largely absent in such studies.

Two important studies have, however, been conducted by Weeramunda (1989, 1993). The first is a study of knowledge, attitudes and practices in relation to HIV and AIDS, the second is an unpublished report on child prostitution in a selected district in the tourist belt. As far as studies of sexual behaviour are concerned, the latter is one of the best surveys so far undertaken, although it is based entirely on questionnaire responses, which understandably limits the validity of responses to intimate questions such as those on child sexual abuse. A symposium on child sex work was held in 1992, sponsored by the Terres des Hommes and Kindern in Die Knel, and organized by the Department of Child Care and Peace. Another study on child sex work was subsequently conducted for the Department of Probation and Child Care on Child Prostitution (Ratnapala, 1995).

Other than these few studies specifically focusing on sex and sexual behaviour, occasional reference to sex and sex work can be found in various writings. Modern Sinhala literature, novels, short stories and poems contain references to sex and sex workers which remain to be systematically analyzed. Such work would add much to our knowledge of sex workers, and attitudes towards them.

Contextual Concerns

Sex work in Sri Lanka cannot be discussed properly without reference to Buddhist attitudes to sex and sex work. In Buddhist teachings, sex is recognized as a fundamental urge. The sexual organs are treated like any other bodily organs, and should not be looked down on or treated with contempt. A monk leading a celibate life should refrain from sexual intercourse (that is basically penetrative sexual activity with a woman, man, animal or inanimate object), and penetrative sexual acts automatically result in the loss of monkhood. 'As a man with his head cut off cannot become one to live with that bodily connection, so is a monk indulging in sexual intercourse' (Oldenberg, 1883, p. 48). Non-penetrative sexual activity is a lesser offence punishable by probation, confiscation or forfeiture (Ratnapala, 1993).

Lay people, on the other hand, may enjoy sex within the family where ideas of 'one man, one woman' prevail. Like taking others' life and property, telling lies and taking alcohol or drugs, sexual intercourse with other women or men, and leaving ones' husband or wife, are regarded as wrongful forms of behaviour. However, since Buddhist teachings were practical and understanding of human nature, the power of sex did not bar men or women from seeking more than one wife, or one husband. If that is the local custom, such systems were accepted. But the general principle was, even in this context, that those involved in polygamy and polyandry should try to remain faithful to their partner(s). Visiting a sex worker was not considered a 'sin', but it could be costly. In one text, *Parabhava Sutta*, in the book *Sutta Nipata* (Anderson and Smith, 1948), for example, it is said that one loses one's hard-earned wealth on account of visits to sex workers.

Two types of female sex workers are portrayed in the Buddhist texts: *Vesi* or *Vesiya*, who conduct business from their homes; and *Ganika*, or high-class urban sex workers, the 'common property of the whole body of men associated together by a common bond' (Chakladar, 1954, p. 400). In Sri Lanka, there has never been a clear distinction between these two types. Sinhala literary sources, particularly the *Sandesa Kavyas* of the sixteenth and seventeenth centuries provide details of such female sex workers. According to these descriptions, such women were exceedingly beautiful. They frequented the city in search of customers, most often at the fall of darkness.

There is little direct reference to male sex work in the past. Individual instances of homosexual activity, as well as the role of some males as male sex workers are, however, referred to in a number of Buddhist texts and folklore. Additionally, eunuchs who served in the king's court may have been involved in sex work. But as an institution, hardly any reference to male sex work can be found, either in literary or folklore sources.

Male Sex Work Today

In Sri Lanka, homosexual behaviour between men takes place from a very early age in the family or community life (Ratnapala, 1996a). Young men frequently work together with adult males in agriculture, fishing and gem-mining work. In such situations, which require spending a considerable time away from home, there are plenty of opportunities for homosexual activity. It is not unknown in gem-mining areas, for example, for young children to be kept in temporary quarters to assist adults. Ostensibly, this is to assist in physical work, but actually these young children may be 'kept' for sexual activity.

Transvestite Sex Workers

Of male sex workers, perhaps the best known are the *Ponnaya*, transvestites in the city of Colombo. They are openly visible, moving about in small groups. Wearing female attire and make-up, they frequent the roads in Colombo by shady trees, parks and street junctions. Here, they wait for their clients at a place not observed by others. Clients normally arrive in motor vehicles, taking away chosen (and often already contacted) individuals. After driving to a solitary place, client and sex worker usually engage in petting leading to oral sex. Thereafter, the client drops the transvestite at the place where he was picked up. In the case of clients who need more time and want to have other forms of sex, the sex worker is normally taken to a known hotel, guest-house or private flat. The entire night is often spent together and anal sex may take place.

Clients are mostly young or middle-aged unmarried men, divorcees or men whose wives have died. Pimps, street children and female sex workers consider the transvestites as undesirable, and often pick quarrels with them. They stay nearby or a little distance away.

Beyond sex work, the transvestites often engage in odd jobs. Some become entertainers, taking part in religious processions. In Colombo there are probably 260 to 270 transvestites involved in sex work today. This includes a group of 35 to 40 individuals who live in the south of Colombo and who are devotees of a particular god in the area, Kataragama, also known as Skandha. Their 'leader' is the lay priest there, and the majority work in or around the shrine.

Transvestites also have a key role to play in certain other activities. They may appear at weddings and religious rituals, where they sometimes cook the food. Additionally, when there is a wedding, they come to the house for several days to assist in preparations and dressing the bride. Such stays provide opportunities to engage in sex. In this kind of situation, their sex work is thus subsumed in the more socially accepted role of 'helpers' in ceremonies.

Child Sex Workers

Children are also involved in sex work in Sri Lanka. Male children are often procured for this purpose in rural areas and brought to Colombo, Negombo,

Kalutara and such other locations in the tourist belt. This is organized by local pimps catering for European paedophiles. Houses are rented out and children are brought there by cheating them, or by using force. In 1995–96, an estimated 1500 children were involved in this kind of work. Of them, nearly two-thirds were boys (Ratnapala, 1995). Local pimps provide boys according to the particular client's taste. Sometimes, drugs are given to these children in order to arouse them. Some such encounters are videotaped, perhaps so that clients can see them, or share the experiences with their friends or colleagues, later.

Paedophile clients comprise two age groups: those aged from 20 to 35, and those who are middle-aged. Some members of the latter group tend to have visited the country many times, bought property and even involved themselves in local social and economic activities.

Boy sex work is highly organized so as to ensure that members of the chain do not get caught, and that the principal organizers remain anonymous. The latter are often protected by the political or legal powers. Boys engaged in the business may range in age from 16 to 18, and often come from the poorest strata of society. Their parents are uneducated and socially powerless, with large numbers of children. The business is lucrative, with the organizers earning a large fee, of which very little is given to the child.

In well known tourist areas, groups of boys, aged 14 to 16, work as 'freelance' male sex workers unattached to any group or powerful local individual, or any pimps or middlemen. The unwritten rule for these boys is to 'serve' the tourists up to the age of 16 and thereafter leave the locality. The usual service offered is anal sex. The boys thereafter move to other areas of the tourist belt, or to Colombo and work as male sex workers there.

Sex Work with Women

The growth of the tourist trade has also encouraged some young men to offer sexual services to women visitors. Such men are found in or near tourist hotels, often operating as tour guides or such innocent-looking jobs. Those employed in the hotels as bell-boys, waiters, and so on, as well taxi drivers, may also provide such services. Since sex workers are socially ostracized, they often conceal their real work beneath a more socially acceptable role.

Such male sex workers find their clientele among two types of foreign women: young women and those who are middle-aged. Both come to Sri Lanka looking for sexual adventure. The young sex workers can easily recognize those women who are seeking sexual adventures. Sexual activity takes place in hotels, on the beach, on an arranged trip, or even in the houses of sex workers themselves.

Local women may also be approached through advertisements in popular newspapers. Very often such advertisements carry innocent-looking offers of body massage and such other activities. The language used offers the key to what is really being offered. In addition, word of mouth information from one client to another helps sex workers establish networks of regular clients or customers.

Intervention Implications

No intervention strategy is useful unless it takes into account the sexual behaviour of the targeted group in the cultural context in which it occurs, and formulates the strategy accordingly. A range of possible interventions for HIV prevention among male sex workers and their clients suggest themselves. Male workers could, for example, be encouraged to practise safer sex with an emphasis on non-penetrative intercourse. This form of sex is already practised by some. A particular challenge exists, however, in relation to oral sex. Many sex workers object to using condoms for this because of their 'awful' taste, and some clients believe that condoms dull sensation. Additionally, some sex workers also like to swallow the semen and resist using condoms because of this.

Traditionally, anal intercourse has not been widely practised in Sri Lanka because of the association of the anus with faecal matter. Instead, the two thighs are used to rub the penis until ejaculation is reached. Increases in tourism has contributed to an increased prevalence of anal intercourse. There are now areas, for example, where the most frequently provided sexual service to tourists is anal intercourse. Past efforts to introduce condoms here have not been successful because the condoms supplied were not durable. Efforts to promote the use of KY lubricant did not succeed either, as it was only available locally in large quantities. The only alternative was to get the boys to persuade clients to bring strong condoms with them. This was done by careful observation of the 'bond relationship' between sex worker and client, and by introducing the idea as a means of cementing an already existing relationship. Information is valued on the basis of whether it contributes to the increase or decrease of the bond relationship with the foreigner they chose.

Various indicators signal this increase in commitment. The client may give the boys valuable gifts. Such gifts may also be given to his family members, to assist the building of a house, to buy a bicycle or a musical instrument. Or a client may come and live in the boy's own house as a member of his family. Finally, the foreigner may take the boy on a trip abroad. Bringing strong condoms was carefully introduced to fit in with pre-existing patterns of bonding. The strategy succeeded, and tourists who came began to bring such condoms. This was done by spreading word of the need for condoms to the tourists, who then told friends who planned to visit that they should bring the required condoms with them.

Several reasons can be advanced for the success of this intervention. Often, clients were rich and educated foreigners who had a good knowledge of HIV/AIDS. Many had long associations with individual boys and had developed a concern and even affection for them. The boys themselves were all from the same locality, and therefore among themselves had a strong community spirit. The tourist trade in the locality had a tacit understanding of what was going on and did not unduly interfere with the use of condoms. Such interference by state and police authorities was identified in earlier interventions with female sex workers as a major obstacle to HIV prevention. The police had used the carrying of condoms as evidence to 'prove' that the woman concerned was a sex worker. As a result, sex workers became afraid to carry condoms with them.

In the case of male sex workers, this problem was resolved by the project taking up the matter with the senior police officers. Thereafter, as many police stations as possible were visited and education about HIV/AIDS was undertaken. Condoms were given to the police, who were asked to distribute them among the sex workers. We knew that at least some police officers would use them, and it was our belief that with the passage of time, the police would develop a more healthy attitude towards condom use.

This attitude towards condom use is not peculiar to the police, but is held by society as a whole. Unlike in the past, sex is nowadays treated as a 'dirty' thing and condoms are considered symbolic of an obscene or permissive sex life. This attitude could be changed by intensive public education and through work that emphasizes the non-judgmentalism implicit in much Buddhist teaching. Work done by *Sarvodaya*, a local NGO, engaged in HIV/AIDS intervention from a Buddhistic perspective, has been a considerable success.

One-to-one and small group communication is another strategy that can be used with male sex workers. Except for pornography, most male sex workers do not read any other type of literature. They do, however, have close friendship networks. Friends spend long hours in conversation with one another, and by using these small groups as a starting point, much headway could be made in developing an intervention strategy.

The social 'geography' of these small groups, how and where they operate, in what social contexts they are recognized, and the processes through which they learn about sex, were all carefully analyzed. The hypothesis here is that there may be a link between what is talked about in friendship networks and patterns of behaviour. It was also possible to identify leaders in most groups and to use such individuals as linchpins in the oral communication strategy. In this case, male sex workers were informally organized under the local lay religious priest. Getting to know this person was the 'open sesame' to reach the others. Once this had taken place, approaching small groups and getting them involved was far easier.

Male sex workers' dedication to religious activities provides another focus for intervention. In dedicating themselves to religious work, they follow a given set of religious rituals and beliefs. For example, on two days of each week, special ceremonies to honour the gods are carried out. Each small group of male sex workers visits the shrine and takes part in performing certain aspects of this ritual. This is a good moment to intervene, but any health promotion must, of course, be undertaken with due regard to religious sensitivities.

Sex workers enjoy telling erotic stories and describing sexual incidents to one another. By carefully identifying the literature they read, and perhaps getting such publications to include HIV/AIDS-related concerns, prevention messages could be got across. Alternatively, such a goal could be achieved orally using the idioms, contexts and incidents that figure in the discussions that take place in friendship groups. Success here would be predicated upon prior study of the sexual language used, and the contexts in which meanings associated with sex are placed.

Male sex workers employed in hotels and engaged in other minor jobs could also be contacted through their primary groups, their peers. By identifying a number of influential individuals and training them in peer communication, many men could be reached. A close socio-cultural mapping of primary groups, and the development of techniques to find out whether the particular piece of information had reached targeted individuals, will be necessary here. Constant surveillance and an awareness of changing life-patterns are very important. Without close rapport, a strategy such as this will not be successful.

Condom availability has a significant effect on the promotion of safe sex. Availability in a pharmacy alone will not motivate sex workers to go and buy them openly. Condom vending machines need to be discreetly made available in locations which fit their needs, their group life and their patterns of behaviour. Pharmacies can also be persuaded to exhibit condoms attractively and place them so that they could be seen by customers. Shop assistants can be trained to look at customers without embarrassment and confine their 'conversation' to nods and symbolic acts. Trained to communicate in this way, they will be more effective when it comes to marketing condoms in a culturally appropriate way. In Sri Lanka, condoms are always associated with 'illicit' sex, and it is a stigma for anyone to carry a condom and be seen with it. Pharmacists consider it immoral to sell condoms, and may need persuasion to do so. Broader societal attitudes, and those in the immediate community, will need to be taken into account when condoms are marketed.

References

ANDERSON, D. and SMITH, R. (Eds) (1948) *Sutta Nipata*, London: Pali Text Society (reprint).

BOND, T. (1980a) *Boy Prostitution in Sri Lanka*, mimeograph, Colombo.

BOND, T. (1980b) *Hello, What's Your Name? The Tourist Boys and Sri Lanka*, mimeograph, Colombo.

CHAKLADAR, S.C. (1954) *Social Life in Ancient India*, 2nd edn, Calcutta: Sunil Gupta.

DEPARTMENT OF CENSUS AND STATISTICS (1991) *Statistical Pocket Book*, Colombo: Department of Census and Statistics.

DEPARTMENT OF NATIONAL PLANNING (1991) *Report of the National Symposium on the Plan of Action for the Children of Sri Lanka*, Colombo: Ministry of Policy Planning and Implementation.

GEIGER, W. (Ed.) (1912) *Mahavansa*, vols i–ii, London: Pali Text Society.

GODAKUMBURA, C.E. (1958) *Sinhalese Literature*, Colombo: Apothecaries Ltd.

OLDENBERG, H. (1883) *Vinaya Pitaka*, vols i–v, trans. (1938–52) I.B. Horner as The Book of Discipline, vols i–v, London: Pali Text Society.

RATNAPALA, N. (1993) *Crime and Punishment in the Buddhist Tradition*, New Delhi: Mittal.

RATNAPALA, N. (1995) *Behaviour Modification among Commercial Sex Workers of Sri Lanka*, Colombo: Dipanee Press.

RATNAPALA, N. (1996a) 'Intervention-linked research on the sexual behaviour of young people in Sri Lanka in the context of the HIV/AIDS infection', unpublished report for NORAD.

SAVE THE CHILDREN OVERSEAS DEPARTMENT (1993) *Working Paper No 7*, London: Save the Children.

TAKAKUSU, J. and NAGAI, M. (Eds) (1938) *Samanta-Pasadika*, vols i–v, London: Pali Text Society.

WEERAMUNDA, A.J. (1989) 'Unpublished report on the Sri Lankan survey on knowledge, attitude and behaviour relating to HIV/AIDS', Geneva: World Health Organization.

WEERAMUNDA, A.J. (1993) 'Unpublished report on the pilot study on child prostitution in a selected area of the Kalutara District'.

Chapter 13

Bar Talk: Thai Male Sex Workers and Their Customers

Graeme Storer

In Thailand, the male sex industry is extensive in the four cities of Bangkok, Chiang Mai, Pattaya and Phuket. In Bangkok, for example, as many as 50 venues are scattered throughout the city (Allyn, 1992; Jackson, 1995). There are male bar workers, masseurs in saunas and gyms, 'singers' in karaoke bars and male escorts. In addition, freelance workers are found walking the streets (Poshyachinda and Danthamrongkul, 1996; Narvilai, 1994) or cruising the discos, pubs and cinemas frequented by homosexually active men. In this chapter, I will focus attention on male bar workers in Bangkok. There are a number of reasons for being concerned with this particular group. First, the sexual network for the male bar workers is complex and can include homosexually active men (both gay and non gay-identified), *kathoey* (transgendered persons) and women. Second, the relationships among the bar workers, customers and bar operators are characterized by a lack of personal reflection and the workers' ability to negotiate sex is constrained by the power exerted by the customers and management. And third, the customers may be either Thai or non-Thai; this provides a further complication for the sex workers who may be called on to negotiate the sex session (the *off*) either in their first language, Thai, or in a second language, usually English (Storer, 1996).[1]

In examining the interactions among Thai male bar workers, their customers and the owners and managers of the bars in which they work, I will seek an understanding of the discursive and sexual practices associated with the bars. More specifically, how do the male sex workers and their customers negotiate the *off*? What (if any) differences exist when the negotiation takes place in Thai or English? What are the critical moments in these interactions and how are they discursively resolved? I will include a discussion of how the data generated in a series of in-depth interviews and group discussions with Thai male sex workers and their customers are informing a process of 'triangulation as intervention'. I will also discuss the implications for promoting safe sex behaviours among homosexually active men.

Background

Epidemiological data from Thailand indicate that HIV incidence rates may be slowing among young Thai men. This may be related to an increase in condom use and a decrease in the frequency of sex with female sex workers (Natpratan, 1995; Mastro and Limpakarnjanarat, 1995, p. 524; Mason *et al.*, 1995). However, similar behavioural changes have not been seen among the population of homosexually active men (Beyrer *et al.*, 1995; Kunawararak *et al.*, 1995; Sittitrai, Sakondhavat and Brown, 1992; McCamish and Sittitrai, 1996). Because of a 'general reluctance' to talk openly about same-sex behaviours (Sittitrai, Sakondhavat and Brown, 1992; Alexander, 1995) and because reported same-sex behaviour can vary considerably with data collection techniques (Beyrer *et al.*, 1995), it seems likely that there has been under-reporting of male–male sex. With male sex workers, there is an even greater chance of under-reporting because of the high turnover of workers (Sittitrai, Phanuphak and Roddy, 1994). These findings indicate the need to broaden HIV prevention strategies, giving greater emphasis to male–male sex behaviours.

Studies of Thai male sex workers have shown that the majority of the workers are behaviourally bisexual (*haa sip*, *haa sip*) and do not identify as gay (Sittitrai, Brown and Virulrak, 1991; Nopekesorn, Sungkarom and Somlum, 1991; Sittitrai, Sakondhavat and Brown, 1992; Narvilai, 1994; Kunawararak *et al.*, 1995; Sriwatjana, 1995). It seems that many of the customers of the Thai male sex worker are also bisexual and that some are married. In addition, customers may be either Thai or non-Thai, a further challenge for the workers who may be required to interact in a second language. Outside the workplace, the bar workers may have commercial encounters as well as casual and regular partners. The scope of the industry and the complex sexual and social networks suggest that interventions directed through male bar workers could potentially reach a wide audience of homosexually active men.

In this chapter, I will scrutinize the interactions between Thai male bar workers, their customers and management in an attempt to clarify the discursive and sexual practices associated with the bars. I will look in turn at three filters – the socio-historical constructions of HIV/AIDS and gender and sexuality, an ethnography of the bar sites (situated practice), and lived experiences as reported by the research informants – and will map each of these representations onto a discussion of the negotiation of sexual practice. I will then show how triangulation of the data makes explicit critical moments in the interactions between Thai male bar workers and their customers and clarifies the strategies developed by the workers to negotiate the *off*.[2] But, first, I will describe the research methodology in detail.

Methodology

The work I am reporting here is part of an ongoing study and draws on a series of in-depth interviews which I carried out over a two-year period (from

December 1994 to November 1996) with male bar workers in Bangkok and with regular male customers of the workers. The customers were both Thai and non-Thai (either resident in Thailand or visitors to Thailand). I carried out the interviews with the bar workers in Thai at times convenient to the workers, usually late afternoons or early evenings. The interviews were typically one-to-one and were tape-recorded. I wrote up notes immediately after each interview and transcribed the tapes into English within 24 hours. I later confirmed the translations with English-speaking Thai men. The interviews with customers were carried out at a place chosen by the informants, either in the privacy of their homes or at some 'neutral' venue. Interviews with non-Thai informants were carried out in English. In addition, I conducted group interviews with gay-identified Thai men and with *kathoey*. All informants were able to contact me for a follow-up discussion if they so wished and I met with some of the informants two to four times over the two-year period.

The male sex workers informing this study were recruited from either the inner-city bars in the Patpong area or from suburban bars in the Saphan Kwai area of Bangkok and ranged in age from 19 to 28, with the majority between 19 and 22. Twenty-five male bar workers participated in the interviews. In addition, there were 13 customers and six bar employees. All names of informants and venues given in this chapter have been changed to maintain anonymity. The use of italics in the transcripts indicates either a transliteration of the Thai or words borrowed from English. Bracketed ellipses (. . .) indicate pauses of greater than half a second.[3]

A Framework for an Integrated Data Analysis

Before approaching the complex theme of negotiation we need to understand better the discursive constructions of 'reality' and talk. I begin with the view that language is a mode of action that is historically situated; language is socially shaping but it is also socially shaped (Fairclough, 1995). An assumption I make is that the narratives related by the research informants verbalize and situate their experiences as text (Schriffen, 1996); in this way, they transform and displace stretches of experience from the past into linguistically represented episodes, events, processes and states (Labov, 1972).

In developing the research methodology, I have been guided by two concerns related to the interview process. First, the structure of any linguistic production depends on the symbolic power relations between speakers and on their ability to access and control the 'language of authority' (Bourdieu, 1977, p. 648). For a person to be able to contribute equally in a discussion, he or she must have equal status which presumes 'having equal discoursal and pragmatic rights and obligations' (Fairclough, 1995, p. 47). But while interlocutors of equal status have access to the same kinds of meanings, interlocutors of unequal status take up semantic choices of different kinds (Poynton, 1989). Thus, the tenor of my discussions with the research informants – as enacted through the dimensions of power and solidarity (Poynton, 1989) – is shaped by the dynamics of the interaction between myself as a middle-class, non-Thai, gay researcher and young Thai male sex workers of quite different educational and socio-economic backgrounds.[4] Though we do share certain concerns relating to homosexuality, safe sex practices and health, I remain aware that the informants may engage in a process of self-surveillance (Bourdieu, 1977, pp. 658–62) in order to maintain face (*naa*) and to satisfy their wish to be seen as regular guys, rather than one of *those* guys.

My second concern rests with the nature of reported data, which is often construed as 'proof' even though it is secondary and mediated (Lane-Mercier, 1991; Bloor, 1995, pp. 92–4). In the bars where the men work, the background music and chatter do not allow for a recording to be made of the actual talk between the workers and customers. In addition, I am never present at the time of the sex session. Reported speech is always 'shaped' in the retelling and while it may be close to the original, it can never correspond exactly to what happened.

I have attempted to address these two concerns by drawing on a methodological framework in which a process of reflection is central to the data analysis. The framework comprises four approaches: (1) a socio-historical perspective – the socio-historical conditions within which the discursive and sexual practices occur and which frame male sex work and male–male sex;[5] (2) an ethnography of the bar sites – the local practices of the bars as these are encoded and legitimized in the 'rules' of the bars, the way that resources are regulated, and the power relations among the participants; (3) an ethnography based on lived experiences – the experiences related by the participants as they attempt to make sense of their lives, verbalize and situate their experiences as text and thereby explicate the 'bar talk' (what goes on in the bars); and (4) triangulation as intervention – engaging the participants in a process of reflexivity provides the text analysis central to understanding how culture, power and discourse interact, reinforce and subvert one another. The intention here is to make explicit the ensemble of procedures that constitute the everyday practices of the bars, as they are located in discourses (Foucault, 1984), in the acquired (Bourdieu's *habitus*, 1991), or in the form of time or occasion (de Certeau, 1984).

In the next section, I will discuss the institutional and social organizational conditions around which the discursive and sexual practices of the bar occur. I will begin by looking at how HIV/AIDS has been represented in Thai public media and, in particular, in the Thai press and then turn to a discussion of gender and sexual identity.

Public Voices/Private Lives

Foucault in his *History of Sexuality* described the 'discursive explosion' that occurred around the subject of sexuality in the West as 'an apparatus for producing an ever greater quantity of discourse about sex, capable of functioning and taking effect in its very economy' (Foucault, 1979, p. 23). But this valorization of the discourse of sex has not been as apparent in other parts of the world and I would suggest that there has been only reluctant discussion of sexuality and sexual behaviour in some Asian countries, a reluctance often framed by arguments about 'appropriateness' and 'cultural norms' (see, for example, Alexander, 1995; Caraël *et al.*, 1995). Such cultural screening has not been the case in Thailand and HIV/AIDS is a public concern in local Thai newspapers and magazines (Fordham, 1996). Nevertheless, cultural models continue to shape shared meanings and public warning messages are not uniformly recognized (Lyttleton, 1995, p. 178; Fordham, 1996, 1998).

In Thailand, HIV/AIDS has been largely constructed around male promiscuity and, in particular, promiscuity in the sphere of sex work. The female sex worker remains a scapegoat and is seen as the primary source of infection for men (Fordham, 1996). These representations have resulted in understandings of pools of infection that exclude non-commercial sex. In addition, references to male–male sex behaviours when found in Thai print media are usually 'funny', sensational and about the *kathoey*. Male sex work rarely appears in this public discourse. Unfortunately, local gay publications have not taken a lead here and a quick glance at Thai gay magazines, shows that many of the articles are translations lifted out of Western magazines, and as such bear little relation to Thai gay men or contemporary Thai lifestyles. Because homosexuality has been a muted presence in the Thai HIV/AIDS campaign and in the discourse surrounding HIV/AIDS (Lyttleton, 1996), Thai male sex workers must respond to and ascribe meanings to HIV/AIDS campaigns largely directed at the family man or heterosexually active youth. This has, in effect, silenced the male sex workers.

Studies of Thai male sex work indicate that the majority of the workers are behaviourally bisexual (*haa sip, haa sip* or 50–50) and define their work in economic rather than sexual terms (Sittitrai, Brown and Virulrak, 1991; Nopekesorn, Sungkarom and Somlum, 1991; Sittitrai, Sakondhavat and Brown, 1992; Narvilai, 1994; Kunawararak *et al.*, 1995; Sriwatjana, 1995). However, the sexual identity of male sex workers is reified in their work and sexual behaviours (Boles and Elifson, 1994, p. 39) and issues of identity are significant in understanding occupational practice among male sex workers (Bloor *et al.*, 1993; de Graaf *et al.*, 1994). It will be useful to examine how sociohistorical constructions of gender and sexuality frame the interactions between Thai male bar workers and their customers and affect behavioural norms and group identification.

Rehearsing Masculinity

It seems like Thai society accepts. But I don't think they do. I think they are beginning to now but I still have to be careful. I can't be *over.* It's like there are rules that I have to follow. But really, Thai society is not that accepting. They don't show it, but it's in their hearts. And I don't show them how I feel either. (Pom, 28 November 1995)

I have argued elsewhere (Storer, in press) that Thai society is tolerant rather than accepting of homosexuality and that gay identification is constrained by a traditional gender role bifurcation. The only indigenous Thai word to name homosexual is *kathoey* and, more often than not, the language of homosexuality is English. But while terms like *gay, gay king* and *gay queen* have been appropriated into the Thai vernacular, they seem to mean different things to different people. For some, *gay* has been used as a label for 'modern' and 'egalitarian' homosexuality through a process of 'stigma transformation' (Murray, 1994). But for others, 'the new word has become a euphemism for those men who are homosexually penetrated' in an instance of 'relexification' (Murray, 1994, p. 297). The presumption remains that masculinity and homosexuality cannot coexist and, in the traditional scheme of things, the insertee is an inferiorized kind of man while the inserter is relatively unstigmatized and generally maintains his masculinity in homosexual encounters (de Lind van Wijngaarden, 1995).[6] Thus, a homosexually active Thai man may deny being gay, associating it with behaviour expected of a *kathoey* (Allyn, 1991, p. 144). But not all Thai men buy into these heterosexual presumptions:

> [Male sex workers] can't say that they are men when they sleep with other men and have feelings. At the most, they might be 80 per cent men and 20 per cent gay. They are men (. . .) They just won't show they are gay. Some have a wife and children, but they work in the bar. If you're 100 per cent man, then you can't sleep with another man. (Sam, 23 January 1996)

While it may not be immediately apparent what social sanctions exist in Thailand for those men who openly admit to sex with men (Sittitrai, Sakondhavat and Brown, 1992), gossip is pervasive and there is a definite 'reluctance and delay in applying stigmatized labels to oneself' (Murray, 1992, p. 31).[7] As in other parts of the world, the perception that homosexuality negates or violates family roles can inhibit disclosure of homosexual (or bisexual) behaviour. For the male sex worker there is also the fear that his family or friends will learn that he is selling sex to men and that he will then become subject to the discourses which stereotype masculinity and stigmatize prostitution (Browne and Minichiello, 1995). Understandably, then, a major concern of the bar workers is their ability to 'pass', and the workers with whom I talked were quick to distinguish the group norms that governed the interaction between fellow sex workers and customers.

> I can do this for the money (. . .) It's very good money. We sell a service. What they want, we do. If they want to be *fucked*, then I will

fuck them. But I never let them do it to me. I'm a *man*. I'm a *man* who sells a service. (Chart, 1 February 1995)

Thus, we can see that identity, as manifest in public appearances and behaviours, is readily separated from private practice (Morris, 1994) and there is a definite opposition to naming oneself as one's sexuality. Maintaining a masculine 'image' (*phap-phot*) and preserving face are paramount here. My research suggests that the Thai male bar workers do not readily talk among themselves about sex with their customers and that this management of impressions (Goffman, 1969) can inhibit frank discussions with them about male–male sex and associated risk behaviours. Additionally, it is difficult to target customers when their homosexuality is hidden or where their contact with male bar workers is a fleeting 'night out with the boys' (Storer, 1996).

It has been my intention in this section to not assign a *homosexual* identity to the Thai male bar workers and to challenge representations of gender and sexuality as these relate to male sex work and male–male sex. My position is that a single focus on identity moves attention away from discussions of *homosexual behaviours* and encourages the reluctance to talk about same-gender sex. Questions that ask, for example, 'Are you gay?' or 'Do you prefer to have sex with men?' invite denial when gender and sexuality are defined through binary oppositions and when terms like *phuchai neung roi per sen* (100 per cent man) or *phuchai dtem dtua* ('complete' man) retain currency. While there is evidence of an emerging middle-class gay lifestyle in some parts of Thailand (Jackson, 1995, 1996b; Altman, 1995), it would be wrong to assume that there is a readily identifiable community of men who have sex with men. This is particularly so for the Thai male bar workers, whose support networks are fragmented and whose friendships are usually confined to one or two other men who come from the same village or region (McCamish and Sittitrai, 1996). It is necessary then to problematize the concept of community when planning interventions with male bar workers and to focus attention on both work-related sexual networks and those that extend beyond the bar.

Playing the Game (an Economy of Pleasure)

Though highly visible, both male and female sex work remain illegal in Thailand; thus, the bars provide a 'safe' haven for the workers and their customers beyond the surveillance of the law. But for the male bar worker, this 'protection' involves working within a set of regulatory codes, and he remains the other within the very culture that assimilates him when he agrees to participate in a performance in which he is objectified: he may be 'handled', or required to undress in public. Some managers 'try out' the workers when they first start in the bar, a practice that is often couched in terms of needing to be able to make recommendations to customers (Storer, 1996). In addition, a subtle hierarchy exists in the bars, with the uniformed doormen and waiters seeing themselves as being superior to the sex workers (McCamish and Sittitrai, 1995), and negotiation of the *off* may be constrained before it even begins. In some bars, the workers can cruise the customers; but in others, they must sit to one side and wait to be 'called over' or for the *kaptan* (captain) or *mama-san* to intervene. In bars operating a call-out service, it is the manager or *kaptan* who takes the phone call and who is in a position to 'favour' certain workers. The rules of the game are made clear to the new recruits:

TOON: At first [the manager] will tell the new boy the rules. Like this (...) What time to come. Please the customers. Like this (...) A customer has to pay the *off* fee to the bar before you can leave with the customer. (...) Like this. They tell all the rules.
GS: Does he tell them anything else?
TOON: No, nothing. (Toon, 22; 18 December 1995)

The majority of the inner-city bars in Bangkok pay the workers a retainer of 50 baht (US$2.00) per night for turning up, though this is not paid if they *off*. They also get commission on the drinks a customer orders for them and for performing in the shows. However, an elaborate system of fines means that the workers may end up owing the bar money. For example, if they do not turn up, they are fined 150 to 200 baht per evening (equivalent to the *off* fee). Some bars cut payment if the workers do not get enough *offs*. There is also a hierarchy among the workers themselves and San, for example, felt excluded from the inner circle:

If a boy doesn't *off* for a week, he is advised to try his chances somewhere else. We have to arrive by 8:00 p.m. If we come after 8:30 we might get fined 40 baht. If we come after 9:00 p.m. we are fined 150 baht (...) [The manager] has three or four boys in the bar that he looks after. The rest he doesn't care about. Even the bar staff are not with us. That's how he controls us. (San, 27 December 1994)

The rules applying to the customer involve a series of payments: he may be required to pay an entry fee at the door; he must order a drink on entering the bar; he will be expected to buy another drink if a worker sits with him; and he must pay the *off* fee to secure the worker's services.

For the male bar workers, a 'protocol of service' demands that they please the customers (*ao jai khaek*; *dtaam jai khaek*). But some workers, especially those with less experience or no self-esteem, believe that the protocol of service does not allow them to negotiate with the customer – the customer is always right. The situation is further complicated when the worker does not have the necessary language skills to speak for himself. Here Lao tells us about his difficulties with a *farang* customer:

What I didn't like was when I met with a sadist (...) He didn't go (...) He didn't go gently. He pushed it right in (...) pushed it right in and then bit me here, bit me there [indicating shoulders and chest]. It really hurt. I couldn't stand it. *Okay,* I couldn't stand but I had to put up with it (. . .) because he was a customer. If I really couldn't stand it (. . .) If it was a Thai, then I would be angry. I would have (. . .) I would have a fight for sure. But this is a *farang* customer. And another thing, I'm worried that the bar will get a bad name. I have to put up with it. (Lao, 21 December 1995)

It appears that little or no negotiation takes place in the bar itself and that the main concern of the workers is to get their customers *off* as quickly as possible and thereby secure payment:

This is the idea of the boys, okay? If a customer asks, 'Can I fuck you?' (. . .) Well, first, you have to get them out of the bar. As soon as you *off* from the bar (. . .) The bar will not accept any responsibility [if the customer complains]. Outside, it's up to your ability. If you can do it, then do it. Right? You can try it with me but I can trick you. (Tong, 18 December 1995)

The examples given above point to the bars as a critical site in the determination of regulatory practices. In the next section, I will focus attention on what the workers and customers have to say about negotiating the *off*.

Negotiating the *Off*

Being in the business of sex, one might reasonably assume that sex workers would be among the best informed about sexual health. But while, generally, the bar workers' knowledge levels were high and they expressed concern about their health and risk at work, there was considerable confusion and mis-information about HIV and no distinction was made between HIV and AIDS. I found the male bar workers from the suburban bars to be less sure of health issues and less prepared to negotiate the *off* with their customers than those from the Patpong bars. This may reflect the fact that many younger men apprentice themselves in the suburban bars before moving to the more competitive inner-city bars. In both groups, decisions about unsafe sex continue to include the perceived ability to 'know' a person's HIV status (Storer, 1996).

I have to always look at the customer carefully. I have to see who is clean, who is not. And then I decide what I am going to do with him. If he doesn't look clean, then I don't do much – maybe just jerk him off. If I had a customer that I didn't like the look of and he wanted me to *smoke* [give head], I would tell him I could not as I had an ulcer in my mouth. (San, 27 December 1994)

In a study of male sex workers in northern Thailand, de Lind van Wijngaarden (1995) suggested that *farang* customers are less likely to insist on anal sex. My own research supports this finding:

> With Thai customers it is difficult. They expect us to do everything they want. With *farangs* it is easier. We can agree. Usually the Thai want to have anal sex (. . .) With Thai it is necessary to agree everything before leaving the bar. With the *farangs* you can just go. (Chai, 27 December 1995)

A possible explanation here is that the bar workers are less able to negotiate sexual practice with Thai customers because they remain aware of and constrained by Thai social strata or by the value given to maintaining 'smooth interactions', 'image' and 'appearance', or to acceptance 'at face value' (see Komin, 1990; Morris, 1994). But the workers were quick to point out that 'not all *farang* are good' and the experience related by Lao earlier shows that it would be incorrect to assume that *farang* customers are not exploitive.

Most bars programme safe sex by giving their workers one condom and a sachet of lube when they *off* with a customer. However, this attempt to promote safe sex practices may have resulted in complacency. Reg, for example, did not see himself as the target of interventions:

GS: Do you think that there is a safe sex culture among the Thai men?
REG: Well the bars programme safe sex through the boys. They supply them with condoms and lube and the boys have regular checks, every week or every month (. . .) I don't know which one.
GS: But what about customers? Why not give condoms to the customers?
REG: [Grimacing] Well I don't know about that. (Reg, 9 January 1996)

It appears also that the workers do not carry extra condoms and that difficulties often arise because the customers do not come prepared. For a worker, there is a constant juggle to please the customer (*ao jai khaek*), negotiate safety and ensure payment. But the worker still needs to pay the rent and, as with female sex workers, economic livelihood for a male sex worker may be improved by a willingness to engage in high risk sexual activities.

LAO: Mostly (*suan maak*) when I go with the customer I always have to use a condom (*dtorng chai took krang*).
GS: Mostly you use a condom (. . .) but a few times you do not? (. . .)
LAO: Well (. . .) yes, there are some times.
GS: How do you decide when to use and when not to use a condom?
LAO: Mostly I have to use a condom every time.
GS: Right. [I understand that]
LAO: [Right]
GS: But sometimes we forget (. . .) Why is that? Why do we decide one day not to use a condom?

LAO: Because, if I go and sleep with a customer (...) Suppose I go with a customer and I have one condom with me. Suppose the customer wants to do it twice (...) There's no condom. This is me. So, for the money I do it (...) I work like this for the money. (Lao, 21 December 1996)

Negotiation is indeed a complicated business and for bar workers it means two things – negotiating safety and ensuring payment. A worker's ability to negotiate safety with a customer is influenced by his knowledge, his language skills and how confident he is. In the next section, I will look at how triangulation of the data provides an opportunity for the bar workers to address their personal strategies for managing risk.

Reflecting on Experience

An obvious critical moment in the interaction between a bar worker and his customer occurs if the customer tries to pressure the worker to engage in unprotected anal sex against his will. At this critical juncture, the worker calls on a set of semantic strategies in order to try to manage the interaction. Such choices are often made unconsciously, but triangulation of the data provides a technique for making these choices explicit and thereby open to analysis. Sam shows the way:

GS: Sam, some of the boys I talked with told me that the customers say things like: 'You don't have to worry. I'm clean. I go to check my blood often. There's nothing wrong with me.'

SAM: I've met this many times. I think that 70 per cent of my customers speak like this. *Pee sa-aat. Pee pae condom. Sai laew khorng my kheun. Pee my chorp chak wao. Pee chorp ao. Dtorng ao sot. Took khon ja poot yaang nee.* (Older brother is clean. I am allergic to condoms. When I put a condom on, I don't get a hard on. I don't like to jerk off. I like to do it. It has to be fresh. They all talk like this.) (Sam, 23 January 1996)

I would point to two features of the discourse. First, note the repetition of *pee* (older brother or sister); *pee–nong* (older–younger) are commonly used to substitute for 'I' and 'you' and can express familiarity. However, they also reinforce an age difference and thereby retain the hierarchal structures implicit in the more formal pronouns in the Bangkok–Thai language (see, for example, Charoensin-o-larn, 1988). Second, note how Sam's customers reportedly focus on their personal needs rather than on risk assessment. Thus, Sam has to construct a reply that will challenge his customer's status as well as explain to him that he has got it wrong. Fortunately, Sam's response is well rehearsed:

GS: And what do you say when this happens?

SAM: What I say is, 'How many people do you have sex with and not use a condom? And if I say yes to you, how do you know I won't say "yes" to another person. I just have to meet one person who is HIV positive and it will spread to many others.'

What makes Sam's strategy so effective, I think, is the way that he positions himself in relation to the customer. He first asks how often the customer has unprotected sex (a gentle reproach, perhaps?), but then quickly switches responsibility to himself: 'If I say yes', and 'I just have to meet ... and it will spread.' Sam makes his point and 'smooth interaction' is maintained. This is a non-face-threatening speech act (Brown and Levinson, 1987) and so gives the customer room to back down.

In my discussion with Sam, I began by asking him to confirm stories told to me by other bar workers. This elicited a strategy Sam had used to negotiate safe sex and to secure payment. But the process of self-reflection and analysis need not stop here. I can now draw on Sam's reply with less experienced workers who are still learning their way around the bar scene: 'Does this happen? Does this talk point to an effective interaction? How would you deal with this kind of situation?' Asking bar workers to analyze each other's talk in this way allows them to make sense of their lives and provides them with an opportunity to verbalize and rehearse their own negotiation skills.

Implications for HIV Interventions

For Thai male bar workers, the ability to negotiate 'freely' is constrained by the power exerted by their customers and management. In addition to status (class, regionalism, age and wealth), power relations are defined by value systems, the protocol of service and the language of negotiation (either Thai or English). There are implications here for designing interventions to promote safe sex among bar workers and their customers.

First, there needs to be a stronger bar endorsement for safe sex which actively supports the workers. Second, greater attention could be given to developing strategies that will encourage bar operators to more pro-actively promote safe sex among their workers *and* their customers. For example, safe sex messages could be given in both Thai and English to strengthen the idea that all customers (Thai and non-Thai) have a role to play in negotiating safety, and customers could be given condoms when the pay the *off* fee. Third, programmes to ensure that all bar workers have the necessary language and skills to negotiate terms and prices prior to the *off* should be implemented and should incorporate issues relating to self-esteem. Fourth, in addition to being placed in the context of sexual negotiation and unequal relationships, health messages should address the decision-making strategies used by the workers for personal risk assessment both inside and outside the workplace, and include both male–male and male–female sex practices. The triangulation process described here draws on reserves of knowledge and skills among the male bar worker population. It also provides workers with an opportunity to reflect on their experiences and to verbalize and refine their own strategies for managing risk in an environment of peer support. This is particularly important given the lack of community among the male bar workers.

The challenge for future work will be to locate new ways of understanding the discursive and sexual practices within the bars, the everyday ways of operating or doing things, and the critical nexus that brings together workers, customers and management.

Conclusion

In this chapter, I have described how analysis of interview transcripts can help to identify the discourse strategies developed by the bar workers to negotiate the *off* with their customers. These in turn provide the researcher with texts for further interventions when the texts are returned to the bar workers for elaboration and clarification. Ongoing analysis of the reported discourse strategies and triangulation of the data with the informants provide researchers with a tool to address the critical moments in the interactions between the male bar workers and their customers and the decision-making processes used by the workers for personal risk assessment. Additionally, there are broader implications for promoting safe sex among homosexually active men.

Acknowledgements

This work would not have been possible without the input of a number of people. First and foremost, I would like to thank all the bar workers who gave their time to inform the research and who agreed to openly discuss their life stories. Second, I would like to thank the following people with whom I have had extensive discussions: Dr Anthony Pramualratna (UNDP HIV/AIDS Management Specialist, Bangkok), Greg Carl (Research Associate at the Thai Red Cross, Bangkok), and Khun Promboon Panitchthakdi (Country Director for CARE Thailand).

Notes

1 I use the term 'homosexually active men' as a category to include all male–male sex behaviours. The term 'gay' will only be used to refer to men who self-identify as gay. Thai male sex workers, irrespective of their age, are referred to as *dek* (literally child or boy), a term which reflects their lower status and (generally) younger age. Considerable control is, of course, exercised in this naming and I will use 'boy' only in direct quotation. Otherwise, I will use 'male bar workers', 'workers' or 'the men'. The word *khaek* (literally 'guest') is used to refer to customers. The term *farang* is used in

Thai to name Westerners (non-Asians) and will also be used here. The term *off* is part of the vernacular of the bars and is used by the workers when they 'go off' with a customer. It also describes the *off* fee paid to the bar by the customer when he takes a worker out.

2 I define 'critical moments' as points in an interaction when one of the participants is required to make a decision about how to direct or manage the discourse. He then selects, often unconsciously, from a set of semantic strategies in order to accomplish this goal. Compare Bourdieu's description of 'critical situations' that can arise when communication occurs between different classes, where the language is 'charged with social connotations' (Bourdieu, 1991, p. 40).

3 While the findings presented in this chapter relate to a specific population, male bar workers in Bangkok, there is a high degree of concurrence between my own conclusions and those drawn by other researchers in Chiang Mai (de Lind van Wijngaarden, 1995); Pattaya (McCamish and Sittitrai, 1996); and Bangkok (Sittitrai, Phanuphak and Roddy, 1994 and Greg Carl, Thai Red Cross, personal communication).

4 Tenor refers to the negotiation of social relationships among participants and the projection of interpersonal meaning (Eggins, 1994, pp. 63–5; Martin, 1992, pp. 523–6).

5 I use the term 'frame' partly to signify the 'alignments' people bring to their interactions with each other (Goffman, 1974); partly to signify the set of expectations and associated 'scripts' they bring to these interactions (Schank and Ableson, 1977); and partly to signify their own interpretive acts (MacLachlan and Reid, 1994).

6 As de Lind van Wijngaarden (1995) notes further, it would be taboo for a man to admit to being anally penetrated, as it would directly affect his social representation. This suggests that there is a gap between the public performance of masculinity and what actually takes place behind closed doors.

7 Peter Jackson has suggested that Thai academia and areas of the public sector support anti-gay, anti-lesbian and anti-*kathoey* attitudes and practices that are out of step with the more tolerant attitudes of the general public. Jackson's analysis of 207 Thai language academic publications on transgenderism and male and female homosexuality reveals that the dominant paradigm in Thai academic literature views homosexuality as pathology and seeks causes in order to cure. Academic discourses are given considerable authority and prestige in Thailand, and, as a result, are largely unchallenged (Jackson, 1996a, p. 83).

References

ALEXANDER, M. (1995) 'Special conference report: Third International Congress on AIDS in Asia and the Pacific', *National AIDS Bulletin*, **16**, 1, pp. 34–41.

ALLYN, E. (1991) *Trees in the Same Forest: Thailand's Cultures and Subcultures*, Bangkok: Bua Luang.

ALTMAN, D. (1995) 'The new world of gay Asia', in S. PERERA (Ed.) *Asian and Pacific Identities: Identities, Ethnicities, Nationalities*, Sydney: Meridian.

BEYRER, C., EIUMTRAKUL, S., CELENTANO, D.D., NELSON, K.E., RUCKPHAOPUNT, S. and KHAMBOONRUANG, C. (1995) 'Same sex behaviour, sexually transmitted diseases and HIV risks among northern Thai men', *AIDS*, **9**, pp. 171–6.

BLOOR, M. (1995) *The Sociology of HIV Transmission*, London: Sage Publications.

BLOOR, M.J., McKEGANEY, N.P., FINLAY, A. and BARNARD, M.A. (1993) 'HIV-related risk practices among Glasgow male prostitutes: reframing concepts of risk behaviour', *Medical Anthropology Quarterly*, **7**, 2, pp. 1–19.

BOLES, J. and ELIFSON, K.W. (1994) 'Sexual identity and HIV: the male prostitute', *Journal of Sex Research*, **31**, 1, pp. 39–46.

BOURDIEU, P. (1977) 'The economics of linguistic exchanges', *Social Science Information*, **16**, 6, pp. 645–68.

BOURDIEU, P. (1991) *Language and Symbolic Power*, ed. and intro. J.B. THOMPSON, trans. G. RAYMOND and M. ADAMSON, London: Polity Press.

BROWN, P. and LEVINSON, S. (1987) *Politeness: Some Universals in Language Usage*, Cambridge: Cambridge University Press.

BROWNE, J. and MINICHIELLO, V. (1995) 'The social meanings behind male sex work: implications for sexual interactions', *British Journal of Sociology*, **46**, 4, pp. 598–633.

CARAËL, M., CLELAND, J., DEHENETTE, J.-C., FERRY, B. and INGHAM, R. (1995) 'Sexual behaviour in developing countries: implications for HIV control', *AIDS*, **9**, 10, pp. 1171–5.

DE CERTEAU, M. (1984) *The Practice of Everyday Life*, trans. S.F. Rendall, Berkeley: University of California Press.

CHAROENSIN-O-LARN, C. (1988) *Understanding Postwar Reformism in Thailand*, Thailand: Duang Kamol Editions.

EGGINS, S. (1994) *An Introduction to Systemic Functional Linguistics*, London: Pinter Publishers.

FAIRCLOUGH, N. (1995) *Critical Discourse Analysis: The Critical Study of Language*, London and New York: Longman.

FORDHAM, G. (1996) 'The construction of HIV/AIDS as a disease threat in the northern Thai (print) media', presented at the Sixth International Conference on Thai Studies, 14–17 October, Chiang Mai, Thailand.

FORDHAM, G. (1998) 'Northern Thai culture and the assessment of HIV/AIDS risk: a new approach', *Crossroads*, **10**, 2.

FOUCAULT, M. (1979) *The History of Sexuality, Vol. 3: The Care of the Self*, Harmondsworth: Penguin Books.

FOUCAULT, M. (1984) 'The order of discourse', in M. SHAPIRO (Ed.) *Language and Politics*, Oxford: Blackwell.

GOFFMAN, E. (1969) *The Presentation of Self in Everyday Life*, Harmondsworth: Penguin Books.

GOFFMAN, E. (1974) *Frame Analysis*, New York: Harper and Row.

DE GRAAF, R., VANWESENBEECK, I., VAN ZEESEN, G., STRAVER, C.J. and VISSER, J.H. (1994) 'Male prostitutes and safe sex: different settings, different risks', *AIDS Care*, **6**, 3, pp. 277–88.

JACKSON, P. (1995) *Dear Uncle Go: Male Homosexuality in Thailand*, Thailand: Bua Luang Books.

JACKSON, P. (1996a) 'Thai academic studies of *kathoeys* and gay men: a brief critical history', Proceedings of the Sixth International Conference on Thai Studies, Theme III: Family, Community and Sexual Sub-Cultures in the AIDS Era, 14–17 October, Chiang Mai, Thailand.

JACKSON, P. (1996b) 'The persistence of gender', *Meanjin: Australian Queer*, **5**, 5, pp. 110–20.

KOMIN, S. (1990) 'Culture and work-related values in Thai organizations', *International Journal of Psychology*, **25**, pp. 681–704.

KUNAWARARAK, P., BEYRER, C., NATPRATAN, C., FENG, W., CELENTANO, D.D., DE BOER, M., NELSON, K.E. and KHAMBOONRUANG, C. (1995) 'The epidemiology of HIV and syphilis among male commercial sex workers in northern Thailand', *AIDS*, **9**, pp. 517–21.

LABOV, W. (1972) 'The transformation of experience in narrative syntax', in W. LABOV, *Language in the Inner City*, Philadelphia: University of Pennsylvania Press.

LANE-MERCIER, G. (1991) 'Reported discourses: strategy of reproduction, construction, or deconstruction', *Bulletin of the Canadian Applied Linguistics Association*, **13**, 1, pp. 21–34.

DE LIND VAN WIJNGAARDEN, J.W. (1995) *A Social Geography of Male Homosexual Desire: Locations, Individuals and Networks in the Context of HIV/AIDS in Chiang Mai, Northern Thailand*, unpublished Master's thesis, Department of Anthropology, University of Amsterdam.

LYTTLETON, C. (1995) 'Storm warnings: responding to messages of danger in Isan', *TAJA*, **6**, 3, pp. 178–96.

LYTTLETON, C. (1996) 'Messages of distinction: the HIV/AIDS media campaign in Thailand', *Medical Anthropology*, **16**, pp. 363–89.

McCAMISH, M. and SITTITRAI, W. (1995) 'Social context of safe and unsafe behaviour among Thai male sex workers: implications for prevention', presentation at the Third International Conference on AIDS in Asia and the Pacific, 17–22 September, Chiang Mai, Thailand.

McCAMISH, M. and SITTITRAI, W. (1996) *The Context of Safety: Life Stories of Male Sex Workers in Pattaya*, Thai Red Cross Society, Bangkok: Program on AIDS, Research Report No. 19.

MacLACHLAN, G. and REID, I. (1994) *Framing and Interpretation*, Melbourne: Melbourne University Press.

MARTIN, J.R. (1992) *English Text: Systems and Structure*, Philadelphia/Amsterdam: John Benjamins Publishing Company.

MASON, C.J., MARKOWITZ, L.E., KITSIRIPORNCHAI, S., JUGSUDEE, A., SIRISOPONA, N., TORUGSA, K., CARR, J.K., MICHAEL, R.A., NITAYAPHON, S. and McNEIL, J.G. (1995) 'Declining prevalence of HIV-infections in young Thai men', *AIDS*, **9**, 9, pp. 1061–5.

MASTRO, T.D. and LIMPAKARNJANARAT, K. (1995) 'Condom use in Thailand: how much is it slowing the HIV/AIDS epidemic?', *AIDS*, **9**, pp. 523–5.

MORRIS, R.C. (1994) 'Three sexes and four sexualities: redressing the discourse on gender and sexuality in contemporary Thailand', *Positions*, **2**, 1, pp. 15–43.

MURRAY, S.O. (1992) 'The "underdevelopment" of modern/gay homosexuality in Meso-America', in K. PLUMMER (Ed.) *Modern Homosexualities: Fragments of Lesbian and Gay Experience*, London and New York: Routledge.

MURRAY, S.O. (1994) 'Stigma transformation and relexification in the international diffusion of gay', in W.L. LEAP (Ed.) *Beyond the Lavender Lexicon: Authenticity, Imagination and Appropriation in Lesbian and Gay Languages*, New York: Gordon and Breach Publishers.

NARVILAI, A. (1994) '*Phuchai kai dtua* (male sex work in urban cultures)', summary (in Thai) of an academic conference on urban cultures, Urban Communities and their Transformation in Bangkok and its Environs, 7–8 December, Sirinthorn Anthropology Centre, Silpakorn University, Bangkok.

NATPRATAN, C. (1995) 'Signs of hope in the north of Thailand', *AIDS Analysis Asia*, **1**, 5, pp. 10–11.

NOPEKESORN, T., SUNGKAROM, S. and SOMLUM, R. (1991) *HIV Prevalence and Sexual Behaviours Among Thai Men Aged 21 In Northern Thailand*, Program on AIDS, Thailand: Thai Red Cross Society, Bangkok, Report No. 3.

POSHYACHINDA, V. and DANTHAMRONGKUL, V. (1996) 'Shifting borders, shifting identities: new perspectives on Thai homosexuality', presentation at the Sixth International Conference on Thai Studies, 14–17 October, Chiang Mai, Thailand.

POYNTON, C. (1989) *Language and Lender: Making the difference*, Oxford: Oxford University Press.

SCHRIFFEN, D. (1996) 'Narrative as self-portrait: sociolinguistic constructions of identity', *Language in Society*, **25**, pp. 167–203.

SCHANK, R.C. and ABLESON, R.P. (1977) *Scripts, Plans, Goals and Understanding*, Hillsdale, N.J.: Lawrence Erlbaum Associates.

SITTITRAI, W., BROWN, T. and VIRULRAK, S. (1991) 'Patterns of bisexuality in Thailand', in R.A.P. TIELMAN, M. CARBALLO and A.C. HENDRICKS (Eds) *Bisexuality and HIV/AIDS: A Global Perspective*, Buffalo, New York: Prometheus Books.

SITTITRAI, W., PHANUPHAK, P. and RODDY, R. (1994) *Male Bar Workers in Bangkok: An Intervention*, Thai Red Cross Society: Program on AIDS, Research Report No. 10.

SITTITRAI, W., SAKONDHAVAT, C. and BROWN, T. (1992) *A Survey of Men Having Sex with Men in a North-Eastern Thai Province*, Thai Red Cross Society: Program on AIDS, Research Report No. 5.

SRIWATJANA, P. (1995) 'Life styles and health behaviour of male prostitutes in the Patpong area', presentation at the Third International Conference on AIDS in Asia and the Pacific and Fifth National AIDS Conference in Thailand, September.

STORER, G. (1996) 'Interactions: Thai male sex workers and their customers', presentation at Knowledge and Discourse: Changing relationships across academic disciplines and professional practices, June 18–21, University of Hong Kong.

STORER, G. (in press) 'Productions of gender and sexuality in modern Thailand', in P.A. JACKSON and G. SULLIVAN (Eds) *Lady Boys, Tom Boys, Rent Boys*, Special Edition of *Journal of Gay and Lesbian Social Services*, **9**.

Chapter 14

Walking the Tightrope: Sexual Risk and Male Sex Work in the Philippines

Michael L. Tan

To the public, they are known usually as 'call-boys'. Local gay slang has developed different descriptors, usually a play on the term call-boy: *callbam*, *shobam* and *sholing*. Other terms have emerged, sometimes coined among sex workers themselves, terms such as escorts, guest relations officers and entertainers. Public awareness of male sex work in the Philippines comes from media coverage, in print as well as on television.

Academic work about male sex workers has been sparse, coming mainly from non-Filipino researchers. Whitham and Mathy's study of homosexuality in four societies (1986) included the Philippines, with several pages devoted to descriptions of call-boys based on fieldwork in the late 1970s. More recently, Mathews (1987) has published the results of fieldwork conducted in the 1980s. Both studies, however, describe male sex work in relation to foreign gay tourists.

Unfortunately, both popular and academic writing about male sex workers tend toward sensationalism. There is, for example, the genre represented by the late John Stamford and his *Spartacus* gay guides, in which Filipino males are depicted as having no qualms about sex for payment. In 1979, Stamford wrote that 'practically all' adolescent males in the town of Pagsanjan (about 100 kilometres south of Manila) were involved in sex work. Pagsanjan was, in fact, a haven for pederasts, but Stamford's claim is greatly exaggerated.[1] While Stamford represents an extreme, his descriptions tend to be repeated in other articles by foreign gay writers and researchers, who see the Philippines as a place where there is little anti-gay discrimination and, ironically, by Filipino journalists, writers and non-government organizations (NGOs) who see the Philippines as a paradise for Caucasian pederast tourists preying on helpless rural communities or male migrants coming to the big city.

These descriptions distort the picture, with serious implications for public policy and interventions, especially in the area of HIV/AIDS prevention. Understanding the problems that come with male sex work requires an analysis of its context. In particular, we need to analyze the demand for male sex work, and how this demand affects risk perceptions and risk behaviour. This demand ties in closely to sexual ideologies, particularly constructions of gender. While Mathews (1987) has described some of the linkages between sex work and gender ideologies, his work needs updating and deepening in this era of HIV/AIDS, especially in the ways sexual risks are created.

In this chapter, I will first present an overview of 'formal' male sex work in the Philippines to show the diversity of male sex workers. This is followed by a socio-historical review to show how sexual ideologies, in particular the construction of *bakla* (loosely translated: homosexual men) relates to male sex work. I will describe how risk perceptions are shaped and reshaped through the interactions between sex workers and clients, again with sexual ideologies forming an important cultural context in affecting both risk-taking as well as risk-reduction behaviour. In the last section I discuss some of the implications of this study for policy and practice.

Sources of Information

This chapter is mainly based on interviews with male sex workers as part of interventions launched by Health Action Information Network (HAIN), a non-governmental organization (NGO) in the Philippines. These interventions date back to 1986 when we were first approached by Gabriela, a women's NGO, to help with HIV/AIDS education for male child sex workers in Pagsanjan (the area described by John Stamford in *Spartacus*). Eventually, Gabriela asked us to help with health education for older sex workers, both male and female. All these projects were informal and *ad hoc*, consisting largely of talks whenever a request was made and occasional outreach activities in cruising areas. Since 1995, for reasons that will be explained later, HAIN has withdrawn from participation in formal, structured projects with male sex workers and has limited its work to occasional visits to their work areas for short workshops.

Despite the wealth of information that has emerged through our projects, I do not claim that this chapter is comprehensive. First, because of the nature of our HIV education projects, the information we have is skewed more towards establishment-based sex workers. Second, the emphasis here is on sex work with male clients who self-identify as gay or bisexual. While we have interviewed some women clients, the data here remains quite limited. It is also important to stress that the clientele for the male sex work described in this chapter came mainly from upper-income backgrounds. Third, there are still important information gaps, particularly in relation to the client/sex worker relationship. The gap comes mainly because the number of clients we have interviewed is much smaller than that of male sex workers. While we have data from questionnaires completed by 204 male sex workers over the years and notes for some 65 workshops with the sex workers, documenting their views about male sex work, HIV/AIDS and other concerns, we only have notes based on very informal interviews with about 16 clients.

Finally, we have to recognize that male sex work evolves quite rapidly. Reading earlier academic work about male sex work, it is striking how many of the terms are no longer in use, and how the 'rules' have changed. Cruising areas, establishments and the sex workers themselves come and go. The cruising area for freelance workers that HAIN studied in 1992 no longer exists. Between July 1996, when I was first asked to write this chapter, and April 1997, when I completed final revisions, at least three new male sex worker establishments have been set up in Manila while two have closed down. As will be described later, the average stay of male sex workers in these establishments is about three months, which means that over this period there could have been three generations of male sex workers in some of these bars and massage parlours.

The emphasis here will not be on sexual acts, the traditional focus of ethnographies about sex work. Instead, the concern is to identify the social and cultural contexts that shape risk perceptions and behaviour. No names of existing establishments or cruising areas are given, and the names of sex workers and managers are either not mentioned or are changed. Sex work – male or female – is illegal in the Philippines and the publicity generated about male sex work, whether through journalistic or academic accounts, has all too often further stigmatized and endangered sex workers.

Types of Formal Male Sex Work

In the Philippines, it is important to distinguish 'formal' sex work from another arrangement, that of neighbourhood or community cruising. Formal here refers to the presence of an organizational network of managers and workers, as well as a fee structure. This definition is of course not rigid, since the organizational network can be quite flexible, as in the case of freelance workers. Broadly, we can identify six categories of male sex workers: (1) transsexuals and transvestites, (2) 'dance instructors', (3) child sex workers, (4) massage parlour attendants, (5) bar-based workers, and (6) freelance workers. The categories are not always discrete, but there are enough differences among them for them to be discussed separately. Much more information will be described for the last three categories, partly because our work, as well as that of other NGOs, has been concentrated with these sub-groups.

Transsexuals and Transvestites

It is striking that the Philippines has only a small number of transvestite and transsexual sex workers. While public cross-dressing *bakla* are widespread, only a small number of such *bakla* engage in sex work, limited in fact to two streets in Metro Manila (one each in the cities of Manila and Makati). The customers of this small number of transvestite and transsexual sex workers tend to be male tourists who self-identify as heterosexual. There are, however, fairly large numbers of *bakla* who work as female impersonators, both in the

Philippines and in Japan, with occasional sex work involved. To date no work has been done – in terms of education or research – with this group.

Dance Instructors

Dance instructors (or DIs) are men in their twenties and thirties who, as their name suggests, provide lessons in ballroom dancing to wealthy middle-aged women or *matronas*. Besides the ballroom dancing lessons, the men become constant companions, which may involve the provision of sexual services. Dance instructors resemble more closely the American gigolo. Neither they, nor the public, would use the term 'call-boy' here, mainly because their primary identity corresponds to a legitimate profession. Ballroom dancing is offered now on television and in events sponsored by groups like the Catholic Women's League.

Child Sex Workers

Together with Thailand and Sri Lanka, the Philippines acquired a reputation in the 1980s for child sex work, involving both males and females. The sex trade here has been associated mainly with foreign tourists, although there is no doubt that Filipino clients also exist. The trade in both male and female children used to be quite visible, with open solicitation by pimps in particular streets in Manila and in resorts around the country. Stricter laws have resulted in the prosecution of at least three foreigners and two Filipino congressmen, which have now driven this aspect of the sex trade underground.

Massage Parlours

Massage parlours are a known front for sex work throughout the Philippines, but parlours with male sex workers are found only in Metro Manila. As of April 1997, nine such establishments could be identified, with about 300 attendants. Most clients come at night but the parlours are supposed to operate 24 hours a day. The establishments are licensed as massage parlours and the attendants are supposed to have received training as masseurs. Clients receive a standard massage and are then asked if they want 'extra service'. Sex work is done in the massage parlour itself, although 'take-outs' are also available, with clients coming in to pick-up an attendant or phoning in to request a particular attendant for home service.

Massage parlour attendants tend to be rural migrants, although there are also those who grew up in the city. Attendants tend to come closest to physical 'real male' ideals: often being well-built hunks. As one client put it: 'It's all very physical. You can go through the whole process without saying anything.'

Transactions are simple and impersonal. A client peers into a room where the attendants are sitting and makes his pick. He goes to his room and receives his massage and the extra services and leaves. The average stay is about an hour. The relationship between the attendant and the client is quite feudal. The sex workers call their clients 'sir' and do not usually talk unless they are talked to. Many live in the massage parlour itself and are bound strictly by establishment rules.

Bar-based Sex Work

Bar-based sex work, like that in the massage parlours, is confined to Metro Manila. There are occasional attempts in other Philippine cities such as Cebu and Angeles to set up such bars but they tend to close down rather quickly, for reasons that will be explained later. In April 1997, there were five such bars with a roster of about 400 sex workers reporting for work on a regular or irregular basis. Usually called 'gay bars', these contexts offer some entertainment with 'macho dancers' and female impersonators. The male sex workers mill around the bar. They are not allowed to approach clients on their own; instead there are managers who act as pimps. Clients can 'table' a sex worker by requesting a sex worker to sit with him and talk. 'Tabling' itself is already a transaction, since the client is charged per hour, with a cut for the escort. Clients who take out an escort have to pay a 'bar fine'. Sex with an escort takes place in motels or in the client's home and can be for a short time – a few hours – or overnight.

The sex workers in these bars tend to be raised in the city. Bar-based workers have to be able to conduct a conversation with their clients. The clients are also quite mixed, including Filipinos and foreigners, gay men and 'bisexuals', middle-aged women and young women sex workers, although the bulk of the clients are males.

Freelance Sex Work

Freelance male sex workers are found in a variety of cruising areas in larger Philippine cities: public parks, shopping malls, public toilets and cinemas. These cruising areas often overlap those used by gay men looking for other gay partners. Much of the sex work is carried out on a part-time basis in between jobs or during periods when extra cash is needed (for example paying for tuition fees). Cruising usually takes place at night, but there are areas, such as cinemas, where 'pick-ups' can occur during the day. Freelance workers do not have pimps and tend to work alone, sometimes with fierce competition over turf. Sex takes place sometimes in the cruising area itself or in one of the many motels available in Philippine cities for 'short-time' sex.

There is a range of male sex work in the Philippines although sex workers do move from one category to another. One sex worker interviewed had, for example, first worked as a freelance in Davao City in the southern part of the Philippines. He was then recruited by friends, also former freelance workers in Davao, to move to Manila. In Manila, he worked first in a massage parlour, moving on to a freelance area and finally ending up in a bar. In a sense, then, a network connects the different categories, although the different establishments see each other as competition and there is an unspoken rule that a sex worker cannot be affiliated to two establishments at the same time.

Historical Context and Sexual Ideologies

Most Filipinos are nominally Roman Catholic and will thus agree with statements such as 'homosexuality is a sin'. However, there is also a secular view that looks at 'homosexuals' as a 'third sex', almost as if homosexuality were innate. This 'third sex' is called the *bakla*, described as 'a man with a woman's heart'. The *bakla* pairs off with a *tunay na lalake* or 'real male'. A real male should self-identify as heterosexual,[2] and should be masculine or macho in his behaviour. A *bakla* having sex with another *bakla* is described as 'lesbianism', or *pompyangan*, a clash of cymbals.

The male libido (*libog*) is considered to be strong and needs to be satisfied. It is considered acceptable for a 'real man' to have sex with a *bakla* as long as he himself does not become *bakla*. This is especially the case for *binata* or unmarried males, who are not allowed access to their girlfriends because girlfriends have to be 'respected' and female virginity retained intact until marriage. Young men's access to women sex workers is also limited because of economic factors. This leaves the *bakla* as a 'sexual outlet' (a term used by one man interviewed). As *baklas* often joke about themselves: '*May mga prostitute at may mga substitute.*' ('There are prostitutes, and then there are substitutes.') Some *baklas* have married men as their partners; in fact, *mga tatay* (daddies) are considered a special conquest, since a married male is even more of a real male than single men, having proven himself through marriage and having children.

Men do not have to pay *baklas* to have sex; instead, they may sometimes be paid by the *bakla*. I say 'may', because there will be times when sex is 't.y.' (thank you, or free). As one 'real male' described it: '*Depende na yan. Minsan five-o; minsan dalawang beer. At minsan, kung mabait ang bakla, t.y. na lang.*' ('It depends. Sometimes five-o [fifty pesos] and sometimes it is two beers. Sometimes, if the *bakla* is kind, then it's t.y. [thank you]'.) A 'real man' can also enter a longer-term relationship with a *bakla*, becoming a 'boyfriend' in exchange for gifts and financial incentives. Note that the relationship is not seen as commercial. It is either a casual fling or one of a *bakla* and a boyfriend. The terms used – *hada* for a casual fling and 'boyfriend' or *asawa* (spouse) for someone with whom a relationship is being built – are the same terms used for gay dating and partnerships. At the same time, some form of material benefit – in cash or in kind – is required, and becomes an important marker for the 'real man' to retain his masculinity. This applies even to a casual fling, which often takes place after a session of drinking paid for by the *bakla*. The beer, and the 'real man's' becoming *lasing* (drunk) can be described as a kind of distancing. It is not important whether the male was drunk or not; invoking the beer, paid for by the *bakla*, 'legitimizes' the sexual encounter, as will other gifts and benefits if a relationship is pursued. Many *baklas* interviewed talk about the dilemma here: 'One-way *ang* relationship. *Kami ang nagmamahal, kami ang nagbabayad, nagsusustento. E, hindi naman sila makaka-reciprocate. Oras kasi na minahal tayo, hindi na sila lalake.*' ('The relationship is one-way. We love, we pay, we support. They ['real men'] cannot reciprocate. Once they love us, they are no longer male.')

Remaining a 'real male' is covered by other gender roles. 'Real men' are not supposed to do the laundry, or even to iron clothes. 'Real men' will 'protect' their *asawang bakla* (*bakla* spouse) from other men. 'Real men' can also go into fits of jealous and violent rage if their *bakla* partner flirts with other men, although this rage does not necessarily mean that love is involved. '*Territoriyo lang yan*', says one *bakla*, with a smile that explains how territory interfaces with economic benefits. Both the *bakla* and the 'real man' know that nothing binds either party in their relationship. The measure of the 'real male' is his philandering, while the *bakla* is seen as 'still' being male and therefore also a potential philanderer, although his philandering is described by the term *malandi* (a term stronger than flirtatious, with connotations of a bitch in heat).

'Real men' are emphatic in saying that they will never 'sing' (give oral sex) or 'dance' (receive anal sex). Once they give oral sex, there is the possibility that one is 'becoming' *bakla* or gay, while receiving anal sex is anathema, practically equated to becoming *bakla*. These notions tie in closely to the idea that being *bakla* is *nakakahawa* or contagious. The relationship between the *bakla* and a 'real male' is therefore transient and, in a way, tense as the 'real man' tries to remain a 'real man', because gender ideology is such that once he becomes *bakla*, he will no longer be desirable. As one *bakla* described the 'transformation': '*Dati asawa ko, ngayon ate na lang.*' ('He used to be my husband, but now he's my elder sister.')

These arrangements between a *bakla* and a 'real man' have a long history. This can be confirmed not only in interviews with older *bakla*, but also with older 'real men' who can be quite candid in describing the 'flings' they had with *bakla* in their youth. For example Carlo, a leader in an urban poor community in Manila, is in his fifties and has many stories about life in the early 1960s. There were no gay bars then, he said. The *bakla* were found mainly in 'carnivals' (fairs), working as female impersonators. *Baklas* would 'adopt' younger males. Carlos was in such a relationship for two years and was put through two years of high school by one of these *baklas*. He later married and now has children and grandchildren. Yet he has retained friendships with the *baklas* and offered to bring to interview some of the 'survivors', now in their sixties and seventies.

Three characteristics are especially important in these *bakla*/boyfriend arrangements. First, such arrangements are mainly found in low-income districts of towns and cities, usually involving a neighborhood *parlorista* – *bakla* working in or owning a small beauty parlour or a dress shop – and local men. Second, the *bakla* and his boyfriend are usually from the same socio-economic class. In fact, there may be cases where the *bakla* is actually from a lower income background, but because he has a steady source of income, he ends up supporting someone who comes from a more affluent family but without any regular income. Third, such relationships are not stigmatized for reasons that have been explained earlier. It is 'natural' for men with sexual needs to seek out the *bakla* since *walang nawawala* (nothing is lost by doing so). Thus, arrangements between a *bakla* and his boyfriend can be quite public.

There is a historical antecedent for male sex work in the *bakla*/boyfriend arrangement, one that takes on greater similarities to gift exchange based on reciprocity: the 'real male' gives sex in exchange for money or other economic benefits, but in the absence of fixed fee structures. These arrangements also build on the potential of there being a longer, albeit transient, relationship, with economic benefits for the 'real man'. Such interactions remain quite common in cities and towns throughout the Philippines.

It is hard to determine when formal male sex work first started in the Philippines. Documentation on female sex work dates back to the Spanish period (Tan *et al.*, 1990; Camagay, 1995) but similar documentation for male sex work is absent. Formal male sex work is probably fairly recent, considering that a Sanitation Code passed shortly after the Second World War specifies tests for 'venereal diseases' only for 'hospitality girls', a euphemism for women sex workers.

Interviews with older gay men, however, yielded information about male brothels existing in Manila's ghettos around the 1960s. The brothels – called *casa*, the Spanish word for house, which is also used for brothels with women – were quite spartan: '*Wala, katre lang. Bibigyan ka ng twalyang may tatak na Good Morning. Hay, at walang lubricant. Kung kailangan, Crisco ang inaabot sa iyo.*' ('There was nothing: just a wooden cot. They'd give you a towel with Good Morning printed on it. [Referring to a cheap brand of towel.] And no lubricants. If you needed something, they'd give you Crisco [cooking lard].')

None of the original brothels from the 1960s have survived, but they seem to have been replaced by massage parlours, which began to proliferate in the 1970s. The massage parlours have come a long way, now offering air-conditioned rooms, a bed with a mattress, massage lotion, condoms and lubricants.

Curiously, 'gay bars' were the other type of establishment that became a venue for male sex work. The term 'gay' came into public use in the 1970s, obviously imported from the West. Young upper-class Filipinos, many of whom had studied in the United States, now talked about being 'gay'. Being gay took different meanings. For some, gay carried with it connotations of liberation, which included a reorientation in sexual preferences. Gay men talked about having sex with other gay men, something which shocked (and continues to shock) other Filipino homosexuals. For others, however, and I believe this continues to be the 'mainstream', the term 'gay' was simply appropriated for local use, interchanged quite often with *bakla*. Thus, many Filipinos still perceive gay as an effeminate cross-dressing male, the same way a *bakla* is constructed.

Formal sex work, particularly in bars and massage parlours, is a commodity transaction, involving fixed fees and social interaction limited to the exchange of money for services, which are very different from the *bakla*'s encounters with 'real men'. In the latter arrangement, we find gift exchange based on a form of reciprocity, and the 'real male' gives sex in exchange for money or other economic benefits, but without fixed fee structures. There is, too, the potential of a continuing relationship of reciprocity, in a *bakla/ boyfriend* relationship.

Analyzing Demand: Desiring Males and Being Male

We need now to analyze the demand for male sex work. This means moving into the field of intersubjectivity, where sexual ideologies are operationalized. I have mentioned the importance of *bakla* ideology, one which carries over into male sex work in creating a demand for 'real men'. This also creates, on the part of the sex worker, a preoccupation with 'being male'.

Male sex workers must satisfy the demand for 'real males'. This comes with physical characteristics – the 'hunk' is desirable, so sex workers need to work out. But being male involves more than the physical. There is a very strong element of performance here, with male sex workers constantly talking about their escapades with women. Many have live-in partners or are married, and boast incessantly about how many children they have (typically, *tatlong anak, tatlong nanay*: three children with three mothers). One male sex worker told me they talk this way because the *bakla* client expects this.

This is not to say that all male sex workers 'are' or 'self-identify' as heterosexuals. There are quite a few male sex workers who self-identify as bisexual, gay or even *bakla*, but such admissions are rarely made except to close friends. The 'camouflage' here can be quite effective. Ramon, one of the most popular escorts in one of Manila's gay bars, derived great pleasure in demonstrating how he could move very quickly from what he called his Marlboro Man routine into a Miss Philippines stance, in the way he would cross his legs or hold his cigarette. He would do the Marlboro Man when there were 'guests' in the bar, but if the coast was clear, he would shift to being Miss Philippines.

Gender ideology also shapes demand in terms of age and physical appearance. For example, unlike women sex workers, male sex workers span a wider age range. While most male sex workers are aged about 18 to 24 (already quite old if applied to women sex workers), we have found some who are older than 30. The older sex workers actually fit into a particular market niche that I have mentioned earlier: men who are 'daddies' or who look like fathers. Note how 'father' is in fact a derived gender role. The beer belly – a prerequisite for such types – is seen as 'evidence' of the sex worker's being a father, and a 'real man' at that.

The relationships between gender ideology and sex work extend beyond *bakla* ideology. Included here are notions of what is male, as well as female. These ideologies influence notions of male sex work itself, as well as the self-images that male sex workers have. For example, male sex workers feel their work is demeaning because traditionally, *babae lang*, only women, are seen as having to do such work. In the Philippines, people generally refer to sex as *gamit* (to use), with the male 'using' the female. For example, men say *Ginamit ko siya* (I used her) to refer to sex with a woman, while women say *Ginamit ako* (I was used) for sex with a man. Only in the case of male sex workers do we find men being described as *ginagamit* or used. Not surprisingly, this is often cited by male sex workers as an example of their devaluation: '*Saan bang may lalakeng nagpapagamit?*' ('Where do you have men being used?'). It is not just a matter of sex here; some sex workers complain about how degrading it is to be 'tabled' or to dance on stage since these are activities are also done by women sex workers.

Trabaho Lang Yan (It's only Work).

So far, the focus has been on sexual ideologies and the way these structure role expectations. We will turn now to look at how role expectations establish a framework for risk perception. To do this, we have to look at how the 'actors' – sex workers and clients – look at male sex work itself. These perceptions relate to self-image as well as views of 'the other' – the client's perceptions of the sex worker, and the sex worker's views about the clients, both on the part of the sex workers as well as the clients. To do this, I will discuss important client and sex worker perceptions separately, emphasizing 'rationalizing' processes and then showing how these converge in perception of risks.

A frequent remark from male sex workers is '*Trabaho lang*' ('It's just work'). While the remark seems self-explanatory, the context in which this is said shows *trabaho lang* to be much more complex. The sex workers' discourse about *trabaho lang* includes resentment, almost as if there were no choices left. '*Wala akong mapasukan*' ('I could not get any other job') is a frequent explanation. Resentment often interfaces with guilt, including strong notions that having sex with another male is *kasalanan* or sin. Since many of our workshops involve gay male facilitators, such 'morally correct' views about homosexuality were not made to 'please' the facilitators: the sex workers would in fact preface their comments with 'Sorry, but ...' as they made very strong anti-gay remarks. The sentiments are not just homophobic; as explained earlier, there is also the perception of male sex work as degrading because it reduces one to the status of women.

Given these negative feelings about male sex work, *trabaho lang* carries important components of justifying sex work as *hanap-buhay*, the Tagalog word for employment, which literally translated means 'searching for life'. Typically, sex workers cite their families as the reason for their work. In our interviews, sex workers would bring out their wallets to show pictures of girlfriends, wives, children, explaining that their work is for 'them'. With women sex workers, dependents tend to be siblings or parents. With the male sex workers, the role is that of a breadwinner, described by the sex workers as *padre de pamilya*, the head of the family, again fulfilling a gender role expectation.

Trabaho lang also means desexualizing sex. '*Pinipikit ko na lang ang mata ko at iisipin ko babae siya.*' ('I close my eyes and think [of the client] as a woman.') Yet, male sex workers, particularly the bar-based 'escorts', are aware too that they must play male roles of courtship, of making the client feel desirable: '*Yan ang mahirap sa trabaho. Biro mo naman, kung mas malaki siyang tao, tapos bad breath pa. Kahit ano ang gawiin mo, mahirap magkunwari.*' ('That's what's hard about the work. Imagine if he's bigger than you are, and has bad breath. No matter what you do, it's difficult to pretend.') *Trabaho lang* desexualizes sex through pretence and denial.

Another way of rationalizing is to see sex work as temporary. Quite often, sex work is done in between jobs or waiting for another job. 'Another job' will include, in some cases, becoming an entertainer in Japan, which will often mean sex work as well. Sex workers do not generally remain in the same establishment or in sex work for more than a few months. There are of course extremes, such as three sex workers who have been working for more than seven years, but our research generally shows that male sex workers have more mobility than their women counterparts in terms of moving among the different establishments, or working intermittently as sex workers, or simply moving out of sex work.

While the rhetoric about *trabaho lang* is strong, we were surprised to find that male sex work is not quite as lucrative as public perceptions may have it. Our interviews suggest that income from male sex work may be limited. Male sex workers generally get lower pay than their female counterparts because of the idea that males do not lose anything (*walang mawawala*), although we will see that the male sex workers themselves, while repeating this *walang mawawala* assertion, also describe what they 'lose'. In our study of one upmarket bar, fewer than half of the sex workers had monthly incomes higher than P5000 (US$200), which would be the average pay for a clerk in Metro Manila.

The reason here is that competition can be quite tight, with supply often outstripping demand. Typically, on a weekend, a bar can have as many as 50 customers taking home a sex worker, but there will also be sex workers with two or three clients and sex workers without any. Weekend nights usually attract about 70 sex workers, which means at least 20 will go home with only the P50 (US$2) allowance given by the establishment.

The motives for entering sex work cannot be reduced to economics. Our interviews suggest that male sex workers, particularly those working in bars, have other expectations of facilitated social mobility. In a feudal society such as the Philippines, connections are important. Sex work is therefore not just meeting wealthy clients, but clients who have the connections, who might be the key to another job. Other sex workers talk about the possibilities of shacking up with the client (*ginagarahe*, or to be put in the garage). Here, we find an interesting overlap with the older institution of the *bakla* and the neighbourhood *tambay* ('stand-by') except that the transaction now takes place in a formal sex work setting, one which is much less personal because it is *trabaho lang*.

How, then, does *trabaho lang* relate to risk perceptions? *Trabaho lang* rationalizes one's involvement in sex work, mainly by distancing or even dichotomizing the personal (for example sexual identity) with the professional. *Trabaho lang* also recognizes the importance of the male body as capital: '*Puhanan ang katawan namin.*' ('Our bodies are our capital.') The male sex workers' health concerns are systemic and generic: how to keep healthy; how not to eat too much; how not to get sleepy. There is a fixation over vitamins, which are perceived to keep one healthy and to ward off diseases, including HIV/AIDS and sexually transmitted diseases (STDs). Condoms are not popular for many reasons: 'they reduce sensitivity' or 'they don't work'. But most importantly, HIV and STDs are not seen as immediate risks.

The perceived risks are not diseases, but of not being able to earn money, and of not being able to get a client for the night. Given the way supply outstrips demand, it not surprising that sex workers try to outdo each other with their 'performance', even as they try to balance what they will do in bed with the ideology of 'being male'. While the sex workers claim they adhere to safer sex practices, jamming sessions with beer also lead to their talking about how, if the price is right, one can take on the receiver's role in anal sex.

Gender ideologies are still important as we look into risk frameworks. One important 'risk' seen in sex work is the possibility that one might eventually become 'gay'. In our workshops, sex workers who self-identify as 'real men' ask us repeatedly if homosexuality is *nakakahawa* or contagious, and cite stories about other male sex workers who 'became' gay after working for a year or two. Some are convinced that it is sex work that eventually turns a 'real man' into a *bakla*. The fear, then, is that sex work may no longer be just work: '*hahanapin mo na*' ('you start looking for it').

Trabaho lang plays on many aspects of gender and sexual ideologies, on being male, and on being the breadwinner. *Trabaho lang* actually distinguishes formal sex work from the older institution of community *bakla* cruising – in the latter, the 'real men' never say *trabaho lang* to refer to their encounters with the *bakla*. *Trabaho lang* defines the boundaries, for as long as one does it only to earn money 'for now', then it becomes acceptable. The perceived risks here revolve around the work not generating the money one needs, as well as the work producing new desires that transform the sex worker from a 'real man' into a *bakla*.

Client Perspectives: Trick or Trade

While male sex workers perceive their clients as being varied – *baklas* and *matronas*, or 'gay' and 'bisexual' for example – client perceptions often focus on the maleness of the sex worker: '*Kailangan lalake siya.*' ('He has to be male.') How do these expectations translate into perceptions of male sex work and male sex workers? On one hand, there is an acceptance that since sex workers are 'real males', the only role they will play in bed is that of Leila D.,[3] someone who just lies there and plays a passive role.

At the same time, clients speak strongly about their expectations that male sex workers be more active, and even take 'girl' roles in bed. Typically, clients ask managers if a sex worker 'sings' (gives blow jobs) or dances (takes the recipient role for anal sex). Despite HIV and AIDS, it seems that song and dance expectations may actually have risen over the years. Ironically, a challenging of gender roles may also have created new forms of risks. Some *bakla* interviewed say that they also like insertive anal sex with male sex workers because, as one explains it, '*may thrill sa role reversal. Ayoko naman na ako lagi ang girl. At biro mo, ang laki laking mama, kayang kaya mo.*' ('There's thrill in role reversal. I don't want to always be the girl. And imagine, you're able to control such a huge man.')

Dissonance in gender roles is sometimes 'resolved' linguistically; for example, a blow job from a male sex worker is described as *brocha*, the term used to refer to a male giving oral sex to a female (that is cunnilingus). I have not yet heard of a similar translation to 'masculinize' the recipient role in anal sex. A more important rationalization is the argument that male sex workers are probably gay, or have 'gay tendencies': '*Imposible naman na magagawa nila ang ginagawa nila kung wala silang feeling para sa kapwa lalake.*' ('It's impossible that they can do what they do if they don't have feelings for other men.') Such 'suspicions' have a rationalizing function: '*Gusto naman nila. Wala namang namimilit sa kanila.*' ('They want it anyway. No one forces them.') Such rationalizations are a variation on the *trabaho lang* argument, that this is only work with the added qualifier that one chooses work.

We see that while the rhetoric moves on stereotypes, actual behaviour may be much more flexible. There is a desire for 'real men', and yet there are suspicions that male sex workers are probably gay, which then justifies their being able to 'sing' and 'dance'. This flexibility emerges as well in sexual discourse. Both sex workers and clients admit that much of male sex work is often one of fantasy or *pantasya*, and that 'male control' on the part of the male sex worker is often role-play.

On one hand, the male sex worker is desirable because he is masculine and, more importantly, one might be able to get a 'real man' to do things that 'real men' do not, such as receive anal sex. On the other hand, there is a fear that today's trade might become tomorrow's trick. After all, one pays to have sex with a 'real man'. Several gay men I interviewed, as well as bar managers, have stories about former male sex workers who 'turned gay'. The following story is typical: 'You should have seen him when he was working at *Spartacus*: a real Adonis, tall, well-built. Ay, but after a year I saw him again, imagine, he was competing with me in a beauty pageant. He had heels higher than mine and lipstick redder than the girls on Mabini.' Fears of 'turning gay' are shared both by the sex worker and the client, but take on different forms.

On the surface, the fears clients have are expressed in *bakla* discourse as 'today's spouse, tomorrow's sister'. Deeper analysis shows, however, that in formal male sex work, the tensions take a different direction. There is almost an acceptance that a male sex worker might be gay: 'as long as he doesn't start flicking his wrist at me', quips one client. How does this happen? The male sex worker's desirability – his 'maleness' – carries the connotations of 'badness' described earlier. The male sex worker has *bisyo* or vices, similar to the *tambay* described earlier, idle young males who attach themselves to the neighbourhood *bakla*.

One bar manager asserts: '*Hindi naman sila papasok sa pagka-call boy kung hindi sila delinquente. Siguradong may mga bisyo yan. Ayaw mag-aral. Titigas ng ulo.*' ('They would not have become call-boys if they were not delinquents. They're sure to have vices. They don't like studying. They're hard-headed.') It is striking how often clients and managers refer to the sex workers as 'boys'. The usage of the term approximates the use of 'girls' when referring to women sex workers: there is condescension, a suggestion of immaturity and the need for discipline. With male sex workers, the metaphor moves on to that of 'bad boys', boys whose badness is part of their being fun.

Being hard-headed becomes part of being male, together with all the connotations of being dangerous. This is especially the case with freelance workers. Gay men usually have stories about unpleasant encounters with freelance workers, ranging from small-time extortion to murder. The point about extortion is important because it relates to the fear of disclosure. This is especially important for gay men who are not 'out'. Male sex workers are often aware of this vulnerability: '*Mga big time kasi sila: politico; negosyante; artista; pari. Madaling ma-blackmail.*' ('They are big time: politicians; businessmen; actors; priests. Easy to blackmail.') These risks are reduced through establishment-based sex work. The bar fine paid to the establishment is not just for opportunity costs, but also becomes a kind of insurance. One bar owner showed me a stack of index cards, where each sex worker had, on file, an address, names of relatives and other personal information in case they needed to be tracked down.

Client perceptions about sex workers therefore focus on masculinity, which is both desirable and dangerous. The ideal is to have control over this masculinity, one achieved through the security of bars and massage parlours and the use of intermediaries such as pimps and managers. The formalization of male sex work becomes clearer here, in the way it functions to offer customized masculinity from a 'stable' of men whose masculinity is assured, yet affording control over that very masculinity.

The Guest, Cellphones and Calvin Klein: Class Ideologies and Male Sex Work

So far, the emphasis has been on the contribution of sexual and gender ideologies to risk perceptions and risk-taking. We have seen, too, that these ideologies are important in the way they affect power relations, in the way some of the rules are 'breached', as in the *bakla* expecting to wield control over a *malaking mama* (a huge man). These ideologies spill over into a deconstruction of 'sex work' itself, as in the dichotomization of sex and work, or in the denial of sex work as sex. The discussions eventually move into the issue of power and control. It is clear that male sex work is different from the *bakla*/boyfriend relationship in that the client asserts more control. But this power relationship does not derive from gender ideologies alone. In fact, I would assert that male sex work builds on class as well as gender ideologies.

Formal male sex work seems to have emerged with an upper-class urban clientele that has disposable income. Even paying the entrance fee to one of the lower-end 'gay bars' with macho dancers would cost P40 (about US$1.50). Without sex, tabling charges and drinks can add up. In upmarket 'gay bars', one can spend up to P5000 (US$200) in one night without any sex, for a private room and several rounds of 'macho drinks'. All this occurs in a country where the highest daily minimum wage is currently about P180 (US$7). Bars and massage parlours are not accessible to many *parlorista*, the *bakla* working in beauty parlours. My point is that the class differences between the client and sex worker can be quite sharp, which explains why both Filipino and foreign clients (as well as researchers on male sex work) often think the sex workers are all 'poor' when in fact the sex worker's background may be middle-class.

Class differences shape intersubjectivities, even definitions of 'masculinity'. Male-ness is sometimes described as '*katawan ng construction worker*', a construction worker's body. But it is not just physical assets that contribute to maleness. There is also the element of 'badness'. Yet this badness is feared, projected into fears that one might get robbed, get killed, get HIV/AIDS.

Many gay men I talked with want mandatory testing of male sex workers for HIV. The fears here are often class-based, for example 'I'm sure many of them have AIDS because they haven't had any education. *Ignorante sila* (they are ignorant).' Note how this again builds on the idea that sex workers are poor and uneducated.

Client fears are also translated into preferences for particular sex work venues. Thus, massage parlours may be preferred because rooms are already available for sex, without having to worry about security. Yet other gay men argue that the upmarket bars are safer because the sex workers are more middle-class, educated and 'more disciplined'. The discipline comes from strict establishment rules about how the sex worker should behave. Here, the concept of the 'guest' is important: the guest must be pleased; the guest's needs are paramount.

Transactions can be extremely feudal in such establishments, particularly massage parlours, where the sex worker address the client as 'sir'. This is not a trivial formality: conversations are littered with the honorific terms such as *po* (a sign of respect used for elder people) and the use of the plural pronouns. For example, if the client asks how much the sex worker charges, he will answer, '*Sila na po ang bahala*' which translates as 'It is up to them', 'them' substituted for 'you' when referring to the client. Sex workers have complained, in our interviews, about how they can be reprimanded for being 'rude to the guest'. When I asked for an example of being rude, one sex worker quipped, 'not getting an erection'.

In formal male sex work, gender ideologies converge with class ideologies and in the process are reshaped. For example, desire and masculinity are clearly being reformulated. In the last two years, macho dancers have taken to strutting out with Ray-ban sunglasses and Levi jeans with beepers or cellphones conspicuously clipped on the belt. The dancers eventually strip off their Levi's to show – and this is strangely uniform in all the bars – Calvin Klein underwear. The brand names and cellphones are of course the usual status symbols – the sex workers tell me they share these 'decorations' (*pang-decoration*) but it is clear, too, that the 'outfits' create a different kind of 'real male', certainly not the construction worker. When I ask the sex workers what image they try to project, they answer '*estudyante*' ('a student'). One of them laughs, '*Para sa bakla din yan. Tipong may tinutulungang estudyante. Estudyante kasi, mabait, nag-aaral.*' ('That's for the *bakla*. It's like they're helping a student. Students are supposed to be good, studying.') The student sex worker does not just function to assuage guilt (helping someone through school) but also projects a domesticated male, the antithesis of the 'bad boy' that goes with the *bakla*.

Some bars have strict rules – including job termination for 'independent bookings' made outside the establishment. But even in situations where independent negotiations are possible, power relations are skewed. This is summarized well in the construction of the 'guest', as a client to whom all forms of hospitality must be extended. '*Kung ano ang gusto niya*' ('whatever he wants'). One can see how negotiations will be limited in such settings. The sex workers themselves recognize this: '*mahirap na kung may kapangyarihan*' ('It is difficult if the client is powerful'). The situation is more difficult in massage parlours and bars because sex workers here have less autonomy: the pimp-manager is a powerful intermediary. Not surprisingly, sex workers do not like 'home service', especially with new clients. They describe this as risky, not just because they are unfamiliar with the client, but because entering the home of someone more powerful further reduces their ability to protect themselves: '*Pagpasok mo sa bahay niya, wala na, territoriyo niya.*' ('Once you enter his home, that's it. It's his territory.')

Feelings about wealthy 'guests' are ambivalent. On one hand, there is intimidation and fear of the power that such clients wield. Yet many sex workers also say they prefer wealthier clients, not just because they pay more but also because they are perceived as possible connections for better jobs. Moreover, wealthy clients are perceived as 'safer'. This relates to the concept of *decente* or decent. A potential sex partner is evaluated as being clean and decent based on external attributes. Wealthier clients are given this tag of decent: '*Propesyonal kasi. Mga iba nga, doktor*' ('They're professionals. Others are even medical doctors') or '*Edukado sila*' ('They're educated'), which is then projected to the client's sexual health: '*Malinis sigurado*' ('They're sure to be clean'). This is accompanied by contempt for lower-class *bakla*: '*Marumi sila . . . mga iba, ang babaho, maingay, at ang bastos.*' (They're dirty, others smell, they're noisy and are vulgar.')

Male sex work allows for a playing out of traditional sexual and gender ideologies, but in a new setting, where the variables come under strict control. In particular, the very source of desire – masculinity – is itself recast and domesticated. We see here how sexuality overlaps with concerns of power and control that move beyond gender. The most striking remarks that I have obtained from clients reflect this interface: 'If I am going to pay, then I expect singing and dancing' and 'That's stupid: why should anyone pay to give a blow job or to get screwed?' These remarks capture what I mean by a commodity transaction. A consumerist perspective is present in this consciousness: that one pays for a certain type of sex and that one must get his money's worth. It is a 'simple' transaction with few expectations, unlike an encounter between a *bakla* and a neighbourhood 'stand-by', where there are rituals of flirtation and courtship, and a recognition that a potential relationship might develop. In formal sex work, such expectations may be present, but for the most part, a call-boy is there for a paid performance for a fairly fixed period of time: an hour of tabling, three hours of sex. One manager actually used the term *arki* (to rent) to describe these longer-term arrangements, such as during Easter holidays when wealthy clients take out the sex workers for an entire week. No talk of boyfriends or *asawa* here. The arrangement is, precisely, a rental.

Implications for Interventions

In this chapter I have tried to show that stereotypes about male sex work (and about sex work in general) need to be challenged. Male sex workers are quite varied, even within specific categories (for example bar-based workers). The context of risk in sex work builds around 'actors', of clients and sex workers with interacting ideologies. Ethnographies of space, place, actors and motives are needed to guide future interventions for male sex workers. Without such information, priorities may be misplaced. For example, funding agencies have been known to pour money into interventions in Manila cinemas because these venues were believed to be 'high risk' for HIV/AIDS among 'men who have sex with men' and male sex workers. Cinemas and parks also draw attention because they are considered lurid and sleazy, with connotations of 'unsafe sex', yet common sense would suggest that such sites are not exactly convenient for unsafe sex. Neither are such sites conducive for interactive HIV/AIDS education.

Another example of the consequences of a gap between research and practice comes with the fad for training peer educators among sex workers. This presumes that peer relationships exist. Our research suggests that peer groups do not exist – in the bars or in Philippine society in general – beyond small groups of four or five people. Male sex workers in fact can be quite individualistic, seeing others as threats. HAIN has dropped peer education for other practical reasons, mainly the fact that male sex workers drift in and out of their work, and many are in it only for short periods. A more targeted approach is necessary, one which ensures a constant stream of information because of the rapid turnover, while providing referrals for the more serious problems that sex workers may have, whether biomedical or psychosocial. We have tried to establish such referrals but have found it easier for the biomedical linkages. Handling psychosocial needs becomes more difficult since the sex workers' situations vary, from the almost chattel-like conditions of massage parlours to the fairly autonomous freelance workers.

Interactive sessions are important for sex workers to identify their concerns and questions. HIV/AIDS is rarely a 'top-of-the-mind' concern. Few male sex workers know, or even know of, someone with HIV/AIDS. The Department of Health's figures in fact do not show any recorded cases of HIV positive male sex workers, and HIV/AIDS remains invisible. In addition, HIV is perceived as a disease transmitted by women to men; thus, sex with other males is not seen as particularly dangerous. All these perceptions, and the allied constructions of risk, are hardly investigated by the Health Department or NGOs. This means that present interventions may do more harm than good. Already, the emphasis on syndromic management of sexually transmitted diseases (STDs) – using signs and symptoms to diagnose and treat STDs – has created conflicting messages among the sex workers. 'If you can use this for gonorrhea, why can't you use this for AIDS?' asked a sex worker during one of our lectures.

If simple research on health perceptions and health-seeking behaviour is absent, then the gaps are even greater in terms of understanding the ideological context of sex work. I have argued for the importance of a socio-historical approach that looks at the way sex work is shaped in relation to sexual and gender ideologies. I have shown how the demand for male sex workers in the Philippines centres on *bakla* desire for 'real men', one which has been transformed from informal settings involving gift exchanges for a 'boyfriend' into a formal setting of commodity transactions where one pays for sex. At the same time, I have shown how even in formal settings, many aspects of the 'older' ideology remain, such as certain gender roles as well as expectations such as a search for companionship and potential relationships. Male sex work ties in closely to the way 'gay life' evolves in the Philippines.

The interaction between ideology and action moves both ways and is crucial in shaping perceptions about, and responses to, risk. While male sex workers – by virtue of their being 'male' – often have more autonomy than their female counterparts, there is also growing regimentation and 'discipline' in the industry that limits negotiation. This regimentation emerges in formal sex work settings such as bars and massage parlours, with class differences playing a vital role in the transformation. Much rhetoric about masculinity – both its desirability and its danger – is actually class-based. Masculinity needs to be transformed and domesticated to assure the 'guest's' safety and security, to assuage his fears of someone who might be too 'masculine'. This explains current male sex work venues with a growing set of rules about what sex workers should and should not do, and a system of bar fines where clients pay for some 'insurance' that an errant sex worker can be tracked down.

Further complicating the sex workers' ability to negotiate is the way supply outstrips demand. It is not surprising that sex workers try to outdo each other with their 'performance', even as they try to balance what they will do in bed with the ideology of 'being male'. *Tumatawid ng alambre*, or walking the tightrope, is one way the sex workers describe their 'versatility' without compromising their maleness since, after all, this is all *trabaho lang*. It's just work means that singing (giving oral sex) and dancing (receiving anal sex) is all right, especially if the price is right.

A social historical perspective also means being able to monitor trends in sex work and to respond to new needs. For example, we see more self-identified gay men entering sex work. I am particularly concerned with this sub-population. For them, male sex work is not *trabaho lang*. The problems and risks here are different. There have been problems of discrimination from among fellow sex workers, as well as from clients who discover they are gay. Last year, one such gay sex worker committed suicide, despondent over a client who was no longer interested in him.

On the day I finished a second draft of this chapter, I went off with friends to Tondo, a district in Manila with a mixture of low- and middle-income households, to interview some *baklas* about gay life. The interviews were conducted on a Saturday night and we had difficulties getting people to interview, the reason being that many *baklas* were out making *hada* (cruising). I realized that Tondo represented, in many ways, the transition between the 'gift exchange' between the *bakla* and a boyfriend, and the 'commodity transactions' of formal male sex work. I would venture that formal male sex work in fact continues to constitute only a small portion of 'sex work' in its broadest sense. But little is being done to reach the informal sectors of 'occasional' sex work or of 'men having sex with *baklas*'.

My feelings continue to be quite mixed. Where are the risks most serious? One Tondo *bakla* I was interviewing scoffed at the idea of using condoms: '*Hindi naman ako nagdu-do sa call boy. Kilala ko naman sila at kung saan silang nagtatrabaho. Sila lang naman ang nakikipag-do sa mga Kano at sa mga mayayamang bakla. Ayan, yan ang AIDS na yan, hindi sa mga binata dito.*' ('I don't do it with call-boys. I know who they are and where they work. They go out with foreign guests and rich *baklas*. That's where you find AIDS, not with the men here [in the community].') And then I remembered an interview with one of those 'rich *baklas*' in a bar: 'It's safe here. I don't take the skinny young ones here. They're the ones who go with foreigners. Besides, the boys here get AIDS lectures and get tested regularly. It's safe.'

My feelings remain ambivalent. I know we need to intensify programmes with the community *bakla*, but at the same time, are we perhaps falling into the trap of labelling the *bakla* and his street cruising as dangerous when in fact the controlled conditions of upmarket bars – where sex workers must learn to be versatile and to cross the tightrope – may yet prove to be more dangerous? What are the implications of sporadic one-hour AIDS lectures accompanied by HIV testing in these establishments, testing requested by bar owners and clients themselves?

Whose securities, whose risks, are being addressed? *Pagtatawid ng alambre*, walking the tightrope, becomes an appropriate metaphor here for male sex work, describing not just the sex that 'needs' to be done, but also the many balancing acts relating to self-image, sexual identity, understanding 'the other', and of risk itself. Ultimately, one needs to ask: just who is walking the tightrope?

Notes

1 Curiously, he refers to 'adolescent males' when in fact the market was for children. Adolescents were considered too old by pederasts.
2 That is, be attracted to women. As in most cultures, there is no equivalent for 'heterosexual' in Philippine languages.
3 D. is an abbreviation for 'dead'.

References

CAMAGAY, M.L. (1995) *Working Women of Manila in the 19th Century*, Philippine, Quezon City: University of the Philippines Press and University Center for Women's Studies.

MATHEWS, P.W. (1987) 'Some preliminary observations of male prostitution in Manila', *Philippines Sociological Review*, **35**, 3–4, pp. 55–74.

STAMFORD, J.D. (Ed.) (1979) 'Your Spartacus holiday portfolio: Philippine Provinces', Amsterdam: Spartacus, in F.L. WHITAM and R. MATHY (Eds.) *Male Homosexuality in Four Societies*, New York: Praeger.

TAN, M.L., DE LEON, A. and STULFUZ, B. (1990) 'Philippines: focusing on the hospitality women', in PANOS INSTITUTE (Ed.) *The Third Epidemic: Repercussions of the Fear of AIDS*, London: Panos Institute.

WHITAM, F.L. and MATHY, R. (1986) *Male Homosexuality in Four Societies*, New York: Praeger.

Chapter 15

Marginalization and Vulnerability: Male Sex Work in Morocco

*Amine Boushaba, Oussama Tawil, Latéfa Imane and
Hakima Himmich*

I sometimes feel good after spending time with a nice guy ... but afterwards I regret what I've done. I start to ask myself questions: why am I like this? (H)

The problems never go away. If you go out on the street you have to be ready to take a risk. You need to watch out for everything. Everyone is after you ... the police, muggers, the lot. It's a great relief when you return home safe and sound. (O)

When I see the new guys arriving in the park, I advise them to go home before it's too late. They think I'm jealous and don't listen. It [sex work] can appear very attractive at the start, but things change quickly afterwards ... the first thug or client who beats you up [makes you] get disenchanted very fast. (C)

Until about ten years ago, little had been written about male sex work in Morocco. While male sex work, or paid sexual activity with other men, was known about and often linked with tourism, it was rarely mentioned in official discourse. In 1988, a report in the local press by two journalists was the first piece of writing to lift the veil on this taboo subject (Imane and Taârji, 1988). This report, which took the form of a series of testimonies from young men involved in sex work, revealed a disturbing reality and precipitated a swift reaction of denial.

It was only in the early 1990s that the first systematic contacts began to be made with men involved in sex work, and their sexual partners. Worried by the number of cases of HIV transmission through sex between men, the Association de Lutte Contre le SIDA (ALCS) began its first work among homosexually active men (1995, 1996). The aim was to provide HIV prevention services, but a major problem was how to establish contact with those at greatest risk. Because no gay scene in a Western sense existed, the decision was made to focus on one of the most visible aspects of male homosexuality in Morocco, namely male sex work.

Initial contacts suggested that as well as being clandestine, male sex work was also fairly widespread. Male sex workers were to be found in tourist centres such as Marrakech, Agadir and Tangier, as well as in cities such as Casablanca. But sex work was by no means restricted to tourist destinations, and forms of sex work catering for a local clientele exist in these and other places.

Context

A range of young men provide sexual services in Morocco, and in order to understand why this is the case it is helpful to know something about sexual beliefs, perceptions and identities. Western concepts such as homosexuality, bisexuality and heterosexuality have little meaning in this society. While people often talk about 'normal' sex (implying sex between a man and a woman), there are no words in Moroccan Arabic to describe either hetero-sexuality or bisexuality. Phrases in Arabic such as *Al Chouzouz Al Jinsi* (loosely translated as 'sexual deviance') do exist, however, and there are numerous euphemisms to describe the receptive partners in homosexual sex. But men who have sex with other men are not defined as homosexual, bisexual or gay. Instead they are 'active' or 'passive', and it is from the role taken in sexual penetration that sexual identity flows: as either a 'man' or a 'woman'.

While sex between men is widely acknowledged as taking place, male sex work is rarely, if ever, referred to in official discourse, and it is not recognized by the law. Instead, male sex workers most usually find themselves prosecuted in relation to their participation in homosexual acts which are forbidden by law and punishable by imprisonment.

Broadly speaking, it is possible to distinguish between two distinct sub-populations of male sex workers – *gigolos* or hustlers, and *prostitués homosexuels* or homosexual or gay men who regularly or occasionally sell sex. These two groups differ from one another in perceived identity, sexual experience and motivation. On the whole, *gigolos* tend to define them-selves as heterosexual, report having sexual contacts with women, and have a preference for foreign male partners. While the rationale given for involve-ment in sex work with other men is ambivalent, many perceive sex work as a way to make money or to gain other advantages. However, for some, such justifications may be a cover for feelings of eroticism and/or desire for other men.

Prostitués homosexuels, on the other hand, more often see themselves as homosexual or gay, although this does not imply that they have the same kind of identity as is understood in the West. Because of their sexual orientation, many have experienced rejection by their families and communities of origin. Selling sex may offer a refuge from the hostility of others as well as a way to make a living, and some adopt sex work as an 'occupation', particularly in the absence of other kinds of financial support.

Research Process

In order to better understand the social and behavioural profile of these two groups of men, and as a prelude to the development of a local HIV prevention programme, ALCS volunteers undertook observations and interviews at venues where sex workers meet clients in two cities: Casablanca and Marrakech. This work, conducted in 1992–94, was followed by the administration of a more structured survey in 1995 to provide baseline data from which an HIV prevention programme could be designed. Over a 12-month period, 172 people were interviewed in the two cities, at locations including parks, cafés and main squares. A semi-structured questionnaire developed with members of the population, and modified after pre-test, was used to collect data. A combination of snowball and random sampling techniques were employed in the study, and interviewers had knowledge of, or were part of the same milieu, as respondents. Participation in the study was voluntary and anonymity was assured. At the end of the interview, participants were offered information on local STD services (including free and anonymous HIV testing), and were given condoms and lubricant if they wished. The fact that the interviewers were knowledgeable of the milieu within which the study was carried out may explain the relatively low non-response rate. Detailed analysis was undertaken of both survey findings and qualitative data on the following themes: socio-demographic status, sexual identity, sex work experiences, sexual behaviour, and HIV/AIDS risk perception.

Survey Findings

In order to gain insight into the social situation of respondents and their vulnerability to STD/ HIV/AIDS, it is important to take into account several related sets of factors including the social profile of respondents; their sexual behaviour and risk perception.

Social Profile

The average age at first sexual intercourse among respondents was reported as being 15, and their overall profile is shown in Table 15.1. The majority had not completed secondary education and 5% reported never having been to school. A minority of respondents reported that they lived alone or with friends (21%), relations with parents and other family members were most often strained.

Sixty per cent had no regular source of income outside sex work and of those that did, the financial benefits of this employment, most usually as labourers, artisans or apprentices, were limited.

Table 15.1 Interviewees (n = 172)

Variable	Frequency	Percentage
City/Town		
Casablanca	88	51.2
Marrakech	80	46.5
Others	04	2.3
Site		
Streets, squares	93	54.1
Cafés	57	33.1
Parks	15	8.7
Other	07	4.1
Mean age	24.7	–
Educational level		
Never attended school	9	5.3
Primary	36	21.2
Secondary	93	54.7
Higher	32	18.8
	(n = 170)	
Place of residence		
Family	136	79.5
Friend	13	7.6
Alone	22	12.9
	(n = 171)	
No regular employment	106	61.6

Behavioural Profile

While all those interviewed reported having sex with men, one-third also reported sexual relations with women (Table 15.2). The number of male sexual partners varied widely, with some averaging eight a week. This wide variation in numbers of sexual partners may perhaps be explained by the different kinds of involvement in sex work apparent within the sample. Whereas many practised sex work regularly, 38 per cent did so more occasionally.

It is important to recognize the substantial geographical mobility among members of this population. Seventy-three per cent of those interviewed said they had been involved in sex work in several different Moroccan cities. In relation to the origin of clients, 37 per cent of those interviewed reported only having Moroccan clients, whereas others sold sex primarily to a non-Moroccan clientele. This suggests the existence of well developed local forms of sex work in addition to those linked to tourism.

With respect to sexual practices, almost all those interviewed reported having anal sex (97 per cent). The second most popular practice was oral sex

Table 15.2 Sexual behaviour (n = 172)

Variable	Frequency	Percentage
Sexual orientation		
Man	115	66.9
Woman	1	0.6
Man/woman	56	32.6
Paid sexual activity	145	84.3
Average partners per week	8 (range 1 to 35)	–
Partners in other cities/towns	126	73.3
Origin of partners		
Moroccans	63	37.3
'Foreigners'	04	2.4
Moroccans and 'Foreigners'	102	60.4
	(n = 169)	
Sexual practices*		
Anal sex	166	97.1
Fellatio	133	77.8
Masturbation	87	50.9
Other	4	2.3

*More than one response permissible (n = 171).

(78 per cent). Knowledge about, access to, and the use of condoms provided an indication of the steps being taken to protect against HIV infection. Almost all of those interviewed (Table 15.3) knew about condoms (98 per cent), but 57 per cent reported using them either occasionally or never at all. Among those who reported using condoms regularly, a proportion did so because their partner requested it. The reasons for non-use were diverse. Some of the more frequent reasons included partner refusal, personal dislike and low levels of risk perception. Lack of access to condoms was cited by 24 per cent of the sample as a reason for non-use, which suggests that for this minority of respondents improving access to condoms may be one way of reducing risk.

Risk Perceptions

While it was true that the majority of those interviewed had already heard about AIDS, their knowledge about the subject was often vague and incomplete. Only 24 per cent of men contacted were able to accurately identify the major modes of HIV transmission. Among those who identified sex as a potential mode of transmission, a third did not see themselves as being at risk, and of those who did, the majority did not use condoms regularly. In the light of this information, it is clear that a large number of individual and socio-

Table 15.3 Condom knowledge and use, and risk perception (n = 172)

Variable	Frequency	Percentage
Knows about the condom	168	97.7
Frequency of use		
Always	36	20.9
Often	38	22.1
Rarely	69	40.1
Never	29	16.9
Reason for non-use		
Refusal of partner	36	26.5
Lack of access	32	23.5
Lack of pleasure	22	16.2
Because partner requests	15	11.0
Other	31	22.8
	(n = 136)	
Preferred source of supply*		
Pharmacies	83	52.9
Partners	84	53.5
Friends	30	19.1
Other	29	18.5

*More than one response permissible (n = 157).

contextual factors interact to enhance vulnerability to HIV. These include the multiplicity of partners, the relative rarity of protected sex, geographical mobility and economic marginality, among other variables.

Of all the vulnerability enhancing factors cited above, the most important is probably respondents' dependence on sex work as a means of subsistence.

> N said that it was his life circumstances which had encouraged him to enter sex work. He had done different kinds of work, but the amount of money he could earn was not even enough to cover his bus transport. The only solution for him was to enter prostitution in order to earn a living. He was very afraid of having AIDS and had even considered ending his life. (Fieldnotes)

This financial dependency on sex work encourages men to have a high number of sexual partners, and reduces considerably their capacity to negotiate where, when and how sex takes place. Other factors influencing vulnerability may include age, level of education (Tables 15.4 and 15.5), and family context. It was clear that the youngest members of the population interviewed were those at greatest risk, and those least likely to adopt prevention practices. Similarly,

Table 15.4 Frequency of condom use by age (n = 172)

	15–24 years (n = 93)	25 years and over (n = 79)
Regularly use condoms	28%	57%
Non-regular use of condoms	47%	32%
Never use condoms	25%	11%

Table 15.5 Condom use by level of education (n = 170)

	Higher Education (n = 32)	Secondary Education (n = 92)	Primary Education or less (n = 46)
Regularly use condoms	44%	18%	11%
Non regular use of condoms	47%	67%	63%
Never use condoms	9%	15%	26%

those who had completed higher education were far more likely to adopt preventive practices than those whose education had been more limited.

Qualitative Analysis

In order to further examine the vulnerability of the two groups of sex workers, we explored in interviews and earlier fieldwork self-perceptions, social attitudes, motivations for involvement in sex work, and beliefs and aspirations about the future. Some important differences existed between the two groups of men studied. We will examine each separately.

Gigolos

The vast majority of respondents in this group defined themselves as 'heterosexual'. Their clients were often Europeans and many respondents stated having a strong preference for 'foreigners', partly because they were perceived as being more generous, but also because respondents hoped one day to be able to travel to Europe. Clients were generally perceived as being 'passive' and, as a result, sex workers' sexual identity was not threatened. Their masculinity and sense of being a man was not brought into question so long as they always played the 'active' role in anal sex. Respondents who made up this group often mentioned having female partners as well as male clients. Many of them also exhibited homophobic attitudes and stated they were involved in sex work because of the need for money. A few, however, were more ambivalent in their response, perhaps because sex work allowed them a means of expressing their sexuality: society is more tolerant towards a man who has sex with other men for economic need, than towards one who actively decides to adopt a different sexuality.

On the whole, *gigolos* appeared to be fairly well integrated into society. They generally reported having good relationships with their family. The majority did not feel marginalized. They simply lived a double life without any great feelings of guilt. The only anxiety expressed was the possibility that their family might discover their involvement in sex work. This meant that while many of them provided financially for their family, they had to do so in ways that disguised the true origins of the source of income.

Prostitués Homosexuels

All the members of this group identified themselves as homosexual or gay. A small number took female names and were perceived as behaving femininely. *Prostitués homosexuels* tended to have entered sex work at a younger age than *gigolos*. The majority had begun to sell sex at about the age of 15. Not infrequently, first sexual experiences had taken place by force, often involving members of the family. For many, sex work was not simply a means of economic survival, but also a source of refuge from the hostility of those around them, and particularly their family. It also provided the opportunity to live their own sexuality.

> He doesn't live regularly with his family because there are always problems with the fact that he doesn't work. Because it is difficult for him to find work, every time his parents throw him out of the house he has to find somewhere to stay. This is how he got to know the street . . . He only goes back to his parents when he can't find anywhere else to stay. (Fieldnotes)

Prostitués homosexuels were often rejected by their family because of their visible homosexual identity, and many reported having experienced violence at the hands of their fathers or older brothers.

> My brother is a guide, and I'm sure that he goes out with strangers. It's hard to understand. He never speaks to me, and treats me like dirt even in front of our parents. But otherwise he leaves me alone unless he's drunk, then he hits me. He's abused me for a long time, ever since I was very young. (K)

Violence is part of everyday life for *prostitués homosexuels* who are often the victims of aggression from clients, muggers and others. Some respondents in this group reported having frequently been in prison. The length of imprisonment varied from two to six months. This contributes to their exclusion from the family circle and encourages a greater dependence on sex work as a means of survival. Relationships with other sex workers are very important for members of this group, be they support or rivalry in work. They contribute to an inter-group solidarity in the face of external threat and violence.

Comparisons

Prostitués homosexuels like *gigolos* tend not to have long-term goals. For them, the future is ill-defined and far away. Only a very few men interviewed reported having specific goals and were putting aside money for the future. Instead, the tendency was to live from day to day and not think about what the future might bring. Nevertheless, for *gigolos* one hope remains, the possibility of leaving Morocco to live in Europe, which in spite of economic crises, growing racism and tighter border controls continues to be a mythical *el dorado*. As two interviewees put it:

> While I'm young I can be successful, but I'm not stupid. If I listened to my friends, I would never have saved any money. They spend everything they earn, but I have been saving in order to buy a visa for Italy where I can work. I also have a Danish friend who has asked me to marry him. Can you see me marrying a *pédé*! But I would do it if it's the only way of leaving Morocco and getting official papers there. (M)

> I'm waiting for my Swedish friend. He's going to come over this summer. I hope he will take me back with him. Over there, you can be very successful particularly if you are young, good looking and dark skinned. (O)

Those who have the least opportunity and who are in many ways the most vulnerable, are the *prostitués homosexuels* who, in many cases, have lost contact with their families and who live with each other on the margins of society. They find it hardest to obtain any form of employment. Because of the way they are perceived, few employers are likely to take them on.

> When you are a *pédé* in Morocco you don't have much future. It's not like in Europe where homosexuals have rights and can organize and defend themselves. Here if you are mugged or beaten up you can't go and complain to the police because they will arrest you. Maybe we're not real men, but those who attack us, they're not real men either. The real men live in Europe. There everyone is free to live their own life. (B)

Implications for Prevention

A range of programme and intervention implications flow from the preliminary findings described in this chapter. Perhaps the most important of these concerns the manner in which HIV-related services are best provided to men who sell sex in Morocco. Given the current illegality of homosexual behaviour between men and the social marginality of sex workers, the best model for establishing rapport and building confidence with this population is through persons who are either close to, or previously part of, this milieu. An outreach programme using peer educators has been established in Casablanca in recent years. Work takes place several times a week at a number of key venues in the city and occasional efforts are made to reach more peripheral sites beyond the city centre. This work has been complemented by parallel activities, on a more sporadic basis, in Marrakech's tourist city centre.

The main tasks of outreach workers has been to undertake interpersonal contacts with sex workers and the other men who have sex with men who can be found at these venues. The objectives of the work have been to increase HIV/AIDS awareness, provide counselling for prevention, and distribute condoms and educational material. In order to meet this populations' specific needs for STD care and voluntary HIV counselling and testing, a referral system has been developed using local health services.

While it is too early to evaluate the programme's overall effectiveness, initial reactions from male sex workers attest to the acceptability of this outreach approach. By exhibiting a non-judgemental attitude, outreach workers have been able to establish rapport with members of this hitherto unreached population. A preliminary analysis of outreach contacts suggests that in excess of 500 men can be reached in a period as short as 12 months, although not all of these are involved in sex work. Findings also emphasized the importance of condom distribution through outreach work, which has been much appreciated by male sex workers who tend to avoid more traditional outlets such as pharmacies and health centres.

The preliminary evidence suggests that interpersonal education of this kind offers a viable strategy for channelling prevention messages, as well as for discussion with this marginalized population. Moreover, the intermediary role of the outreach team permits easier access to STD care and HIV counselling and testing. Men who have been contacted frequently expressed the need for a broader dialogue on health matters and their everyday lives, entry into sex work, and sexual identity. There is some, albeit preliminary, evidence from the work conducted so far to suggest that safer sex practices may increase relatively rapidly following a period of sustained outreach activity.

In many parts of the world, HIV and AIDS have brought to the fore dormant social issues. These concerns, which include homosexuality and male sex work, can all too easily be dismissed as being of secondary importance when they involve already marginalized minorities. The growth of the HIV and AIDS epidemic globally has raised important questions about whether this is an appropriate approach to take. In the case of Morocco, the research and outreach described in this chapter offer a rare example of how to address HIV-related concerns in an Arab-Muslim cultural context. It is hoped that this hard-won experience will offer incentives for community outreach work with marginal groups and populations elsewhere in the region.

Acknowledgments

The authors would like to thank the members of the research team which undertook the research described in this chapter – A. Azzam, H. El Ali, A. Faker, A. Khairy and S. Mricha; and Peter Aggleton for assistance with translation.

References

ASSOCIATION DE LUTTE CONTRE LE SIDA (1995) *La prostitution masculine au Maroc: résultats des enquêtes sur Casablanca et Marrakech, 1993/95*, Morocco: ALCS.

ASSOCIATION DE LUTTE CONTRE LE SIDA (1996) 'Prévention de proximité auprès des prostitués masculins au Maroc. Recherche-action 1995 et plan d'action 1997/98', unpublished project document submitted to UNAIDS.

IMANE, L. and TAÂRJI H. (1988) *Prostitution masculine, ces adolescents qui vendent leurs corps*, Morocco: Kalima.

Index

In this index, and for the sake of brevity, male sex workers and men who sell or exchange sex for material reward are denoted by the term 'sex worker.'

As most references in this index relate to sex work or sex workers, the subheadings under these terms have been kept to a minimum. For further information on these topics, use a more specific index term eg clients, health, HIV/AIDS etc.

Printed and bound by CPI Group (UK) Ltd, Croydon, CR0 4YY

25/10/2024

01779632-0001